HANDBOOK OF OCCUPATIONAL THERAPY
for Adults With Physical Disabilities

T0144200

HANDBOOK OF OCCUPATIONAL THERAPY
for Adults With Physical Disabilities

William Sit, PhD, OTR/L, BCPR, CLVST-BIG
Associate Clinical Professor
Texas Woman's University
Denton, Texas

Marsha Neville, OT, PhD
Professor
Texas Woman's University
Denton, Texas

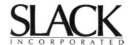

SLACK
INCORPORATED

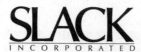

SLACK Incorporated
6900 Grove Road
Thorofare, NJ 08086 USA
856-848-1000   Fax: 856-848-6091
www.Healio.com/books
ISBN: 978-1-63091-442-4
© 2020 by SLACK Incorporated

Senior Vice President: Stephanie Arasim Portnoy
Vice President, Editorial: Jennifer Kilpatrick
Vice President, Marketing: Michelle Gatt
Acquisitions Editor: Brien Cummings
Managing Editor: Allegra Tiver
Creative Director: Thomas Cavallaro
Cover Artist: Katherine Christie
Project Editor: Erin O'Reilly

Drs. William Sit and Marsha Neville have no financial or proprietary interest in the materials presented herein.

The procedures and practices described in this publication should be implemented in a manner consistent with the professional standards set for the circumstances that apply in each specific situation. Every effort has been made to confirm the accuracy of the information presented and to correctly relate generally accepted practices. The authors, editors, and publisher cannot accept responsibility for errors or exclusions or for the outcome of the material presented herein. There is no expressed or implied warranty of this book or information imparted by it. Care has been taken to ensure that drug selection and dosages are in accordance with currently accepted/recommended practice. Off-label uses of drugs may be discussed. Due to continuing research, changes in government policy and regulations, and various effects of drug reactions and interactions, it is recommended that the reader carefully review all materials and literature provided for each drug, especially those that are new or not frequently used. Some drugs or devices in this publication have clearance for use in a restricted research setting by the Food and Drug and Administration or FDA. Each professional should determine the FDA status of any drug or device prior to use in their practice.

Any review or mention of specific companies or products is not intended as an endorsement by the author or publisher.

SLACK Incorporated uses a review process to evaluate submitted material. Prior to publication, educators or clinicians provide important feedback on the content that we publish. We welcome feedback on this work.

Library of Congress Control Number:2019944247

For permission to reprint material in another publication, contact SLACK Incorporated. Authorization to photocopy items for internal, personal, or academic use is granted by SLACK Incorporated provided that the appropriate fee is paid directly to Copyright Clearance Center. Prior to photocopying items, please contact the Copyright Clearance Center at 222 Rosewood Drive, Danvers, MA 01923 USA; phone: 978-750-8400; website: www.copyright.com; email: info@copyright.com

Printed in the United States of America.

Last digit is print number: 10   9   8   7   6   5   4   3   2   1

Dedication

To my beloved son, Duncan.
An angel who always remains fascinated with music and soccer.
—WS

CONTENTS

Section Two: Central Nervous System 111
Unit 1: Need To Know

Unit 2: Evaluation

Unit 3: Intervention

Section Three: Sensory System, Cranial Nerves, and Peripheral Nervous System 221

Unit 1: Need To Know

Unit 2: Evaluation

Unit 3: Intervention

**Section Five: Cardiovascular, Lymphatic, Respiratory,
           and Integumentary Systems............ 371**

Unit 1: Need To Know

Unit 2: Evaluation

Unit 3: Intervention

Section Six: Endocrine, Digestive, Urinary, and Reproductive Systems

ACKNOWLEDGMENTS

Special thanks to those who contributed their knowledge and insights to this handbook:

Sarah Borsch, OTR
Debbie Buckingham, OTR, MS, CVE, CCM, CRC
Whitney Chapman, DPT
Kevin Felton, CO, LO, FAAOP
Niki Fogg, MSN, RN
Hui-Ting Goh, PT, PhD
(Nel) Rica Kendrick-Palmer, BSN, RN
Lai Yu Leong, Pharm D
Vicki Mason, OTR, PhD
Keith McWilliams, OTR/L, OTD, CBIS, DRS
Amanda (Mandie) Mims, MLS Sciences Librarian
Kimberly Mory, MA,CCC-SLP, CHES
Morris Owens, OTR
Noralyn Pickens, OT, PhD
Shubhangi Sharm, OTR
Brett Simmons, MBA, RN
Isabelle Sislak, BSN, RN
Rene Wren, OTR, OTD
Alan Yam, OTR
Amanda Zerangue, MLS, JD

Graduate Assistants:
Jessica Cline, OTS
Chelsea Low, OTS
Mandi Minzenmeyer, OTS
Allison Pratt, OTS
Sarah Taylor, OTS

ABOUT THE AUTHORS

William Sit, PhD, OTR/L, BCPR, CLVST-BIG is a faculty member at Texas Woman's University and chair of the Trinity North District of the Texas Occupational Therapy Association. For decades, he has worked in physical disabilities settings, including acute care, rehabilitation, outpatient, and home health, and he was unsatisfied with the availability of a single resource that effectively identifies key components of evaluation and intervention. As a result, he became motivated to write a handbook that fosters clinical reasoning development for occupational therapists in an adult practice setting, particularly for entry-level therapists and those newly entering a physical disabilities setting.

Dr. Marsha Neville, OT, PhD began her career in occupational therapy in 1974 as a certified occupational therapy assistant. In 1978 she became a registered occupational therapist after graduating from Eastern Michigan University (Ypsilanti, Michigan). She later completed her PhD in Cognitive Neuroscience at the University of Texas at Dallas. Her long career in occupational therapy has focused on adult rehabilitation and research related to interventions for persons with acquired brain injuries. She is a professor in the School of Occupational Therapy at Texas Woman's University.

INTRODUCTION

How the Handbook of Occupational Therapy for Adults With Physical Disabilities Was Developed

Students in their fieldwork placements and recent graduates frequently ask for recommendations in finding a handbook. When developing this handbook, the goal was to provide quick and essential information in an adult practice setting. Resources utilized for the development of this handbook include occupational therapy textbooks, recent journal articles, and occupational therapists with clinical expertise. The most essential information commonly used in clinical practice was then condensed into a handbook.

How to Use This Handbook

This handbook is not intended to provide comprehensive information that will replace textbooks or academic journals, but it may aid in translating the *Occupational Therapy Practice Framework: Domain and Process* into a clinical setting. The hope is that you will be able to carry this handbook and use it as a resource, particularly if you are a fieldwork student, a new graduate, or an occupational therapist transitioning to an adult practice setting for the first time.

This handbook is primarily organized by body system into six sections. The first section relates to occupational performance as a whole, which integrates various body systems for participation in meaningful activites of daily living, instrumental activities of daily living, and other occupations. The following sections are broken down into the central nervous system (Section Two); sensory, cranial nerves, and peripheral nervous system, (Section Three); musculoskeletal system (Section Four); cardiovascular, lymphatic, respiratory, and integumentary systems (Section Five); and the endocrine, digestive, urinary, and reproductive systems grouped together in the final section (Section Six).

Each section is broken down into three units. Unit 1 contains information that is important to know within each section. Unit 2 is focused on evaluations. Unit 3 describes common interventions. At the beginning of each section, you will find a story from my clinical experience that embodies the chapter subject. Each personal story is called the *Case*. The evaluation and intervention units that follow each case begin with a table listing the most common assessments and types of interventions relevant to the body system. The table notes differences that may exist across adult practice settings (acute/intensive care unit, inpatient rehabilitation/long-term acute care facility, home health, skilled nursing facility, and outpatient). Within each section, information is broken down first into important aspects of the evaluation process, and then followed by the implications of each system on occupational therapy intervention. Assessment topics include a summary chart where you can quickly and easily find the purpose, context, form, cost, and contact information for each assessment.

The *Handbook of Occupational Therapy for Adults With Physical Disabilities* is not diagnosis based. Thus, it is important to note that when working with a client, relevant information may be gained from multiple sections due to the interconnected nature of the body systems. Not every assessment, intervention technique, or precaution is included in this handbook, but it can help guide your thinking in a fast-paced clinical setting.

At the back of this handbook, you will find empty pages that you may use to make additional notes or write down contact information for vendors. Use this handbook in a way that will enhance your occupational therapy skills.

—*William Sit, PhD, OTR/L, BCPR, CLVST-BIG*

SECTION ONE

. . . .

Occupational Performance

Sit W, Neville M.
*Handbook of Occupational Therapy for
Adults With Physical Disabilities* (pp 1-110).
© 2020 SLACK Incorporated.

CASE

DIAGNOSIS: GLIOBLASTOMA

One client I recall was a teenage girl who had been diagnosed with an aggressive brain cancer called glioblastoma. The doctors informed her that she had 6 months to live. As her occupational therapist, I asked her, "What would you like to do in therapy?" She responded that she did not want therapy—she did not see any point in getting stronger through therapeutic intervention if she was just going to die anyway. Instead, she wanted to go to Disney World. As her team, we understood. Her physical therapist, speech therapist, and I figured out what we could do to be truly client centered and help her achieve her goal. We carried out therapy, but chose to organize our sessions differently, focusing on patient safety instead of the typical therapeutic exercises. Rather than prioritizing the performance of typical instrumental activities of daily living (IADLs), we learned about options for skipping the lines at Disney World. We performed simulations, and we planned out the best routine, figuring out which park to attend first and what the best options were. Upon her discharge, these sessions culminated in her visit to Disney World. Sadly, she ended up passing away, but we felt gratified in being able to facilitate her engagement in a meaningful occupation of her choice.

CHART REVIEW

The client's chart is the first source of information available prior to meeting the client, so it is important to review the chart before entering the client's room. Take the information found on the chart with a grain of salt; it may not accurately depict the client's status due to error or change in status.[1] The chart may take the form of a narrative paragraph or bulleted list. Any information not found on the chart can be obtained through client or family interviews. Refer to Section One, Unit 1-3 for information on client interviews.

Always confirm that the client's chart specifies a physician's referral to occupational therapy in compliance with federal and state regulations before rendering services.[2] Information on the chart may include the following:

Client description	• Age
	• Sex
	• Race
	• Ethnicity
	• Religion
	• Culture
	• Dominant hand
History of illness	• Diagnoses
	• Timeline
	• Tests
	• Labs
	• Admitted facilities
	• Past medical diagnoses
	• Comorbidities
Prior level of function	• How did the client function prior to current illness?
	• Consider prior level of function when setting goals
Home environment	• Description of physical environment
	• Two-story home, apartment, ranch-style home, etc
	• Available family support

(continued)

Chart Review (continued)

Prior and current use of medical and assistive devices	• Includes wheelchair, walker, or other ambulatory device • Home modifications (eg, grab bars, ramps) • Glasses, contacts, or hearing aids
Current level of assistance	• Is the client independent or does he or she require assistance? • Includes requiring cues, supervision, or extra time
Precautions	• Swallow precautions • Hip precautions • Cardiac precautions • Back precautions • Sternal precautions
Mental health considerations	• Depression • Suicidal ideation

UNIT 1-2 NEED TO KNOW

CLIENT INTERVIEW

CLIENT INTRODUCTION

The *Occupational Therapy Practice Framework: Domain and Process, 3rd Edition*, asserts that the creation of an occupational profile is the initial step in the occupational therapy evaluation process. The occupational profile informs the clinician of the client's past experiences, occupational history, daily patterns and routines, interests, values, and needs.[3] Information about the occupational profile can be gathered through formal or informal interview techniques.[3] The initial client introduction may be short, sometimes only 5 minutes, but the occupational therapist has much to learn from the brief interaction and can begin to establish rapport with the client.

Upon meeting with a client for the first time:

- Review the chart. Refer to Section One, Unit 1-2 for information on chart review.
- Introduce yourself and explain the purpose of occupational therapy.
- Perform a comprehensive functional screen.
- Begin building the occupational profile using interview techniques.

(continued)

CLIENT INTERVIEW (CONTINUED)

COMPREHENSIVE FUNCTIONAL SCREEN

A comprehensive functional screen is performed during the initial meeting with a client to guide the clinical-reasoning process. Information observed about the client's abilities and impairments will inform the clinician about assessments to use during a formal evaluation. At the beginning of the screen, ask the client to rate his or her level of pain and ask how the client slept the night before. These factors have an impact on how the client feels and performs.[4,5] Ask the client specific questions to obtain the following information:

Type of Screen	Description and Examples
Physical Pain assessment[6]	Ask the client to rate his or her pain on a scale of 0 to 10. Zero indicates no pain, and 10 indicates excruciating pain. You may use a visual pain chart with photos. Refer to Section Three, Unit 2-55, for information on pain assessment.
Physical Sleep assessment[4]	Sleep impacts how the client feels and performs. Ask the client how he or she slept the night before.
Physical Musculoskeletal[7]	Ask the client to perform functional movements in all planes, and check for symmetry and functional range of motion (ROM) bilaterally. The following are example prompts: Shoulder and scapula: • Please raise both arms as if you are reaching for a box on a high shelf. • Please cross each arm in front of you as if you were applying deodorant to the opposite side. • Please place your hand in your back pocket. Elbow: • Please bend your elbow as if you were bringing a cup to your mouth to drink.

(continued)

UNIT 1–3 NEED TO KNOW

CLIENT INTERVIEW (CONTINUED)	
Type of Screen	*Description and Examples*
Physical Musculoskeletal[7]	Forearm: • Please hold your arms straight out in front of you, and turn your palms up toward the ceiling. • Please hold your arms straight out in front of you, and turn your palms down toward the ground. Wrist: • With your arms straight out, please bend your wrist so that your fingers point toward the ceiling. • With your arms straight out, please bend your wrist so that your fingers point toward the floor. • With yours arms straight out and palms parallel to the floor facing down, please point your fingers toward each other, then away from each other. Hand: • Please make a fist. • Please open the fist. • Please touch each finger on one hand to the thumb on that hand. Refer to Section Four, Units 1-66 and 2-68 for information on muscle functions, functional movements, and ROM.
Physical Skin[8]	Check for the presence of rashes, wounds, or lesions. <div align="right">*(continued)*</div>

CLIENT INTERVIEW (CONTINUED)

Type of Screen	Description and Examples
Mental Status Orientation[9]	Talk to the client to find out if he or she is oriented to person, place, time, and situation: • What is your name? Where are we? What time/month/season is it? Why are you here? • Oriented x4: Client is aware of who he or she is, where he or she is, the time/date, and why he or she is receiving health care. • Oriented x3: Client who has knowledge of person, place, and time/date. • Oriented x2: Client who has knowledge of person and place. • Oriented x1: Client who has an awareness only of who he or she is.
Mental Status Speech[9]	Note the client's level of comprehension and the fluency of the client's speech.
Mental Status Long-term memory[9]	*Long-term memory* refers to the client's knowledge of an event that occurred in the past.
Mental Status Short-term memory[9]	*Short-term memory* refers to the client's ability to recall newly learned information: • Instruct the client to repeat 3 words: Peach, rock, flower. • Ask the client to recall those 3 words following a different task (eg, following the problem-solving task). • Note whether the client correctly recalled the 3 words.

(continued)

UNIT 1-3 NEED TO KNOW

CLIENT INTERVIEW (CONTINUED)	
Type of Screen	Description and Examples

Mental Status Problem solving[9]	• Instruct the client to count backwards from 100 by 7s:
	  ○ $100 - 7 = 93$
	  ○ $93 - 7 = 86$
	  ○ $86 - 7 = 79$
	  ○ $79 - 7 = 72$
	  ○ $72 - 7 = 65$
	• Short-term memory recall: Ask the client to recall the 3 words—peach, rock, flower.

Neurological Cranial nerves[10]	• Cranial nerve I: Test the client's sense of smell by blocking the client's vision and blocking one nostril, then presenting an odor to the other nostril. Repeat on other side. • Cranial nerve II: Check visual acuity by asking the client to identify a far away object. Check the visual field by standing behind the client with his or her gaze fixed straight ahead. Slowly move an item, such as a pen, into the client's visual field on each side, from above, and from below. Instruct the client to state when he or she sees the item. *(continued)*

CLIENT INTERVIEW (CONTINUED)	
Type of Screen	*Description and Examples*
Neurological Cranial nerves[10]	• Cranial nerves III, IV, and VI: Check eye motor function by asking the client to hold his or her head still and follow an item, such as a pen, with his or her eyes. Check for pupil symmetry. • Cranial nerve V: Check the client's sensation by applying a stimulus, such as a cotton swab, lightly on the forehead, cheek, and jaw. Ask the client to open and close his or her jaw, and check for symmetry of movement. • Cranial nerve VII: Check for facial asymmetry or droop during movement while asking the client to raise his or her eyebrows, smile, frown, and pucker his or her lips. • Cranial nerve VIII: Test the client's balance by asking the client to stand with his or her eyes open, then closed. Check for sway or loss of balance. • Cranial nerve IX: Check for a gag reflex by swiping a cotton swab on the back of the client's tongue. • Cranial nerve X: Check the client's speech for hoarseness or slurring. • Cranial nerve XI: Ask the client to swallow and check for movement of the Adam's apple. • Cranial nerve XII: Check motor function in the tongue by asking the client to stick out his or her tongue and move it from side to side. Check for muscle wasting on one or both sides, symmetry of movement, and smoothness of movement. Note if tremors were present. Refer to Section Three, Unit 2-52 for information on cranial nerve screening. *(continued)*

UNIT 1-3 NEED TO KNOW

CLIENT INTERVIEW (CONTINUED)	
Type of Screen	*Description and Examples*
Neurological Motor[11]	• Check for tone in the upper extremities. • Perform manual muscle testing in the upper extremities. • Check eye motor function by testing cranial nerves III, IV, and VI. Refer to Section Four, Unit 2-69 for information on manual muscle testing.
Neurological Sensation[11,12]	Check the client's sensation on palms and upper extremities. Refer to Section Three, Unit 1-50 for information on dermatomes.
Neurological Coordination[11]	Ask the client to touch his or her nose with his or her index finger on each hand. Ask the client to touch fingertip to fingertip.
Neurological Standing balance[11]	Ask the client to stand, and lightly touch your hands to the client's so that you are not helping him or her balance. Time how many seconds until the client begins to lose balance. If the client can maintain balance for more than 10 seconds, the client is likely not a high fall risk.
	(continued)

CLIENT INTERVIEW (CONTINUED)

INTERVIEW TOPICS

The following information is important to obtain during the interview process with the client or caregiver to assist with the intervention and discharge plan. Some information may be available on the chart, but it is the practitioner's responsibility to conduct a thorough interview.[3]

Information to Obtain	Description and Examples
Client's current living situation[3]	• Does the client live in a single-story building? • Are there stairs in the home or outside of the home? • Who lives at home with client? • Are there others who live in close proximity and can provide support? • How does the client move around the community? • What type of car does the client or family drive? • How does the client obtain groceries?
Client's prior level of function[3]	• What was the client's level of independence with activities of daily living (ADLs) prior to hospitalization and seeking occupational therapy services? • What was the client's level of independence with meal preparation, driving, shopping, and other daily activities?
Client's current use of devices or equipment[3]	• What medical or accessibility equipment does the client have at home? This may include items such as mobility devices, glasses, hearing aids, and a shower chair.
Summary of the client's typical day[3]	• Consider the client's ADLs and IADLs. • Consider the client's habits, routines, and rituals. • Consider the client's context. • Note areas where the client has difficulty. • Note areas where the client is successful. • Include any current strategies or routines the client uses for medication management.

(continued)

UNIT 1-3 NEED TO KNOW

CLIENT INTERVIEW (CONTINUED)	
Information to Obtain	*Description and Examples*
Client's current and past work responsibilities[3]	• Consider the client's education, volunteer, and work occupations. • Consider the context of these occupations. • Consider the activity demands. • Consider the client's occupational history.
Current and past activities in which the client enjoys participating[3]	• Consider the client's leisure, play, social participation, and rest occupations. • Consider the context of these occupations. • Consider the activity demands. • Consider the client's occupational history.
Client's other occupational roles[3]	• Consider the client's roles. • Consider the demands of those roles.
Client's goals[3]	• What does the client hope to achieve in therapy? • What are the client's priorities? • Goals may include enhancing occupational performance, preventing decline in occupational performance, competence in fulfilling role expectations, improving or maintaining health and wellness, and/or enhancing quality of life. • Practitioner goals for the client must always be client centered.
Client's discharge plans[3]	• Where does the client plan to go after being discharged from therapy? • Who will be the caregiver? Is the caregiver trained and able to provide care? • Consider what the client's daily life will look like after being discharged from your care.

CONTINUUM OF CARE

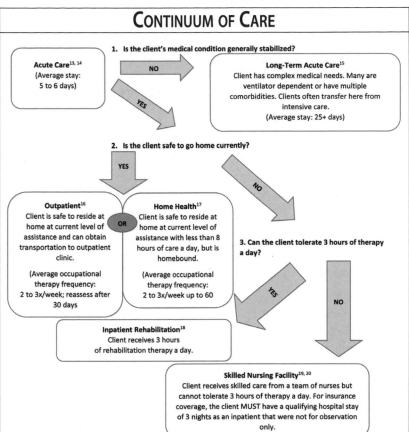

1. Is the client's medical condition generally stabilized?

Acute Care[13, 14]
(Average stay:
5 to 6 days)

NO →

YES ↘

Long-Term Acute Care[15]
Client has complex medical needs. Many are
ventilator dependent or have multiple
comorbidities. Clients often transfer here from
intensive care.
(Average stay: 25+ days)

2. Is the client safe to go home currently?

YES ↓   NO ↘

Outpatient[16]
Client is safe to reside at
home at current level of
assistance and can obtain
transportation to outpatient
clinic.

(Average occupational
therapy frequency:
2 to 3x/week; reassess after
30 days

OR

Home Health[17]
Client is safe to reside at
home at current level of
assistance with less than 8
hours of care a day, but is
homebound.

(Average occupational
therapy frequency:
2 to 3x/week up to 60

**3. Can the client tolerate 3 hours of therapy
a day?**

YES ↙   NO ↓

Inpatient Rehabilitation[18]
Client receives 3 hours
of rehabilitation therapy a day.

Skilled Nursing Facility[19, 20]
Client receives skilled care from a team of nurses but
cannot tolerate 3 hours of therapy a day. For insurance
coverage, the client MUST have a qualifying hospital stay
of 3 nights as an inpatient that were not for observation
only.

**4. Return to Question #2 Following Discharge from inpatient rehabilitation facility/skilled
nursing facility**

UNIT 1-4 NEED TO KNOW

DOCUMENTATION

Documentation is an essential part of occupational therapy practice. Documentation serves to provide important information about the client, explain the rationale for services, and record the client's status chronologically.[21] There is a common saying among faculty: "If you didn't write it down; It didn't happen." Students and new practitioners should strive to develop a working vocabulary to describe the client's abilities and what occurred in therapy. Practitioners may refer to the American Occupational Therapy Association (AOTA) official documents for documentation-specific guidelines and suggested content.[21]

TYPES OF DOCUMENTATION

- Screening report
- Evaluation report
- Reevaluation report
- Intervention plan
- Contact report note
- Progress report note
- Transition plan
- Discharge or discontinuation report

FUNDAMENTALS OF DOCUMENTATION

- Client's name
- Date and type of contact
- Type of documentation, agency, and department name
- Signature at the end of the note
- Countersignature
- Acceptable terminology
- Appropriate abbreviations
- Correct corrections
- Legal disposal of records
- Compliance with confidentiality
- Compliance with agency requirements for storage

(continued)

DOCUMENTATION (CONTINUED)	
SOAP NOTES	
One common method for documentation is to write a SOAP note.[22] SOAP stands for the following: Subjective Objective Assessment Plan	
Subjective	The subjective portion involves a client statement that is relevant to treatment: • Pain • Fatigue • Feelings • Attitudes • Concerns
Objective	The objective portion records items that are measurable, quantifiable, and observable as they relate to function. Begin the objective section by stating the client's participation, the duration of the session, and the purpose of the session. The following is an example: • Client participated in 50 minutes of occupational therapy intervention for the purpose of neuromuscular training and strengthening in preparation for ADLs. The objective section may be organized by functional category or targeted skills: • Function: ADLs, IADLs, etc • Cognition: Attention, memory, problem solving, sequencing, etc • Sensorimotor: Grasp, strength, ROM, tone, endurance, posture, etc • Psychosocial: Communication, behavior modification, etc • Perceptual: Visual scanning, visual spatial, proprioception, etc *(continued)*

UNIT 1-5 NEED TO KNOW

DOCUMENTATION (CONTINUED)	
Objective	Identify the treatments used: • Education: Diagnosis, energy conservation, use of device, etc • Preparatory activities: ROM, weightbearing, modalities, etc • Occupation-based activities: Hygiene, meal preparation, work, etc Indicate any actions by the therapist that were applied to assist the client: • Modifications: Modified tasks, environment, assistive devices, etc • Physical assistance: Tactile cues, positioning, proprioceptive cues, etc • Visual assistance: Visual tools, pointing, demonstrations, etc • Verbal assistance: Instructions, open or closed questions, etc Be sure to use standard abbreviations as well as qualifiers: • SBA, min Ⓐ, mod Ⓐ, max Ⓐ Note what portion of the activity required assistance.

Assessment	The assessment portion states your professional opinion and adjustments:
	• Functional limitations:
	  ◦ Decreased ROM continues to limit independence in upper extremity dressing.
	• Inconsistencies:
	  ◦ Client reports pain during ROM but demonstrates ROM during functional tasks.
	• Justify goals:
	  ◦ As client's ability to interact increases, he will be able to begin modified school tasks.
	<div align="right">*(continued)*</div>

	DOCUMENTATION (CONTINUED)

Assessment	• Discuss emotional state:
	  ◦ Client continues to resist use of an assistive device and states he will make a full recovery and not need it.
	• Identify strengths:
	  ◦ Client is demonstrating increased insight and problem-solving ability related to family interactions. He identified new communication methods with his children, and it is anticipated he will meet his goal to return home in 1 week.
	• Indicate progress in therapy and rehab potential:
	  ◦ Client's increased standing tolerance has enabled her to prepare simple meals in the kitchen. It is anticipated that with increased endurance, she will be independent with daily meal preparation.
	• Justify treatment:
	  ◦ Client will benefit from a home exercise program to increase strength and endurance for IADLs.
	• Demonstrate the skilled need for occupational therapy evaluation, instruction, and treatment.

Plan	The plan portion states specific treatments to achieve the goals. The plan must relate to the information in the objective and assessment parts of the note, and includes what treatments will focus on: • Occupation-based treatments • Purposeful activity • Preparatory activity The plan is followed by goals. *(continued)*

Documentation (Continued)

Goal Writing

Occupational therapists guide treatments and measure their client's progress by writing short- and long-term goals. All goals must be client centered and set in collaboration with the client. Using a frame of reference can assist with phrasing of the goals.[22]

	Purpose	Components	Duration	Examples
Short-Term Goals	• Helps measure effectiveness of interventions in short term • Breaks down long-term goals into small steps for timely gains	• Drives treatment planning for the week • Works toward long-term goals • Can be component or occupation based • Include a time frame • Must be linked to function in the objective or assessment section of the note • Must be measurable • Must document in follow-up whether the goal was met	1 to 2 weeks	• Patient will complete 1 multistep project with minimal supervision in 2 weeks. • Patient will perform chair-to-tub transfer with minimum assistance in 1 week. • Active ROM in wrist will increase 20 degrees to increase grip strength needed for daily activities by end of 2 weeks.

(continued)

DOCUMENTATION (CONTINUED)

	Purpose	Components	Duration	Examples
Long-Term Goals	• Provides a long-range vision for treatment planning • States where the client will be at discharge	• Must be functional and linked to occupation • Must relate to short-term goals • When long-term goals are met, must indicate need for reevaluation or discharge	Dependent on the setting and needs of the client	• Patient will be modified in basic ADLs using adaptive equipment. • Patient will return to work with environmental modifications.

(continued)

TRANSFER CHECKLIST

Practicing proper transfer techniques is important for ensuring practitioner and client safety.[23] The following checklist outlines important aspects of a client transfer and may be used to check your skills. The checklist is designed for a moderate-assist client transfer from bed to wheelchair.

INTRODUCTION

1	Introduce yourself. Include a description of occupational therapy and the purpose of the transfer for plan of care.
2	Clearly and concisely prepare the client for transfer. Obtain client consent, state the goal of transfer, and state the benefits for participation in the transfer.
3	Make sure your voice instills confidence.

BODY MECHANICS

4	Check that the client is within your personal transfer capacity. Review the chart, screen the client, or have assistance available if you are unsure.
5	Position the client or move the client close to you.
6	Position your body to face the client.
7	Keep a neutral spine. Do not bend or arch your back.
8	Bend your knees. Lift with your legs, not your back.
9	Keep a wide base of support.
10	Keep your heels down.
11	Avoid rotating your trunk.

EQUIPMENT

12	Apply the gait belt correctly. Make sure the belt is fastened and located correctly, and identify issues that would the change location of gait belt (eg, surgical incisions, gastric tube, colostomy, drainage tube).
13	Select the appropriate equipment to ensure a safe transfer. Make sure the wheelchair is an appropriate height/width, select removable or fixed armrests, and ensure adequate friction in the client's footwear to prevent slippage.
14	Lock the wheelchair.

(continued)

TRANSFER CHECKLIST (CONTINUED)

15	Check the stability of the transfer surfaces. Make sure the bed brakes are locked.
16	Position the wheelchair appropriately for a pivot transfer. Angle the wheelchair to the transfer surface or parallel to the bed.
17	Position the wheelchair equipment within reach.
18	Demonstrate knowledge of how to manage wheelchair equipment, including brakes, armrests, and footrests.
19	Move unnecessary bedding and equipment (eg, move footrests and armrests out of the way to prevent obstructions).

PATIENT POSITION

20	Bring the client from sitting to supine or supine to sitting in a controlled and safe manner. Use a log roll method and maintain any sternal, spinal, and hip precautions.
21	Guard the client at all times. Keep your hand on the client, provide verbal cues, and increase safety awareness.
22	Protect the client's feet from the wheelchair, and ensure adequate footwear and/or ankle or foot orthotics.
23	Verbally cue the client to symmetrically align posture.
24	Manually assist the client to ensure anterior tilt of the pelvis prior to preparing to bring to stand.
25	Verbally cue the client to position arms appropriately to assist within capacity.
26	Verbally cue the client to facilitate weight shift.
27	Manually assist the client to shift weight.
28	Position the client's feet and your feet with an appropriate base of support. The client's heels should be directed toward the transfer surface.
29	Ensure the client has equal weightbearing on feet prior to bringing the client to stand. Stagger the client's stance with the weak leg slightly behind the other leg.
30	Verbally cue the client to come to a standing position.
31	Manually cue with the gait belt to direct the client's weight shift and movement of feet.
32	Verbally and manually cue to facilitate the client's pivot movement.

(continued)

UNIT 1-6   NEED TO KNOW

UNIT 1-6 NEED TO KNOW

TRANSFER CHECKLIST (CONTINUED)	
33	Provide lower extremity tactile cues to encourage the client to move his or her feet and pivot.
34	Avoid twisting your trunk or your client's trunk.
35	Verbally cue and safely direct the client's movement from stand to sit.

COMMON ASSESSMENTS ACROSS PRACTICE SETTINGS					
ASSESSMENT	ACUTE	INPATIENT	HOME HEALTH	SNF	OUTPATIENT
Common Assessments Across Practice Settings					
Interest Checklist	✓	✓	✓		✓
Australian Therapy Outcome Measure	✓	✓			✓
Kohlman Evaluation of Living Skills	✓	✓			
Assessment of Motor and Process Skills	✓	✓			
Assessment of Living Skills and Resources	✓	✓			
Structured Anchored Approach to Functional Assessment	✓				
Activity Measure for Post Acute Care "6-Clicks"	✓	✓		✓	✓
Activity Card Sort		✓	✓		✓
Community Integration Questionnaire					✓
Craig Hospital Inventory of Environmental Factors					✓
Measure of the Quality of the Environment			✓		✓
Work Environment Impact Scale			✓		✓
Assessment of Work Performance			✓		✓
Cognitive Performance Test		✓			✓
Arnadottir OT-ADL Neurobehavioral Evaluation		✓			✓

(continued)

UNIT 2-7 EVALUATION

UNIT 2-7 EVALUATION

COMMON ASSESSMENTS ACROSS PRACTICE SETTINGS (CONTINUED)

ASSESSMENT	ACUTE	INPATIENT	HOME HEALTH	SNF	OUTPATIENT
Functional Outcome Measures for Acute and Intensive Care Unit Settings					
Katz ADL Index	✓	✓			
Functional Status Score for the Intensive Care Unit (ICU)	✓				
Physical Function ICU Test	✓				
Chelsea Critical Care Physical Assessment Tool	✓				
ICU Mobility Scale	✓				
Surgical ICU Optimal Mobilisation Score	✓				
Manchester Mobility Score	✓				
Perme ICU Mobility Score	✓				
Canadian Occupational Performance Measure	✓	✓	✓	✓	✓
Functional Independence Measure and Quality Measures for Inpatient Rehabilitation Facilities	✓	✓	✓		
Barthel Index	✓	✓		✓	
Executive Function Performance Test		✓			✓

(continued)

COMMON ASSESSMENTS ACROSS PRACTICE SETTINGS (CONTINUED)

ASSESSMENT	ACUTE	INPATIENT	HOME HEALTH	SNF	OUTPATIENT
Home Safety Assessments					
AARP Home Safety Checklist			✓		
Cougar Home Safety Assessment v. 4.0			✓		
Safety Assessment of Function and the Environment for Rehabilitation—Health Outcome Measurement and Evaluation (SAFER-HOME) v. 3			✓		
Home Environment Assessment Protocol			✓		
In-Home Occupational Performance Evaluation (I-HOPE)			✓		
Westmead Home Safety Assessment			✓		
Comprehensive Assessment and Solution Process for Aging Residents (CASPAR)			✓		
Driving and Community Mobility Screening					
Driving for older adults		✓			✓
Available driving self-assessment tools					
AAA-Roadwise					
Drivers 55 Plus					
"Am I a Safe Driver?"					
Driving Habits Questionnaire					
Fitness to Drive Screening Measure					

SNF: skilled nursing facility.

(continued)

UNIT 2-7 EVALUATION

UNIT 2-7 EVALUATION

COMMON ASSESSMENTS
ACROSS PRACTICE SETTINGS (CONTINUED)

INTEREST CHECKLIST[24]

- Purpose: Identifies client's level of interest in leisure activities and past, present, and future participation. Activities can be used to drive treatment and goals.
- Context: Acute, inpatient, and outpatient settings
- Format: Checklist
- Time to administer: Quick
- Materials: Checklist and writing utensil
- Cost: Free
- Website: https://www.moho.uic.edu/products.aspx?type=free

AUSTRALIAN THERAPY OUTCOME MEASURE[25]

- Purpose: Measures therapy outcomes in the areas of impairment, activity, limitations, and well-being
- Context: Clients with any diagnosis at any age
- Format: Performance based
- Time to administer: 10 minutes or more
- Materials: Score card, manual, and writing utensil
- Cost: Free
- Website: www.austoms.com/about

KOHLMAN EVALUATION OF LIVING SKILLS[26]

- Purpose: Assesses client's independence with ADLs, safety, and IADLs money management, transportation, telephone use, work, and leisure
- Context: Clients across settings, such as older adults, acute care clients, clients with traumatic brain injury (TBI), adolescents, etc
- Format: Rating scale or interview
- Time to administer: Less than 45 minutes
- Materials: Manual
- Cost: $99 for AOTA members and $140 for nonmembers
- Website: https://myaota.aota.org/shop_aota/prodview.aspx?TYPE=D&PID=277716288&SKU=900374

(continued)

COMMON ASSESSMENTS
ACROSS PRACTICE SETTINGS (CONTINUED)

ASSESSMENT OF MOTOR AND PROCESS SKILLS[27,28]

- Purpose: Assesses motor and process skills during ADLs and IADLs
- Context: Clients with any diagnosis at any age
- Format: Interview and performance-based observation
- Time to administer: 30 to 40 minutes
- Materials: Does not require special equipment. Five-day certification course required.
- Cost: $65 and up for manual
- Website: http://www.innovativeotsolutions.com/tools/amps

ASSESSMENT OF LIVING SKILLS AND RESOURCES[29,30]

- Purpose: Assesses the client's participation in IADLs related to skills and resources used
- Context: Community-dwelling older adults
- Format: Interview with performance-based observation and rating scale
- Time to administer: Quick; under 10 minutes
- Materials: Score sheet and writing utensil
- Cost: Free
- Source: The revised scoring guidelines can be found in the *Australian Journal of Occupational Therapy* published in 2007.[30]

STRUCTURED ANCHORED APPROACH TO FUNCTIONAL ASSESSMENT[31]

- Purpose: Provides a framework for assessing function in an acute inpatient setting
- Context: Acute physical inpatient setting
- Format: Interview with performance-based observation
- Time to administer: 2 to 4 hours
- Materials: Varies. Materials may include any task item or assessment that provides information about the client's status
- Cost: Free or cost of assessment items
- Source: Described in the *British Journal of Occupational Therapy* published in January 2005[31]

(continued)

UNIT 2-7 EVALUATION

COMMON ASSESSMENTS
ACROSS PRACTICE SETTINGS (CONTINUED)

ACTIVITY MEASURE FOR POST ACUTE CARE "6-CLICKS"[32]

- Purpose: Assesses the amount of help an individual needs to complete ADLs
- Context: Acute, inpatient, and post acute care clients with hip fracture, stroke, and cancer; geriatric populations; orthopedic conditions; and cases that are medically complex.
- Format: Electronic questionnaire
- Time to administer: Quick
- Materials: Computer for computer adapted test
- Cost: Free
- Website: http://am-pac.com/category/home

ACTIVITY CARD SORT[33]

- Purpose: Identifies activities performed by the client across leisure, social, and IADL domains
- Context: All rehabilitation settings
- Format: Card sort or interview
- Time to administer: 20 to 30 minutes
- Materials: Activity cards
- Cost: $99 for AOTA members and $140 for nonmembers
- Website: https://myaota.aota.org/shop_aota/prodview. aspx?Type=D&SKU=1247

(continued)

COMMON ASSESSMENTS
ACROSS PRACTICE SETTINGS (CONTINUED)

COMMUNITY INTEGRATION QUESTIONNAIRE[34]

- Purpose: Assesses a client's reintegration into the community and home
- Context: Clients with TBI, spinal cord injury (SCI), and stroke
- Format: Self-report questionnaire
- Time to administer: Quick; under 10 minutes
- Materials: Score sheet and writing utensil
- Cost: Free
- Website: https://www.sralab.org/rehabilitation-measures/community-integration-questionnaire

CRAIG HOSPITAL INVENTORY OF ENVIRONMENTAL FACTORS[35]

- Purpose: Assesses environmental factors that are facilitators and barriers to participation for clients with disabilities
- Context: Clients with SCI, orthopedic injury, cardiac conditions, and multiple sclerosis (MS)
- Format: Self-report questionnaire or interview
- Time to administer: 5 to 10 minutes
- Materials: Score sheet and writing utensil
- Cost: Free
- Website: https://craighospital.org/programs/research/research-instruments

MEASURE OF THE QUALITY OF THE ENVIRONMENT[36]

- Purpose: Assesses environmental factors that facilitate or inhibit participation in daily activities and role fulfillment
- Context: Clients with stroke
- Format: Self-report questionnaire or interview
- Time to administer: 30 to 60 minutes
- Materials: Score sheet and writing utensil
- Cost: $23.50 for the manual; score sheet can be purchased for an additional fee
- Website: http://ripph.qc.ca/en/documents/mqe/what-is-mqe

(continued)

UNIT 2-7 EVALUATION

COMMON ASSESSMENTS
ACROSS PRACTICE SETTINGS (CONTINUED)

WORK ENVIRONMENT IMPACT SCALE[37]

- Purpose: Assesses the work environment for individuals with disabilities
- Context: Used in a variety of settings for individuals with disabilities who are returning to work or are currently working
- Format: Semi-structured interview and rating scale
- Time to administer: Quick
- Materials: Assessment form and writing utensil
- Cost: $40
- Website: https://www.moho.uic.edu/productDetails.aspx?aid=12

ASSESSMENT OF WORK PERFORMANCE[38]

- Purpose: Assesses the client's motor, process, and communication skills as they relate to the client's efficiency and accuracy completing work activities
- Context: Individuals with disabilities experiencing difficulties with work
- Format: Semi-structured interview and observation-based rating scale
- Time to administer: A few hours to weeks, depending on the practitioner. The person administering the assessment should assess one work task at a time.
- Materials: Assessment and writing utensil
- Cost: $40
- Website: https://moho.uic.edu/productDetails.aspx?aid=17

(continued)

COMMON ASSESSMENTS ACROSS PRACTICE SETTINGS (CONTINUED)
COGNITIVE PERFORMANCE TEST[39]
• Purpose: Assesses deficits of cognitive processing and predicts the impact of deficits on IADL and ADL performance • Context: Individuals with Alzheimer's disease and other conditions that impact executive function and memory • Format: Performance-based observation • Time to administer: 15 minutes to several hours • Materials: Assessment kit, manual, and score sheets • Cost: $617, but cost differs depending on the retailer • Website: http://www.maddak.com/cpt-cognitive-performance-test-p-27823.html
ARNADOTTIR OT-ADL NEUROBEHAVIORAL EVALUATION[40]
• Purpose: Assesses neurobehavioral deficits and their impact on ADL participation • Context: Clients with neurobehavioral disorders or dementia • Format: Performance-based observation • Time to administer: 25 minutes • Materials: Manual and assessment form • Cost: Requires purchase of a textbook containing the measure, in addition to a training course • Website: http://www.a-one.is

UNIT 2-7 EVALUATION

Functional Outcome Measures for Acute and Intensive Care Unit Settings

The following assessment tools can be used to evaluate and reevaluate occupational performance in acute care and ICU settings. This table provides a summary of each tool. Some tools may be described in greater detail in later tables.

Tool	Description
Katz ADL Index[41]	• Purpose: Assesses 6 ADLs (bathing, dressing, toileting, transferring, continence, and feeding) to determine level of functional impairment • Context: Elderly population • Format: Observation questionnaire • Time to administer: Under 30 minutes • Materials: Checklist • Cost: Free • Website: https://www.improvelto.com
Functional Status Score for the ICU[42]	• Purpose: Assesses physical function in the ICU based on 5 functional tasks (rolling, supine-to-sit transfers, unsupported sitting, sit-to-stand transfers, and ambulation). Higher scores indicate better function. • Context: ICU • Format: Seven-point ordinal scale • Time to administer: Under 30 minutes • Materials: Score sheet • Cost: Free • Website: https://www.improvelto.com

(continued)

FUNCTIONAL OUTCOME MEASURES FOR ACUTE AND INTENSIVE CARE UNIT SETTINGS (CONTINUED)	
TOOL	**DESCRIPTION**
Physical Function ICU Test[43]	• Purpose: Assesses heart rate, blood pressure, respiratory rate, and oxygen saturation during strenuous activity • Context: ICU • Format: Ordinal scale • Time to administer: Varies; 10 to 15 minutes • Materials: Stopwatch • Cost: Free • Website: https://www.improvelto.com
Chelsea Critical Care Physical Assessment Tool[44]	• Purpose: Assesses 10 items to determine level of independence. Items include respiratory function, cough, moving within the bed, supine to sitting on the edge of the bed, dynamic sitting, standing balance, sit-to-stand transfers, bed-to-chair transfers, stepping, and grip strength. • Context: ICU • Format: Six-point scale; scores are plotted in a chart • Time to administer: Varies; under 10 minutes • Materials: Dynamometer • Cost: Free; requires online training from http://cpax.ocbmedia.com • Website: https://www.improvelto.com
ICU Mobility Scale[45]	• Purpose: Measures mobility milestones in critically ill clients • Context: ICU • Format: Interview • Time to administer: Quick; 1 minute • Materials: Form and writing utensil • Cost: Free • Website: https://www.improvelto.com

(continued)

FUNCTIONAL OUTCOME MEASURES FOR ACUTE AND INTENSIVE CARE UNIT SETTINGS (CONTINUED)	
TOOL	**DESCRIPTION**
Surgical ICU Optimal Mobilisation Score[46]	• Purpose: Guides early mobilization based on out-of-bed activities • Context: ICU • Format: Observation • Time to administer: Quick; 1 minute • Materials: Form and writing utensil • Cost: Free • Website: https://www.improvelto.com
Manchester Mobility Score[47]	• Purpose: Measures the client's passive movements, active or active-assisted movements, chair position in bed, sitting edge of bed, hoisting out of chair, transfers with standing hoist, 2-person transfers, 1-person transfers, mobilized to end of bed, mobilized 10 meters, and independence with mobility • Context: ICU • Format: Observation • Time to administer: Quick; 1 minute • Materials: Form and writing utensil • Cost: Free • Website: https://www.improvelto.com

(continued)

FUNCTIONAL OUTCOME MEASURES FOR ACUTE AND INTENSIVE CARE UNIT SETTINGS (CONTINUED)	
TOOL	**DESCRIPTION**
Perme ICU Mobility Score[48]	• Purpose: Measures mental status, potential barriers, functional strength, transfers, gait, and endurance • Context: ICU • Format: Performance observation • Time to administer: Varies; up to 1 hour • Materials: Form, writing utensil, bed, chair, and stopwatch • Cost: Free • Website: https://www.improvelto.com; Requires training from http://www.permeicuseminars.com/perme-icu-mobility-score
Canadian Occupational Performance Measure (COPM)	Refer to Unit 2-9 of this section for information on the COPM.
Functional Independence Measure (FIM)	Refer to Unit 2-10 of this section for information on the FIM.
Barthel Index	Refer to Unit 2-11 of this section for information on the Barthel Index.

UNIT 2-8 EVALUATION

CANADIAN OCCUPATIONAL PERFORMANCE MEASURE

SUMMARY

- Purpose: Assesses an individual's perceived occupational performance in the areas of self-care, productivity, and leisure
- Context: Designed for use with all clients
- Format: Semi-structured interview
- Time to administer: Varies; 15 to 45 minutes
- Materials: COPM manual, score sheet, and pen
- Cost: Varies, as forms may be purchased in varied quantities and formats
- Website: http://www.thecopm.ca

The COPM is a 5-step semi-structured interview conducted by an occupational therapist during the evaluation process.[49] The COPM informs the occupational profile and assists in developing therapy goals by identifying activities that the client wants, needs, or is expected to do. The COPM can be used with all clients without regard to diagnosis, and has been validated with patients who have stroke, chronic obstructive pulmonary disease, pain, cerebral palsy, TBI, Parkinson's disease, arthritis, and ankylosing spondylitis, as well as pediatric patients.

IMPLICATIONS FOR THERAPY

Allows meaningful goals to be identified for therapy. Using the COPM in occupational therapy practice is shown to increase clinical knowledge of important client issues, clinical decision making for treatment, ability to state outcomes clearly, and documentation of outcomes.[50]

(continued)

CANADIAN OCCUPATIONAL PERFORMANCE MEASURE (CONTINUED)

STEPS	DESCRIPTION	EXAMPLE PHRASES DURING STEPS
Introduction	Begin by explaining the role of occupational therapy and the purpose of COPM to client.	"Occupations are any activities that you want or need to do. The COPM is a tool that we will use to identify the occupations you may be having trouble with due to _____ so that I can get a better idea of what your goals are and what we can work on during our occupational therapy sessions."
1. Identify problems in occupational performance	The 3 main categories of occupations measured by the COPM are self-care, productivity, and leisure. Within each category is a set of occupations. You will ask clients to identify things they want to do, need to do, or are expected to do in each occupational area.	"The first section of the COPM is focused on identifying problems you are having in performing activities. I am going ask you to describe different areas of your daily routine and write down the problems you identify."
A. Self-Care	• Personal care (eg, dressing, bathing, feeding, hygiene) • Functional mobility (eg, transfers, indoor and outdoor mobility) • Community management (eg, transportation, shopping, finances)	"Tell me about your morning routine. Is there anything related to your personal care, such as dressing or hygiene, that you are having difficulty with?"

(continued)

UNIT 2-9 EVALUATION

UNIT 2-9 EVALUATION

CANADIAN OCCUPATIONAL PERFORMANCE MEASURE (CONTINUED)		
STEPS	**DESCRIPTION**	**EXAMPLE PHRASES DURING STEPS**
B. Productivity	• Paid/unpaid work (eg, finding and keeping a job, volunteering) • Household management (eg, cleaning, laundry, cooking) • Play/school (eg, play skills, homework)	"Is there anything in the community that you need to do, want to do, or are expected to do, such as driving or shopping, that you are having difficulty doing?"
C. Leisure	• Quiet recreation (eg, hobbies, crafts, reading) • Active recreation (eg, sports, outings, travel) • Socialization (eg, visiting, phone calls, parties, correspondence)	"Thank you for sharing that. So far, I have written 'getting ready on time, having energy to play with my kids, and cooking dinner.' Is there anything else I missed or that you want to add?"
2. Rating importance	Show the client the 10-point rating scale for rating importance, and record his or her rating for how important each identified occupation/problem is.	"Now I want to go back through the list we made and get a better sense of how important each item you identified is to you. On a scale of 1 to 10, how important is _____ (cooking dinner) to you?" *(continued)*

CANADIAN OCCUPATIONAL
PERFORMANCE MEASURE (CONTINUED)

STEPS	DESCRIPTION	EXAMPLE PHRASES DURING STEPS
3. Selecting problems for scoring	Ask the client to identify up to 5 of the most important problems. Record the chosen problems and the importance rating for each in the scoring section for Time 1. (Note: If client has only identified 3 problems, these 3 problems can be used instead of listing 5.) The client's 5 most important problems do *not* have to be the 5 problems with the highest importance rating from Step 2.	"Now that you have thought about how important each activity and problem is to you, I would like you to choose the top 5 problems that are most important to you and that you would like to work on in occupational therapy."
4. Scoring performance and satisfaction	Show the client the 10-point rating scales for performance and satisfaction of performance, and record his or her ratings for the 5 problems identified on the back of the form in the scoring section for Time 1.	"You mentioned cooking as one of your top 5 current problems. Using the performance scale, with 1 being not able to do it at all and 10 being able to do it extremely well, how would you rate the way you cook right now? OK, now using the satisfaction scale, how satisfied are you with the way you cook right now, from 1, not satisfied at all, to 10, extremely satisfied?"
		(continued)

UNIT 2-9 EVALUATION

CANADIAN OCCUPATIONAL PERFORMANCE MEASURE (CONTINUED)		
STEPS	DESCRIPTION	EXAMPLE PHRASES DURING STEPS
5. Client reassessment	Explain to the client that you will use the problems they identified to plan ways to address them during occupational therapy sessions. Then, at a later date after occupational therapy treatment, re-score the client's performance and satisfaction for the 5 problems identified under Time 2. (Note: During re-assessment, generally it is not advised to show the client his or her previous rating scores.)	"Thank you for being open and sharing these concerns with me. These scores will help me plan what we can work on during occupational therapy, and in a few weeks we will look back and compare your scores to see if we have made progress toward your goals."

CALCULATING SCORES

- Add up all of the scores in the performance column for problems 1 to 5. Calculate the average score (total score / number of problems in the top 5).
- Add up all of the scores in the satisfaction column for problems 1 to 5. Calculate the average score (total score / number of problems in the top 5).
- To compare the change in scores:
  - Time 2 performance average – time 1 performance average (eg, $8.0 - 3.5 = +4.5$)
  - Time 2 satisfaction average – time 1 satisfaction average
  - A change in 2 points or more is clinically significant.

(continued)

CANADIAN OCCUPATIONAL
PERFORMANCE MEASURE (CONTINUED)

TIPS FOR USING THE CANADIAN OCCUPATIONAL PERFORMANCE MEASURE WITH PATIENTS WHO HAVE IMPAIRMENTS

- Administer the COPM in an environment free from distractions if the client has cognitive impairments.
- The COPM may be administered across multiple sessions if fatigue or distraction is a challenge for the client.
- If the client has communication difficulties, then consider using picture cards and allow the client to point. Another strategy is to ask simple "yes" and "no" questions. You may find it helpful to involve the client's family, but be aware that the goals chosen by a caregiver may not be client centered. Consider administering a recently developed aphasia-friendly version of the COPM that uses photographs of activities with text labels.[51]

FIM AND QUALITY MEASURES FOR INPATIENT REHABILITATION FACILITIES

FUNCTIONAL INDEPENDENCE MEASURE

Note: These guidelines do not replace becoming credentialed in the use of the FIM instrument.

Summary

- Purpose: Measures the client's functional ability related to physical dysfunction
- Context: Inpatient rehabilitation, TBI, stroke, MS, SCI, etc
- Format: Performance-based observation
- Time to administer: 30 to 45 minutes to administer; may be administered over multiple sessions
- Materials: The FIM System software
- Cost: Certification course and exam is $799; retesting and recertification carry additional costs
- Website: www.udsmr.org/WebModules/FIM/Fim_About.aspx

The FIM assesses the severity of disability by measuring the functional ability of the client. The FIM is used to track progress and describe the burden of care.[52]

Areas of performance measured by the FIM include eating, grooming, bathing, upper body dressing, lower body dressing, toileting, bladder management, bowel management, transfers (bed, chair, or wheelchair), toilet transfer, tub or shower transfer, locomotion, and stair usage. Areas of communication and social cognition measured by the FIM include comprehension, expression, social interaction, problem solving, and memory.[52,53]

Each area of performance is scored on a 7-point ordinal scale with 7 indicating independence and 1 indicating total dependence. The score is based on the number of specified steps that the client completes. Guidelines for scoring are outlined below.[1-53]

Examples are provided in each section to help you prepare for the FIM certification exam.

(continued)

FIM AND QUALITY MEASURES FOR
INPATIENT REHABILITATION FACILITIES (CONTINUED)

General Guidelines

Score		Requirements for Client Completion
7	Independent	100% of the task was completed by the client in a safe and timely manner.
6	Modified independent	100% of the task was completed by the client, and the client used an assistive device, required excess time (3 times the usual time required to complete), or demonstrated safety concerns (balance, weight bearing precautions, history of falls).
5	Setup/ supervision/ cueing	90% to 100% of the task was completed by the client, and help was required with setup, supervision, cueing, or coaxing.
4	Minimum assistance	75% to 89% of the task was completed by the client, and the client required contact or incidental assistance.
3	Moderate assistance	50% to 74% of the task was completed by the client.
2	Maximum assistance	25% to 49% of the task was completed by the client.
1	Dependent	0% to 24% of the task was completed by client.
0	Does not occur	Performance was unsafe or contraindicated, or the client refused.

(continued)

UNIT 2-10 EVALUATION

UNIT 2-10 EVALUATION

FIM AND QUALITY MEASURES FOR INPATIENT REHABILITATION FACILITIES (CONTINUED)

Calculating Percentage of Completion

Number of Steps in the Functional Independence Measure Category

Number of Steps the Client Completes	1	2	3	4	5	6	7	8	9	10	11	12	13	14	15
1	100	50	33	25	20	17	14	13	11	10	9	8	8	7	7
2		100	67	50	40	33	29	25	22	20	18	17	15	14	13
3			100	75	60	50	43	38	33	30	27	25	23	21	20
4				100	80	67	57	50	44	40	36	33	31	29	27
5					100	83	71	63	56	50	45	42	38	36	33
6						100	86	75	67	60	55	50	46	43	40
7							100	88	78	70	64	58	54	50	47
8	Independent/modified independent (6 to 7)							100	89	80	73	67	62	57	53
9	Setup/supervision (5)								100	90	82	75	69	64	60
10	Minimum assist (4)									100	91	83	77	71	67
11	Moderate assist (3)										100	92	85	79	73
12	Maximum assist (2)											100	92	86	80
13	Total assist/dependent (1)												100	92	87
14														100	93
15															100

(continued)

FIM AND QUALITY MEASURES FOR INPATIENT REHABILITATION FACILITIES (CONTINUED)

Eating: Five Parts

(1) Drink from cup. (2) Pick up appropriate utensil. (3) Scoop food. (4) Bring food to mouth. (5) Chew and swallow.

Scoring begins when food tray is placed in front of the client.

Score	Eating
7	All 5 parts were completed independently and safely. The client opened packages, cut food, and was on a regular consistency diet (including low sodium, diabetic diet, and prune juice).
6	Client completed the task independently with devices (eg, dentures, adapted utensils) used a swallow technique, consumed modified textures or fluid consistency, or required 3 times the usual time (60 minutes or more).
5	Client required supervision, cues, or setup (ie, staff assisted to open packages, cut the food, set up a splint, or insert the client's dentures).
4	Client required occasional contact assistance by the staff (3 out of 5 tasks; ie, staff assisted to place a utensil in the client's hand, occasionally scooped food, or checked for food pocketing).
3	Client completed 3 out of 5 tasks without assistance (ie, staff assisted to scoop each bite while the client brought the food to his or her mouth).
2	Client completed 3 out of 5 tasks without assistance (ie, staff assisted to scoop food and used hand-over-hand guidance to bring food to the client's mouth, and the client was still able to swallow and drink from a cup).
1	Less than 25% was done by the client, or the staff gave feeding through a tube or intravenous (IV) hydration.
0	Activity did not occur (at admission); cannot be scored 0 at discharge.

(continued)

UNIT 2-10 EVALUATION

FIM AND QUALITY MEASURES FOR
INPATIENT REHABILITATION FACILITIES (CONTINUED)

Eating Example

The client is observed in her room with a tray of food in front of her. The therapist decides this may be a good time to FIM eating. The client has a C6 SCI and uses a universal cuff to hold a fork and a long straw for drinking. The client has not started eating her chicken because she requires help cutting the food. She eats for 15 minutes without assistance. The therapist provides her some tips on how to maximize eating with the cuff. What is her FIM?

Answer and Rationale

The FIM score is a 5, because the client required assistance to cut the food, which is considered setup. She also uses adaptive equipment, but the FIM must score the highest amount of assistance needed. Cueing in eating is also considered a 5 and can be coupled with setting up the task.

(continued)

UNIT 2–10 EVALUATION

FIM AND QUALITY MEASURES FOR INPATIENT REHABILITATION FACILITIES (CONTINUED)

Grooming: Four or Five Parts

(1) Wash, rinse, and dry face. (2) Wash, rinse, and dry hands. (3) Clean teeth/dentures. (4) Brush hair. (5) Shave/apply makeup (optional).

- Washing includes 3 steps each: wash, rinse, and dry.

Not included: flossing, applying deodorant, caring for nails, or washing hair

Score	Grooming
7	Client was independent and safe in retrieving all needed items and completed grooming.
6	Client was independent with the use of devices (eg, tube squeeze, wash mitt, adapted sink handles) or required 3 times the usual amount of time needed. (It is acceptable for a client to use a wheelchair.)
5	Client required supervision, cues, or setup (ie, staff assisted to retrieve the items, handed the items to the client, plugged in devices, or applied toothpaste for the client).
4	Client completed 3 out of 4 or 4 out of 5 tasks (ie, staff assisted to insert or remove dentures, or the client required occasional steadying assistance).
3	Client completed 2 out of 4 or 3 out of 5 tasks.
2	Client completed 1 out of 4 or 2 out of 5 tasks.
1	Client completed 0 out of 4 or 1 out of 5 tasks, or required the assistance of 2 staff members.
0	Activity did not occur (at admission); cannot be scored 0 at discharge.

Grooming Example

The client performs a grooming task and independently brushes his teeth, brushes his hair, shaves, and washes and dries his face in a timely manner. He has limited shoulder abduction due to a recent rotator cuff tear and requires you to put on his deodorant for him. What is his FIM?

Answer and Rationale

The FIM score is a 7. Applying deodorant, flossing teeth, caring for nails, and washing hair are not scored in the grooming FIM. The client is therefore independent in grooming.

(continued)

UNIT 2-10 EVALUATION

FIM AND QUALITY MEASURES FOR INPATIENT REHABILITATION FACILITIES (CONTINUED)

Bathing: Ten Parts

(1) Chest. (2) Abdomen. (3) Perineal area. (4) Buttocks. (5) Right arm. (6) Left arm. (7) Right thigh. (8) Left thigh. (9) Right lower leg/foot. (10) Left lower leg/foot.

- Bathing includes 3 steps for each body part: wash, rinse, and dry.
- For clients with amputations, score according to number of appropriate body parts.
- Bathing must be completed wet, and client must be completely naked. A simulation at a gym is not permitted for scoring.

    Not included: back and hair

Score	Bathing
7	Client was independent and safe in retrieving all needed items and completed bathing.
6	Client was independent with the use of devices (eg, long handle sponge, wash mitt) or required 3 times the amount of usual time needed.
5	Client required supervision, cues, or setup (ie, staff assisted to retrieve items, adjusted the water temperature, or added soap to the washcloth).
4	Client completed 75% or more of the bathing (8 to 9 out of 10 body parts), and/or required assistance to remain steadied (ie, staff assisted to put the washcloth in the client's hand or helped wring the washcloth).
3	Client completed 50% to 74%, or 5 to 7 body parts.
2	Client completed 25% to 49%, or 3 to 4 body parts.
1	Client completed less than 25%, or 0 to 2 body parts, or client required the assistance of 2 staff members.
0	Activity did not occur (at admission); cannot be scored 0 at discharge.

(continued)

FIM AND QUALITY MEASURES FOR
INPATIENT REHABILITATION FACILITIES (CONTINUED)

Bathing Example #1

The client has a left above-the-knee amputation from a motorcycle accident. The therapist observes him bathing. He cannot wash the body parts that he doesn't have. What is the FIM score based on this situation?

Answer and Rationale #1

There are 10 body parts considered in bathing (10% for each part of the task). A person with an above-the-knee amputation does not have a left lower leg to score. That body part will not be counted, and each remaining body part is assigned a higher score. Therefore, each of the 9 remaining body parts represent 11% of the entire task. His FIM score for bathing is a 7 if he can wash all 9 remaining body parts.

Bathing Example #2

Melody received a sink bath upon admission. The staff helped adjust the water temperature and prepared the environment. Melody washed her chest and abdomen with minimal cueing. She required physical assistance to wash her arms, upper legs, perineal area, and buttocks. She has dressings on her right and left lower extremities and was instructed by her doctor and nurses not to wash these. What is her FIM score?

Answer and Rationale #2

Melody's FIM score for bathing is a 1, because she required setup and cueing, and bathed 2 out of 8 areas. Bathing is rated on the number of body parts intended to be washed, and in this instance, Melody washed 2 out of 8 body parts.

(continued)

UNIT 2-10 EVALUATION

	<div align="center">**FIM AND QUALITY MEASURES FOR INPATIENT REHABILITATION FACILITIES (CONTINUED)**</div>

Dressing Upper Body

Shirt with buttons: 4 steps; pullover shirt: 4 steps; bra: 4 steps

- Steps include threading arms (2 steps), pulling over head or around body (1 step), and pulling the garment into place or buttoning/securing the garment (1 step).
- Upper body dressing is not scored with a hospital gown. The client must dress in street clothes.

Score	Dressing and Undressing
7	Client was independent and safe in retrieving all needed items and completed dressing.
6	Client was independent with the use of devices (ie, used prosthesis, reacher, button hook, or side rail of bed, or relied on a walker or wheelchair for balance when retrieving or donning clothing), or client required 3 times the usual amount of time needed.
5	Client required supervision, cues, or setup (ie, staff assisted to retrieve items from the closet, or the staff applied the prosthesis/ orthosis for the client, including the help of one staff member to apply a thoracic lumbar sacral orthosis [TLSO] brace).
4	Client completed 75% or more of upper body dressing and required assistance for closure of buttons or zippers, initiation of tasks, or contact for steadying.
3	Client completed 50% to 74% of the steps required for dressing.
2	Client completed 25 %to 49% of the steps required for dressing.
1	Client completed less than 25%, or 2 helpers were needed to apply TLSO brace.
0	Activity did not occur (at admission); cannot be scored 0 at discharge.

Dressing Upper Body Example

The client is able to thread his arms through both sleeves of the shirt and get his head in, but insufficient internal shoulder rotation, elbow flexion, and long finger opposition restricts him from pulling the shirt down over his torso. The therapist assists by pulling his shirt down. What is his FIM score?

Answer and Rationale

The FIM score is a 4. The client completed ¾ components (75%) of the task.

(continued)

FIM AND QUALITY MEASURES FOR INPATIENT REHABILITATION FACILITIES (CONTINUED)

Dressing Lower Body

Underwear: 3 steps; pants with button/zipper: 4 steps; pants with elastic waist: 3 steps; belt: 2 steps; socks: 1 step (left), 1 step (right); shoes: 1 step (left), 1 step (right); tying shoe: 1 step (left), 1 step (right)

- Steps include threading left leg (1 step), threading right leg (1 step), pulling up (1 step), fastening (if necessary; 1 step)
- Lower body dressing is not scored with a hospital gown. The client must dress in street clothes.

Score	Dressing and Undressing
7	Client was independent and safe in retrieving all needed items and completed dressing.
6	Client was independent with the use of devices (ie, used prosthesis, sock aid, hip kit, reacher, side rail of bed, relied on walker or wheelchair for balance when retrieving or donning clothing), or required 3 times the usual amount of time needed to complete.
5	Client required supervision, cues, coaxing, or setup (ie, staff assisted to retrieve items from the closet, or the staff helped to apply a prosthesis/orthosis or elastic hose for the client).
4	Client completed 75% or more of lower body dressing and required assistance for buttons or zippers, contact for steadying, or help initiating tasks.
3	Client completed 50% to 74% of the steps for dressing.
2	Client completed 25% to 49% of the steps for dressing.
1	Client completed less than 25% of the steps for dressing.
0	Activity did not occur (at admission); cannot be scored 0 at discharge.

Dressing Lower Body Example

The client requires physical assistance putting on her underwear, elastic pants, and socks, but independently dons her slip-on shoes. What is her FIM score?

Answer and Rationale

The FIM score is a 1. The client performed 8 out of 10 tasks. She completed less than 25% of the activity (3 steps for underwear, 3 for pants, 2 for socks, 2 for shoes).

(continued)

UNIT 2-10 EVALUATION

FIM AND QUALITY MEASURES FOR INPATIENT REHABILITATION FACILITIES (CONTINUED)

Toileting: Three Parts

(1) Adjust clothing as needed. (2) Complete toilet hygiene. (3) Readjust clothing afterward.

- Toileting can be scored using a bedside commode or bedpan.
- Must be scored during a continent episode only. If the client is incontinent during every episode in a 3-day assessment period, then the score should be rated 1.
- Catheterization cannot be rated for toileting. This is scored in bladder management.
- Scoring does not include help getting on or off the toilet or bedpan.

Score	Toileting
7	Client was independent and safe for all 3 parts of toileting.
6	Client was independent with devices (ie, grab bars for steadying while adjusting clothing), or client required 3 times the usual amount of time needed.
5	Client required supervision, cues, coaxing, or setup assistance from staff.
4	Client required steadying assistance, needed help initiating tasks, or needed help with zippers or buttons.
3	Client completed 2 out of 3 parts of toileting.
2	Client completed 1 out of 3 parts of toileting.
1	Staff completed all 3 parts of toileting.
0	Activity did not occur (at admission); cannot be scored 0 at discharge.

(continued)

FIM AND QUALITY MEASURES FOR INPATIENT REHABILITATION FACILITIES (CONTINUED)

Toileting Example

The client completed a toileting task during her first week stay. She was able to adjust and readjust her clothing after excretion. She had the capability to wipe herself, but when she laterally lumbar flexed, she became unsteady and almost fell off the toilet. The therapist decided to provide physical support by placing her hand on the client's shoulder during this task. On week 2, the therapist educated the client on use of a raised toilet seat and the use of grab bars around the toilet when bending and shifting on the toilet. The client used the grab bars for support. What is the toileting FIM score on week 1? What is the FIM score on week 2?

Answer and Rationale

The FIM score for week 1 is a 4 because the client required assistance to stay steady and safe. Any time a client is touched for assistance, the maximum score the client can get is a 4. The FIM score for week 2 is a 6, because the client used adaptive equipment.

(continued)

UNIT 2-10 EVALUATION

FIM AND QUALITY MEASURES FOR INPATIENT REHABILITATION FACILITIES (CONTINUED)			
Bladder Management			
Consider level of assistance and frequency of accidents. Score the lower of the 2. Does not include help transferring to or from the toilet Incontinence: Loss of sphincter control Accident: Soiling or wetting of clothes or linens			
Level of Assistance (Past 3 Days)		**Frequency of Accidents (Past 7 Days)** Search documentation of last 4 days prior to rehabilitation admission.	
SCORE	DESCRIPTION	SCORE	DESCRIPTION
7	Client was independent or was on dialysis with no voids. Client was independent with a timed schedule program or raised toilet seat (scored in toilet transfer FIM).	7	Client had no accidents, devices, or medications. Client may be on a timed schedule.
6	Client used medication for bladder control (Lasix [furosemide] for edema is not counted). Client was independent with the use of a pad, Pull-Ups (Kimberly-Clark Corporation), diaper, or self-catheterization. Client emptied the urinal, Foley bag, or bedside commode. Exception: If the client usually wears Pull-Ups as underwear and is not incontinent, do not count as an assistive device.	6	Client had no accidents. Client used devices including a catheter, urinal, bedside commode, disposable pad (not linen pad), or wafer. Client used medications.

(continued)

FIM AND QUALITY MEASURES FOR INPATIENT REHABILITATION FACILITIES (CONTINUED)

SCORE	DESCRIPTION	SCORE	DESCRIPTION
5	Client required supervision, cues, or setup (ie, staff placed equipment within reach of the client, or staff emptied the bedpan/urinal/ bedside commode).	5	Client had 1 accident.
4	Client completed 75% or more of bladder management, and staff positioned the bedpan while the client independently bridged or rolled from side to side to get on and off the bedpan.	4	Client had 2 accidents.
3	Client completed 50% to 74% of bladder management, and staff positioned the bedpan and held it in place while assisting the client to roll on or off the bedpan.	3	Client had 3 accidents.
2	Client completed 25% to 49% of bladder management, and staff positioned the bedpan, held it in place, or assisted the client to roll on and off the bedpan.	2	Client had 4 accidents.
			(continued)

UNIT 2-10 EVALUATION

| \multicolumn{4}{c}{**FIM AND QUALITY MEASURES FOR INPATIENT REHABILITATION FACILITIES (CONTINUED)**} |

FIM AND QUALITY MEASURES FOR INPATIENT REHABILITATION FACILITIES (CONTINUED)

SCORE	DESCRIPTION	SCORE	DESCRIPTION
1	Client completed less than 25% of bladder management. Staff performed catheterization, changed linens or clothing, or rolled the client onto his or her side to position the bedpan; or 2 helpers needed to assist. Staff needed to remind the client every 2 to 3 hours to stay on timed void schedule.	1	Client had 5 or more accidents.
0	Activity did not occur (at admission); cannot be scored 0 at discharge.		

Bladder Management Example

The client has been working on bed mobility and is able to roll independently to use a bedpan. He is on a timed void program and requires reminders (every 3 hours) to void. What is his FIM score?

Answer and Rationale

The FIM score is a 1 because he requires reminders to stay on the timed void schedule. In this instance, the burden of care for bladder management is high.

(continued)

FIM AND QUALITY MEASURES FOR INPATIENT REHABILITATION FACILITIES (CONTINUED)

Bowel Management

Consider level of assistance and frequency of accidents.

Score the lower of the 2.

Does not include help transferring to or from the toilet

Incontinence: Loss of sphincter control

Accident: Soiling or wetting of clothes or linens

Level of Assistance (Past 3 Days)		Frequency of Accidents (Past 7 Days) Search documentation of last 4 days prior to rehabilitation admission	
SCORE	DESCRIPTION	SCORE	DESCRIPTION
7	Client was independent or had no bowel movement. Client may use prunes or fiber.	7	Client had no accidents, devices, or medications. Client may be on a timed schedule.
6	Client used medication for bowel control. Client was independent and used a pad, Pull-Up (Kimberly-Clark Corporation), diaper, or a digital stimulation or suppository. Client emptied ostomy, bedpan, or bedside commode independently. Exception: If the client usually wears Pull-Ups as underwear and is not incontinent, do not count these as assistive devices.	6	Client had no accidents and used devices including colostomy, bedpan, bedside commode, or diaper. Client used medications.
5	Client required supervision, cues, or setup. Staff placed the equipment within reach of the client, or staff emptied the bedpan, ostomy, or bedside commode.	5	Client had 1 accident.

(continued)

UNIT 2-10 EVALUATION

FIM AND QUALITY MEASURES FOR INPATIENT REHABILITATION FACILITIES (CONTINUED)			
SCORE	DESCRIPTION	SCORE	DESCRIPTION
4	Client completed 75% or more of bowel management. Client completed bowel care or clothes/linens cleanup. Staff assisted with suppository (lube and insertion).	4	Client had 2 accidents.
3	Client completed 50% to 74% of bowel care or clothes/linens cleanup. Staff positioned the bedpan, held it in place, and assisted client to roll on or off the bedpan.	3	Client had 3 accidents.
2	Client completed 25% to 49% of bowel care or clothes/linens cleanup. Staff positioned the bedpan, held it in place, and assisted the client to roll on and off the bedpan.	2	Client had 4 accidents.
1	Client completed less than 25% of bowel management. Staff cleaned clothes/linens. Staff gave client an enema or disimpaction. Staff rolled client, or 2 staff members were needed.	1	Client had 5 or more accidents.
0	Activity did not occur (at admission); cannot be scored 0 at discharge.		

Bowel Management Example

The client is taking medicine for bowel control and wears adult diapers. The therapist goes to his room to begin his therapy for the day, and he tells the therapist that he soiled himself earlier that day. This is the only time he has had an accident this week. What is the client's FIM score?

Answer and Rationale

The FIM score is a 5 because the client had one accident in a 4-day period.

(continued)

FIM AND QUALITY MEASURES FOR INPATIENT REHABILITATION FACILITIES (CONTINUED)

Bed To/From Chair or Wheelchair Transfer

Includes supine to sit and sit to supine (begin and end in supine)

Score	Bed To/From Chair or Wheelchair Transfer
7	Client transferred independently without devices or help. (A facility that has a no lift policy does not apply to without help.)
6	Client transferred independently with the use of devices (eg, sliding board, walker, rails, chair arms/wheelchair arms, or electric bed), or client required 3 times the usual amount of time. No helper was required to raise the head of client's bed. (TLSO is not counted as a device.)
5	Client required supervision, cues, coaxing, or set-up. Staff helped with footrests, armrests, or brakes.
4	Client required minimum assistance, including assistance for steadying, contact guard assistance, help with one limb, or minimal physical touching.
3	Client required moderate assistance, including help with 2 limbs or assistance with getting up or down.
2	Client required maximum assistance, including assistance for getting up and down.
1	Client required total assistance, including a Hoyer lift, or 2 staff members were needed to help (even just in case); client provided less than 25% of the effort needed.
0	Activity did not occur (at admission); on bed rest, and cannot be scored 0 at discharge.

Bed To/From Chair or Wheelchair Transfer Example

The client is debilitated after surgery and requires assistance transferring to her bed from her wheelchair. The therapist uses a gait belt and assists with lifting her from the chair to perform a stand pivot transfer. Once she has backed up to the bed, she is able to sit without assistance. She wants to lie supine and requires assist bringing her legs onto the bed. What is her transfer FIM score?

Answer and Rationale

The FIM score is a 3. If the client requires lifting or lowering (not both), and/or if a client simply needs help getting both legs into the bed, always rate the FIM as a 3.

(continued)

UNIT 2-10 EVALUATION

UNIT 2-10 EVALUATION

FIM AND QUALITY MEASURES FOR INPATIENT REHABILITATION FACILITIES (CONTINUED)

Toilet Transfer

Transfer only; do not score clothing management for this FIM item. Do not use this FIM if a bedpan is used.

Score	Toilet Transfer
7	Client transferred independently without devices or help on and off a standard 14-inch toilet. (Client may still be considered independent with a wheelchair.)
6	Client transferred independently with devices (eg, a raised toilet seat, grab bars, sliding board, rails, or wheelchair arms), or required 3 times the usual amount of time.
5	Client required supervision, cues, coaxing, or setup. Staff positioned the sliding board, helped lock brakes of wheelchair, helped lift footrests off wheelchair, or provided verbal cues.
4	Client required minimum assistance, including steadying assistance, help with one limb, or minimal physical touching.
3	Client required moderate assistance for help with 2 limbs or assistance with lifting or lowering gently.
2	Client required maximum assistance, including assistance for lifting and lowering.
1	Client required total assistance, including the use of a Hoyer lift, or 2 staff members were needed to help (even just in case). Client provided less than 25% of the effort needed.
0	Activity did not occur (at admission); cannot be scored 0 at discharge.

Toilet Transfer Example

The client sustained a right cerebrovascular accident and has been impulsive during transfers. She is also weak. She requires physical assistance getting out of the chair and lowering to the toilet (and the same for transferring back). She is able to bear weight on her legs and pivot during the transfer. What is her FIM score?

Answer and Rationale

The FIM score is a 2. Remember, in any transfer, the score is a 2 if the client needs assistance both lifting and lowering.

(continued)

FIM AND QUALITY MEASURES FOR INPATIENT REHABILITATION FACILITIES (CONTINUED)

Tub or Shower Transfer

Must be performed wet; no simulation.

Score	Tub or Shower Transfer
7	Client transferred independently without devices or help. (Client may still be considered independent with a wheelchair.)
6	Client transferred independently with devices (eg, sliding board, grab bars, rails, or tub bench), or required 3 times the usual amount of time.
5	Client required supervision, cues, coaxing, or setup. Staff positioned the sliding board, helped lock brakes on wheelchair, or helped lift footrests off wheelchair. Verbal cues were given by staff.
4	Client required minimum assistance, including assistance for steadying, help with one limb (ie, lifting leg into tub), or contact guard assistance.
3	Client required moderate assistance, including help with 2 limbs and assistance for lifting or lowering.
2	Client required maximum assistance for lifting and lowering.
1	Client required total assistance including a Hoyer lift, or 2 staff members were needed to help (even just in case). Staff rolled the client into the shower. Client provided less than 25% of the effort needed.
0	Activity did not occur (at admission); cannot be scored 0 at discharge. Function modifiers: Tub transfer can be scored 0 at admission/discharge. Shower transfer cannot be scored 0 at admission/discharge.

(continued)

UNIT 2-10 EVALUATION

FIM AND QUALITY MEASURES FOR INPATIENT REHABILITATION FACILITIES (CONTINUED)

Tub or Shower Transfer Example

The client wants to take a shower. The therapist assesses him on his first day at the inpatient hospital, and the client reports that he cannot stand. The therapist encourages him to do his best and assures him of help if needed. The therapist assists in getting him to the edge of the bed, sitting on the edge, and then executing the transfer. With maximum effort, the therapist is able to assist in lifting him lift 3 inches off the bed. The therapist performs a squat pivot to transfer him to the shower chair with wheels. The therapist transports the client on the shower chair into the shower. What is his FIM score?

Answer and Rationale

The FIM score is a 1 because a helper performed all aspects of the transfer. If the client needs to be wheeled into the bathroom using a shower chair, then the client requires total assistance.

(continued)

UNIT 2-10 EVALUATION

FIM AND QUALITY MEASURES FOR INPATIENT REHABILITATION FACILITIES (CONTINUED)

Locomotion

Based on expected mode of locomotion at discharge.

Walk: Client is scored on a level surface once he or she is standing.

Wheelchair: Client is scored on a level surface once he or she is seated.

Score	Locomotion
7	Client walked independently and safely 150 feet.
6	Client walked independently with devices (wheelchair on 3% grade across multiple surfaces, walker, cane, or ankle-foot orthosis) for 150 feet. Client was independent with wound vac/IV/oxygen/tubes. TLSO is not counted as a device.
5	Client required supervision, cues, or setup to walk 150 feet.
5E	Household exception: Client was independently mobile for 50 feet with or without a device. Client required one person to hold wound vac/IV/oxygen/tubes.
4	Client traveled 150 feet with one helper. A gait belt or contact guard was needed for balance or safety.
3	Client traveled 150 feet and provided 50% to 74% of the effort needed.
2	Client traveled 50 to 149 feet with one helper and provided 25% to 49% of the effort needed.
1	Client traveled less than 50 feet and provided less than 25% of the effort needed. Two helpers were needed to hold wound vac/IV/oxygen/tubes.
0	Activity did not occur (at admission); cannot be scored 0 at discharge. Function modifiers: Distance walked or distance traveled in a wheelchair may be scored at 0 on admission/discharge.

Locomotion Example

Beth walks distances greater than 150 feet, but the therapy department has safety concerns due to Beth's history of falling. She uses a gait belt with contact guard assistance for safety. What is Beth's FIM score for locomotion?

Answer and Rationale

The FIM score is a 5 for contact guard assistance.

(continued)

FIM AND QUALITY MEASURES FOR INPATIENT REHABILITATION FACILITIES (CONTINUED)

Stairs

Going up and down one flight of indoor stairs

Score	Stairs
7	Client was independent and safe going up and down 12 to 14 stairs.
6	Client was independent with devices (eg, handrail, ankle-foot orthosis, cane) or client required 3 times the usual amount of time. The client is independent with wound vac/IV/oxygen/tubes. TLSO is not counted as a device.
5	Client required supervision, cues, or setup to climb and descend 12 to 14 stairs.
5E	Household exception: Client climbed 4 to 6 stairs independently with or without devices; one-person assistance required with wound vac/IV/oxygen/tubes.
4	Client required minimum assistance, including for steadying, to climb and descend 12 to 14 stairs.
3	Client required moderate assistance; client provided 50% to 74% of the required effort. One helper was required to climb and descend 12 to 14 stairs.
2	Client required maximum assistance. Client climbed and descended 4 to 11 stairs with a helper.
1	Client required total assistance. Client climbed and descended 3 or fewer stairs with 1 or 2 helpers' assistance.
0	Activity did not occur (at admission); cannot be scored 0 at discharge.

Stairs Example

The client is able to climb and descend 6 stairs with 1 helper. What is the FIM score?

Answer and Rationale

The FIM score is a 2 because the client climbed fewer than 11 stairs with the assistance of 1 person.

(continued)

FIM AND QUALITY MEASURES FOR INPATIENT REHABILITATION FACILITIES (CONTINUED)

Communication and Social Cognition Functional Independence Measure Guidelines

Hours Prompting or Assistance Required	Client Participation	Level of Assistance
0	100%	Independent (complete or modified)
1	96%	Supervision/cues/setup: Client requires less than 10% repetition, prompting, or coaxing
2	92%	
3	87%	Minimum assistance
4	83%	
5	79%	
6	75%	
7	71%	Moderate assistance
8	67%	
9	62%	
10	58%	
11	54%	
12	50%	
13	46%	Maximum assistance
14	42%	
15	37%	
16	33%	
17	29%	
18	25%	
More than 18	Less than 25%	Total assistance: Client requires one-on-one supervision

(continued)

UNIT 2-10 EVALUATION

FIM AND QUALITY MEASURES FOR INPATIENT REHABILITATION FACILITIES (CONTINUED)

Comprehension

Comprehension is scored in the client's native language. Record client's primary mode of comprehension, either auditory (in most clients) or visual.

Basic comprehension topics include pain, hunger, thirst, bathroom needs, cold or hot, sleep, and nutrition.

Complex comprehension topics include current events, humor, finances, religion, medical treatment rationale (eg, hip precautions, pressure relief), and discharge planning.

Score	Comprehension
7	Client independently understood complex or abstract conversation and directions.
6	Client was independent with 3 times the usual amount of time or use of devices (ie, glasses if the client's primary comprehension is visual, and hearing aids if client's primary comprehension is auditory) to understand complex or abstract conversations and directions.
5	90% of the time client understood basic communication. Client required cues to understand basic tasks. Staff helped insert or set up hearing aids (auditory comprehension) or put on glasses (visual comprehension). Client required slow speech to understand.
4	75% to 89% of the time the client understood basic communication. Staff needed to repeat words.
3	50% to 74% of the time the client understood basic communication. Staff needed to repeat parts of sentences.
2	25% to 49% of the time the client understood basic communication. Client comprehended only simple expressions, gestures, waves, or hello.
1	Less than 25% of the time the client understood basic communication. Client did not respond appropriately, or client did not understand hello or gestures.
0	Activity did not occur (at admission); cannot be scored 0 at discharge.

(continued)

FIM AND QUALITY MEASURES FOR INPATIENT REHABILITATION FACILITIES (CONTINUED)

Comprehension Example

The client understands about 75% of basic communication. She has difficulty understanding information about her diagnosis or treatment plan, and she often asks you to repeat words. She can repeat back weightbearing precautions, but needs some reminders when in a distracting environment. Her husband stays with her during treatment sessions to receive education about her precautions and other complex information. What is the FIM score?

Answer and Rationale

The FIM score is a 4 because the client understands 75% of basic communication but requires some repetition and relies on her husband for complex information.

(continued)

FIM AND QUALITY MEASURES FOR INPATIENT REHABILITATION FACILITIES (CONTINUED)

Expression

Expression is scored in the client's native language. Record the primary mode of expression, either vocal or non-vocal.

Basic comprehension topics include pain, hunger, thirst, bathroom needs, cold or hot, sleep, and nutrition.

Complex comprehension topics include current events, humor, finances, religion, medical treatment rationale (eg, hip precautions, pressure relief), and discharge planning.

Score	Expression
7	Client independently expressed complex or abstract ideas.
6	Client independently expressed complex or abstract ideas with 3 times the usual amount of time, used a device (augmentative communication device or computer), or slurred. Client had mild problems finding words.
5	Client required cues to express basic needs. Client expressed basic needs and ideas 90% of the time. Staff helped set up communication device (eg, talk tracheostomy valve)
4	75% to 89% of the time client expressed basic needs. Client needed to repeat words. Staff helped occlude tracheostomy for client to express him- or herself.
3	50% to 74% of the time the client expressed basic needs. Client needed to repeat parts of sentences.
2	25% to 49% of the time the client expressed basic needs. Client used single words or gestures only.
1	Less than 25% of the time the client expressed basic needs and was inconsistent.
0	Activity did not occur (at admission); cannot be scored 0 at discharge.

Expression Example

The client is apraxic in his speech pattern. During treatment, the therapist understands about half of the single words communicated. It is much easier to understand single words rather than long phrases. What is his FIM score?

Answer and Rationale

The FIM score is a 2. The client is intelligible about 50% of the time with single words, and phrases are not understood.

(continued)

FIM AND QUALITY MEASURES FOR INPATIENT REHABILITATION FACILITIES (CONTINUED)

Social Interaction

Includes client cooperation, getting along, and participating in social settings with staff, family, and other clients

Score	Social Interaction
7	Client independently interacted appropriately with others. Client could use pain medication or cry for pain.
6	Client needed extra time, structure, or medication to interact appropriately with others. Common anti-anxiety and anti-depressant medications include Celexin, Lexapro (escitalopram oxalate), Prozac (fluoxetine), Zoloft (sertraline), Paxil (paroxetine hydrochloride), and Cymbalta (duloxetine).
5	90% of the time the client interacted appropriately. Client required monitoring by staff or encouragement to attend therapy or eat in dining room.
4	75% to 89% of the time the client interacted appropriately. Staff gave client redirection for appropriate language or needed help to initiate interaction.
3	50% to 74% of the time the client interacted appropriately. Client may be emotionally labile and physically or verbally inappropriate.
2	25% to 49% of the time the client interacted appropriately. Client required frequent redirection.
1	Less than 25% of the time the client interacted appropriately, or the client was withdrawn or combative.
0	Activity did not occur (at admission); cannot be scored 0 at discharge.

Social Interaction Example

The client has an acquired brain injury and requires a low-stimulus environment. He frequently yells from his room, spits, and attempts to hit his nurses and attendants. He responds most appropriately with family about 25% of the time. What is his FIM score?

Answer and Rationale

The FIM score is a 1. The client is agitated and requires a low-stimulus environment. He responds appropriately to family 25% of the time but does not take redirection from others.

(continued)

UNIT 2-10 EVALUATION

FIM AND QUALITY MEASURES FOR INPATIENT REHABILITATION FACILITIES (CONTINUED)

Problem Solving

Ability to make safe and timely decisions, sequence steps, and recognize and solve problems

Basic problem solving includes completing daily tasks and dealing with unplanned events or hazards in daily activities.

Complex problem solving includes balancing a checkbook, participating in discharge plans, and self-administering medications. (There is no need to score finances if a caregiver routinely performed financial management prior to the client's hospitalization.)

Score	Problem Solving
7	Client solved complex problems consistently.
6	Client solved complex problems with extra time or with the use of a device (eg, an alarm clock).
5	90% of the time the client solved basic problems. Client needed help less than 10% of the time under stressful situations for routine problems. Client solved complex problems with cues.
4	75% to 89% of the time the client solved basic problems, indicated by answering 3 simple questions.
3	50% to 74% of the time the client solved basic problems, indicated by answering 2 simple questions
2	25% to 49% of the time the client solved basic problems. Staff gave the client direction more than half the time for initiation, planning, or completion of simple activities, or the client required a restraint for safety.
1	Less than 25% of the time the client solved basic problems. Staff gave the client direction almost constantly. The client did not effectively solve problems, or he or she needed a restraint for safety.
0	Activity did not occur (at admission); cannot be scored 0 at discharge.

(continued)

FIM AND QUALITY MEASURES FOR INPATIENT REHABILITATION FACILITIES (CONTINUED)

Problem Solving Example

The client is hospitalized due to a series of falls that caused a mild brain injury. She enjoys cooking and agrees to make her favorite meal of meatloaf and mashed potatoes. She is able to list all the ingredients for the shopping list. In the kitchen she gathers the needed supplies and ingredients. She becomes distracted by the kitchen setup (not her kitchen) and is disturbed not to have the pan she prefers. The clinic does not have a potato masher, and she requires help problem solving how to adapt to the different kitchen and tools. What is the FIM score?

Answer and Rationale

The FIM score is a 5. The client is able to problem solve basic problems but needs assistance with unfamiliar (more complex) issues.

(continued)

UNIT 2-10 EVALUATION

FIM AND QUALITY MEASURES FOR INPATIENT REHABILITATION FACILITIES (CONTINUED)	

Memory

Includes recognizing familiar faces, recalling routines, and executing tasks or requests without repetition

Examples of multistep requests:

- 1-step request: "Point to the ceiling."
- 2-step request: "Hand me the paper, and pick up the pen."
- 3-step request: "Point to the floor, point to your nose, and hand me the pen."

Score	Memory
7	Client did not need help to recall thoughts. Client independently recognized, recalled, or executed 3 steps of a 3-step request (3 out of 3).
6	Client needed extra time or devices (eg, memory book, calendar for memory, alarm) to recognize, recall, or execute 3 steps of a 3-step request (3 out of 3).
5	90% of the time the client recognized, recalled, or executed 3 steps of a 3-step request and needed prompting only under stress. Cueing and reminders were given, or client lost track of time (3 out of 3).
4	75% to 89% of the time the client recognized, recalled, or executed 2 steps of a 3-step request (2 out of 3).
3	50% to 74% of the time the client recognized, recalled, or executed 2 steps of a 2-step request (2 out of 3).
2	25% to 49% of the time client recognized, recalled, or executed 1 step of a 2-step request (1 out of 2).
1	Less than 25% of the time the client recognized, recalled, or executed a 1-step request (1 out of 1).
0	Activity did not occur (at admission); cannot be scored 0 at discharge.

Memory Example

The client is attempting to transfer from the edge of bed to stand with a walker. She has 90-degree flexion hip precautions and has been instructed to extend out her affected leg prior to standing. In addition, she tries to pull up on her walker when trying to stand. She is instructed to place one hand on the bed and one on the walker. She is unable able to follow the 2 steps of instructions. The steps must be broken down into step 1 then step 2. What is the FIM score?

Answer and Rationale

The FIM score is a 2. She can only follow 1 out of 2 instructions.

(continued)

FIM AND QUALITY MEASURES FOR INPATIENT REHABILITATION FACILITIES (CONTINUED)

QUALITY MEASURES FOR INPATIENT REHABILITATION FACILITIES

Quality measures for inpatient rehabilitation facilities codes are used as payment modifiers in conjunction with the FIM. They measure the safety and quality of performance at admission and are also used to describe discharge goals.

Safety and quality of performance: If assistance from a helper is required due to safety or poor quality of performance, score the amount of assistance required.

6: Independent	No assistance from a helper was needed to complete activities. The task could be completed with or without the use of assistive devices.
5: Setup or cleanup assistance	Helper only assisted before or after the activity.
4: Supervision or touching assistance	Helper provided verbal cues or steadying assistance throughout the activity or intermittently.
3: Partial or moderate assistance	Helper provided less than half the effort.
2: Substantial or maximum assistance	Helper provided more than half the effort.
1: Dependent	Helper provided all the effort, or 2 or more helpers were needed.

If activity is not attempted:

07: Client refused

09: Not applicable

88: Not attempted due to medical condition or safety concerns

(continued)

UNIT 2-10 EVALUATION

UNIT 2-10 EVALUATION

FIM AND QUALITY MEASURES FOR INPATIENT REHABILITATION FACILITIES (CONTINUED)

Sample Headings

Self-Care (3-Day Assessment Period)

1. **Eating**
   - Admission performance
   - Discharge goal
2. **Performing oral hygiene**
   - Admission performance
   - Discharge goal
3. **Toileting hygiene**
   - Admission performance
   - Discharge goal
4. **Showering/bathing self**
   - Admission performance
   - Discharge goal
5. **Upper body dressing**
   - Admission performance
   - Discharge goal
6. **Lower body dressing**
   - Admission performance
   - Discharge goal
7. **Putting on/taking off footwear***
   - Admission performance
   - Discharge goal

Mobility (3-Day Assessment Period)

1. **Rolling left and right**
   - Admission performance
   - Discharge goal
2. **Moving from sitting to lying down**
   - Admission performance
   - Discharge goal
3. **Moving from lying down to sitting on the edge of the bed**
   - Admission performance
   - Discharge goal

*Different from FIM

BARTHEL INDEX

SUMMARY

- Purpose: Assesses the client's ability to care for him- or herself with ADLs
- Context: Neuromuscular or musculoskeletal disorders, stroke, geriatric, TBI
- Format: Self-report or performance-based observation
- Time to administer: Varies; 2 to 5 minutes for a self-report or 20 minutes for observation
- Materials: Barthel Index forms, any items or equipment needed for directly observing ADLs
- Cost: Free
- Website: www.mapi-trust.org

The Barthel Index assesses self-care ADLs and can be administered prior to treatment, as a progress measure during treatment, and prior to discharge. Scores on the Barthel Index are considered when determining if the client will benefit most from long-term care, a SNF, or inpatient rehabilitation, or if the client may return home.[54]

SCORING

The scores in each category may range from 0 to 5, 10, or 15 points. Full credit is not given if the client requires even minor assistance or supervision. The total score is the sum of each category out of 100, and higher scores indicate higher levels of independence.

Additional Guidelines for Scoring

Barthel Index scoring must report the client's actual performance within the past 24 to 48 hours (occasionally longer periods are reviewed), not the client's potential capabilities. The client is considered independent if he or she accomplishes the task in a reasonable amount of time and does not require supervision, cues, or assistance. The client may use assistive devices and assistive aids if necessary, and still be considered independent. Scoring methods may include observing directly, asking the client, and obtaining information from relatives, friends, or nursing staff. Be aware that self-reports may differ from therapist ratings.[54]

(continued)

UNIT 2-11 EVALUATION

BARTHEL INDEX (CONTINUED)

IMPLICATIONS FOR THERAPY

Score less than 60: Client may benefit from long-term care or an SNF (requires full-time care)

Score 60 to 80: Client may benefit from an inpatient rehabilitation setting.

Score greater than 80: Client may function well at home with minimum assistance.

Feeding	0 = Client is unable to feed him- or herself. 5 = Client needs help with cutting or spreading (butter), or requires a modified diet. 10 = Client is independent after the food is placed within reach.
Bathing	0 = Client is dependent with bathing. 5 = Client is independent (includes bathing in a bath tub or shower, or taking a sponge bath)
Grooming Grooming includes washing hands and face, combing hair (styling not included), cleaning teeth, and shaving (including getting a razor from the drawer and plugging it in). For female patients, putting on makeup may be included.	0 = Client needs help with personal care. 5 = Client is independent with grooming.
Dressing Dressing includes putting on and removing clothing. Women do not need to be scored on use of a bra unless it is a prescribed garment.	0 = Client is dependent with dressing. 5 = Client is able to complete half of dressing (50%) unaided. 10 = Client is independent with dressing (eg, any buttons, zippers, shoelaces). *(continued)*

BARTHEL INDEX (CONTINUED)

Bowels	0 = Client is incontinent or needs to be given enemas. 5 = Client has an occasional accident or needs help using a suppository. 10 = Client is continent and may use a suppository.
Bladder	0 = Client is incontinent or unable to manage a catheter. 5 = Client has an occasional accident or needs help with an external device. 10 = Client is continent. If client uses an external device or leg bag, he or she independently puts on the device and cleans and empties the bag.
Toileting Toileting includes getting on and off the toilet, dressing, and wiping. If the client uses a bed pan, he or she must be able to place it on a chair, empty it, and clean it.	0 = Client is dependent with toileting. 5 = Client needs some help but can do a part of toileting alone. 10 = Client is independent with toileting. Client may use bars for stability.
Transfers (Wheelchair to Bed and Return) Transfers include approaching the bed, locking wheelchair brakes, lifting footrests, moving to the bed, lying down, sitting on the edge of the bed, and transferring back to the wheelchair.	0 = Client is unable to transfer and has no sitting balance. 5 = Client requires major help with transfers (physical help with one or two additional people), and client has sitting balance. 10 = Client requires minor help with transfers (assistance may be verbal or physical help). 15 = Client is independent with transfers. *(continued)*

UNIT 2-11 EVALUATION

UNIT 2-11 EVALUATION

BARTHEL INDEX (CONTINUED)

Mobility (Level Surfaces)	0 = Client is immobile or travels less than 150 feet.
	5 = Client is independent traveling in a wheelchair (eg, navigating corners and maneuvering to a table, bed, toilet) and travels more than 150 feet.
	10 = Client walks with assistance (verbal or physical) of one person and travels more than 150 feet.
	15 = Client is independent (use of a device is acceptable) and travels more than 150 feet. Client may wear braces or prostheses, or use crutches, canes, or a walkerette. Client may not be considered independent if a rolling walker is used for mobility. If the client wears braces, then he or she must be able to lock and unlock the braces.
Stairs	0 = Client is unable to climb or descend stairs.
	5 = Client needs help with stairs (help may be physical, verbal, or with a carrying aid).
	10 = Client is independent with stairs. Client may use handrails, canes, or crutches, but must be able to carry canes or crutches while climbing the stairs.

EXECUTIVE FUNCTION PERFORMANCE TEST

SUMMARY

- Purpose: Assesses the impact of executive function on performance, the client's ability to live independently, and the amount of assistance the client requires
- Context: Suspected cognitive impairment, stroke, TBI, or MS
- Format: Performance-based observation
- Time to administer: 45 minutes to more than 1 hour
- Materials: Manual, assessment sheet, writing utensil, 27 inch x 16 inch x 12 inch deep, clear storage box containing assessment materials listed in the manual
- Cost: Free
- Website: http://www.ot.wustl.edu/about/resources/ executive-function-performance-test-efpt-308

The Executive Function Performance Test (EFPT) assesses executive function in clients with potential cognitive impairments and can be used in clients with stroke or MS. The EFPT assessment requires clients to demonstrate performance in the following areas: washing hands, preparing oatmeal, using the telephone, managing medications, and paying bills.[55,56] The practitioner administering the test offers cues in a specific sequence to determine the level of assistance that the client requires to perform the tasks.[55,56] In general, a specific cue should be offered 2 times before moving on to the next cue (unless the client is in danger). A general overview of cues follows. More specific cueing is outlined with the assessment forms.

TYPE OF CUE	DESCRIPTION
No cue	• The client does not require any assistance to perform the task. • The client does not ask questions.
Indirect verbal cue	• The verbal prompt should be phrased as a question. • The question should not tell the client what to do or direct the client to the action.
Gestural cue	• The practitioner points to an item or location. • No words should be paired with the gesture.

(continued)

EXECUTIVE FUNCTION PERFORMANCE TEST (CONTINUED)	
TYPE OF CUE	DESCRIPTION
Direct verbal cue	• The practitioner instructs the client to perform an action, telling the client what to do. • The practitioner may point to or touch an item.
Physical assistance	• The practitioner physically helps the client perform part of the task. • It is not considered physical assistance if the client asks for help because he or she has a motor or visual impairment. (The EFPT is not a motor or visual assessment; it is assessing executive function.)
Cannot do	• The client cannot perform the task or does not continue performing the task after physical assistance has been given.

HOME SAFETY ASSESSMENTS

The client's home environment is an important aspect of occupational participation for practitioners to consider during treatment and prior to discharge. The client must be able to move around his or her home safely, as well as participate in their chosen occupations. Home safety assessments vary in whether they focus on the person, environment, or occupation. Always consider what the client needs to do to function in the home safely.[57]

Aspects of home safety to consider:

- Can the client access the kitchen?
- Can the client utilize the sink, countertops, and cabinets safely?
- Can the client safely do laundry?
- Can the client get the mail safely?
- Can the client reach blinds or curtains to open them safely?
- Does the client have safe reach and access to components of the home?
- Is the client a vulnerable adult who might be at risk?
- Is the client a vulnerable adult who might be taken advantage of?
- Can the client do his or her routine safely when he or she wants and needs to?
- Consider the climate (eg, ice on stairs) and neighborhood safety.

COMMON HOME SAFETY ASSESSMENTS	SUMMARY
AARP Home Safety Checklist[58]	• Purpose: Assesses the safety of the home environment and helps guide recommendations • Context: Designed for use with older adults • Format: Self-checklist • Time to administer: Quick • Materials: Checklist • Cost: Free • Website: https://assets.aarp.org/external_sites/caregiving/checklists/checklist_homeSafety.html *(continued)*

UNIT 2-13 EVALUATION

UNIT 2-13 EVALUATION

HOME SAFETY ASSESSMENTS (CONTINUED)

COMMON HOME SAFETY ASSESSMENTS	SUMMARY
Cougar Home Safety Assessment v. 4.0[56,59]	• Purpose: Assesses the safety of the home environment, including utilities related to fire, water, and electrical safety. The practitioner must be competent in home safety evaluations. • Context: Designed for use with all clients • Format: Checklist, observation, home testing, and interview • Time to administer: Varies; 45 to 60 minutes • Materials: Manual, checklist, thermometer, flashlight, reaching stick/yard stick, and writing utensil • Cost: Free • Website: http://www.misericordia.edu/page.cfm?p=1266
SAFER-HOME v. 3[57,60]	• Purpose: Assesses the client's safety and performance during functional tasks. The SAFER-HOME can also be used as an outcome measure to assess the effectiveness of interventions. • Context: Designed for use with all clients • Format: Client interview and home observation • Time to administer: Varies; 45 to 60 minutes • Materials: Manual, checklist • Cost: $100 for manual; $20 for forms only • Website: http://www.vha.ca/wp-content/uploads/2015/07/SaferHomeOrderForm.pdf

(continued)

Home Safety Assessments (continued)

Common Home Safety Assessments	Summary
Home Environment Assessment Protocol[61]	• Purpose: Assesses safety hazards and comfort in the home for clients with dementia • Context: Designed for use with clients with dementia • Format: Client interview and observation • Time to administer: Varies; 45 to 60 minutes • Materials: Assessment form and writing utensil • Cost: Free • Website: https://ehhi.com/sites/default/files/Toolkit/HEAP_Tool.pdf
I-HOPE[57,62]	• Purpose: Assesses the client's performance quality of activities in the home. The client identifies and prioritizes activities, rates his or her performance satisfaction, and rates barriers to performance. The I-HOPE can be used as an outcome measure to assess the effectiveness of home modifications. • Context: Designed for use with all clients • Format: Card-sort and observation • Time to administer: 60 minutes • Materials: I-HOPE Kit, including a manual, assessment forms, barrier list, activity cards, response cards, and summary score sheets • Cost: $75 • Website: https://starklab.wustl.edu/i-hope-kit

(continued)

UNIT 2-13 EVALUATION

UNIT 2-13 EVALUATION

Home Safety Assessments (continued)	
Common Home Safety Assessments	**Summary**
Westmead Home Safety Assessment[57,63]	• Purpose: Assesses fall safety hazards in the home • Context: Designed for use with clients at risk for falling • Format: Client interview and home observation • Time to administer: 60 minutes • Materials: Manual, assessment form, reporting sheet, and prompt sheet • Cost: $118 • Website: http://www.coordinatespublishing.com.au/home-fall-hazards/4589932185
CASPAR[64]	• Purpose: Assesses the client's task performance in the home for problems. CASPAR may only be used by a home modification specialist. • Context: Designed for use with all clients • Format: Client interview and home observation • Time to administer: Varies; 45 to 60 minutes • Materials: Assessment form, camera, and tape measure • Cost: Free to download • Website: https://www.ehls.com/national-grants

DRIVING AND COMMUNITY MOBILITY SCREENING

OCCUPATIONAL THERAPY ASSESSMENT

Driving and community mobility is an IADL within the occupational therapy scope of practice.[3] Driving provides independence and enables clients to meet occupational needs, so it is important for occupational therapy to assess and provide interventions to assist in successful occupational engagement. Your client's ability and safety to drive can be impacted by illness and disability.

Introduce a conversation about driving with your client, and determine the level of importance that driving holds in meeting your client's occupational needs. Know your state's law regarding driving requirements when considering your client's potential for driving.

The criteria for driving evaluation readiness are outlined here, along with performance skills to evaluate.

Client readiness for a driving evaluation[65]	Clients are ready for a driving evaluation when they have met the following criteria: • Achieved independence/modified independence in basic IADLs • Has good strength and ROM in at least one extremity • Meets the visual acuity requirements set by the state licensing agency • Meets the visual field requirements set by the state licensing agency • Demonstrates adequate visual-perceptual skills • Has minimal to moderate memory impairments • Demonstrates adequate reaction time • Demonstrates limited impulsivity
	(continued)

DRIVING AND COMMUNITY MOBILITY SCREENING (CONTINUED)	
Driving tasks to assess	• Opening and closing doors • Using locks • Transferring to the driver's seat • Storing the wheelchair or scooter • Steering, braking, and accelerating
Performance skills to evaluate and helpful assessments[66-68]	• Vision and visual field Assessment: may include useful field of view test • Cognition and perception assessment: may include Trail Making Test, Motor-Free Visual Perception Test, and cognitive screenings • Hearing screening • Physical and neurological examination • ROM/manual muscle testing • Coordination/proprioception • Sensation • Balance • Tone • The Occupational Therapy Driver Off-Road Assessment Battery can be ordered through AOTA and provides relevant materials for evaluating clients through a general interview/medical history, visual assessment, physical assessment, and cognitive assessment.[67,68]

(continued)

DRIVING AND COMMUNITY MOBILITY SCREENING (CONTINUED)

DRIVING FOR OLDER ADULTS

Some drivers may have poor insight into how their deficits affect their driving ability. Ask your client why he or she has been referred for a driving evaluation to gain an understanding for the client's level of insight. Consider your client's willingness to self-restrict risky driving activities, whether the client is receptive to an alternative method of transportation, the client's motivation to participate in driving training, and the client's awareness of prescription medications that potentially impair driving.

Self-assessment tools and signs of impaired driving are outlined in the following table.

Available driving self-assessment tools[66,68-71]	• AAA Roadwise[68]: This computer-based test includes the useful field of view test and Trails B. • Drivers 55 Plus—Check Your Own Performance[69]: This self-assessment may be found at www.aaafoundation.org • "Am I a Safe Driver?"[70(p201)]: This checklist can be found in the *Physician's Guide to Assessing and Counseling Older Drivers.* • Driving Habits Questionnaire[71]: This questionnaire guides an interview with the client about driving habits. • Fitness to Drive Screening Measure[68,68]: This computer-based test is for caregivers or family members who have observed client's driving in past 3 months; it is located at https://seniordriving.aaa.com/evaluate-your-driving-ability
Signs of impaired driving[72]	• Getting lost in familiar environments • Consistently driving below speed limits and obstructing traffic flow • Hesitating for long periods at intersections • Having difficulty remaining within the lane • Missing or not following traffic signs and/or lights • Utilizing a "follow the leader" approach when maneuvering through traffic

(continued)

UNIT 2-14 EVALUATION

DRIVING AND COMMUNITY MOBILITY SCREENING (CONTINUED)

NEXT STEPS: REFERRAL TO A DRIVER REHABILITATION SPECIALIST

An on-road evaluation is the gold standard for assessing a client's ability to return to driving.[65] Following the clinical evaluation, locate a certified driver rehabilitation specialist in your area and provide them with the information gained from your evaluation. A Certified Driver Rehabilitation Specialist can be located at www.aded.net.

The client must demonstrate adequate skills in the following areas during a typical on-road evaluation (as identified by an occupational therapy specialist).	<ul><li>Using adaptive driving equipment as needed</li><li>Entering and exiting the vehicle</li><li>Adjusting the seat, mirrors, and steering wheel for safety and proper vehicle fit</li><li>Operating the driving controls</li><li>Shifting the vehicle to the appropriate gear</li><li>Residential driving</li><li>Moderate traffic driving</li><li>Highway driving</li><li>Parking</li><li>Navigating the vehicle</li><li>Being aware of road rules and signs</li></ul>

To learn more about occupational therapy roles in driving and community mobility:

Driving and Community Mobility for Older Adults: Occupational Therapy Roles. AOTA Online CEU course. 2010. Available at www.aota-learning.org ($112.50 for members).

Information on the following topics for caregivers can be found at www.thehartford.com/talkwitholderdrivers:

- We Need to Talk: Family Conversations with Older Drivers
- At the Crossroads: A Guide to Alzheimer's Disease, Dementia & Driving
- Your Road Ahead: A Guide to Comprehensive Driver Evaluations

UNIT 2-14 EVALUATION

COMMON INTERVENTIONS ACROSS PRACTICE SETTINGS

INTERVENTION	ACUTE	INPATIENT	HOME HEALTH	SNF	OUTPATIENT
Common Interventions Across Practice Settings					
Medication management			✓		✓
ADL intervention		✓	✓	✓	✓
Fall recovery skills education		✓	✓	✓	
Commonly Used Medical and Adaptive Equipment	✓	✓	✓	✓	✓
Easily Created Adaptive Equipment		✓	✓		✓
Home Modifications		✓	✓		✓
Ergonomic Modifications		✓	✓		✓
Job Accommodations		✓	✓		✓
Driving Rehabilitation and Community Mobility		✓	✓		✓

(continued)

UNIT 3-15 INTERVENTION

COMMON INTERVENTIONS ACROSS PRACTICE SETTINGS (CONTINUED)

MEDICATION MANAGEMENT[73]

- Description: *Medication management* refers to ensuring that the client remembers to take and organize his or her medications appropriately prior to discharge from occupational therapy services.
- Approach: Incorporate medication management into the client's daily routines, store medications in an area that is easily seen, use environmental cues, set alarms or reminders, and use a calendar to plan ahead.
- Precautions: The occupational therapy practitioner may only offer tips for medication management. Ultimately, the physician or pharmacist is responsible for prescribing and answering specific questions regarding the client's medication schedule.
- Significance: The aging population and clients with dementia may require help with remembering to take medications. Medication management prevents harm, illness, injury, or death that may result from taking medications inappropriately.

ACTIVITIES OF DAILY LIVING INTERVENTION[74]

- Description: *Community integration* refers to the process of the client resuming or beginning life in his or her community independently.
- Approach: Create an occupational profile to develop interventions that are client centered. Interventions may include life skills training, money management, home organization and maintenance, domestic skills, and interpersonal skills. Simulations may include trials in the hospital gift shop, cafeteria, or transitional model home. Prior to discharge, the client may benefit from practicing car transfers, training on adaptive equipment or mobility devices, and home modifications.
- Precautions: Utilize safety checklists prior to discharge, especially if the client is discharging to an environment without a caregiver.
- Significance: IADLs and community integration are important components of independent living. Additionally, community integration contributes to the client's sense of well-being and value in his or her abilities.

(continued)

UNIT 3-15 INTERVENTION

COMMON INTERVENTIONS
ACROSS PRACTICE SETTINGS (CONTINUED)

FALL RECOVERY SKILLS EDUCATION[75]

- Description: *Fall recovery skills education* refers to how a client correctly gets up from the floor after a fall.
- Approach: Consider how the psychosocial fear of falling may impact participation. A holistic approach to fall intervention should include education on fall prevention and encourage the client to be functionally independent. Consider medications that the client is taking and their side effects, address any postural concerns, and conduct a vision screen. You may discuss the use of an alerting fall monitor with your client, but be mindful about the client's sense of independence and privacy while wearing a monitor. Fall prevention and recovery exercises may include balance exercises, strengthening, moving from a hands-and-knees to a side-sitting position (and reverse), and practicing floor-to-sit or floor-to-stand maneuvers with emphasis on proper body mechanics. Always use a gait belt when practicing fall recovery skills. You may practice fall recovery skills using a padded mat on the floor if preferable.
- Precautions: Any client who falls needs to be checked by a physician or nurse prior to fall recovery.
- Significance: Falls are a common occurrence that can result in injury, and many older adults who fall have difficulty getting up from the floor even without injury. Occupational therapy practitioners must help clients be as safe and independent as possible following discharge and can do so by addressing fall prevention and recovery.

UNIT 3-15 INTERVENTION

COMMONLY USED MEDICAL AND ADAPTIVE EQUIPMENT

Medical and adaptive equipment facilitate occupational participation across practice settings. The most frequently used types of adaptive equipment reported by elderly clients are devices for functional mobility and bathroom aids.[76] Some common reasons for reported equipment rejection and abandonment are that aids are too cumbersome, are too time consuming, or are perceived to call unwanted attention to clients.

The Centers for Disease Control and Prevention notes that more than 36% of adults in the United States are obese, making it important for the percentage of bariatric equipment in hospitals to reflect this growing number.[77] Hospital employees must be cognizant of the weight limit for standard hospital equipment.

ACTIVITY	ADAPTIVE EQUIPMENT[78,79]
Functional mobility	• Standard wheelchair • Lightweight wheelchair • Heavy-duty wheelchair • Extra heavy-duty wheelchair • Hemi wheelchair • Wheelchair cushions • Rollabout chair • Wheeled walker • Rollator with seat • Hemi walker • Walker without wheels • Bariatric walker • Portable oxygen • Transfer board • Gait belt
Toileting	• Bedside commode • Heavy-duty bedside commode • Drop-arm commode • Raised toilet seat • Toilet aid

(continued)

UNIT 3-16 INTERVENTION

COMMONLY USED MEDICAL AND ADAPTIVE EQUIPMENT (CONTINUED)	
ACTIVITY	**ADAPTIVE EQUIPMENT**[78,79]
Showering	• Shower chair • Tub transfer bench • Long-handled sponge • Leg lifter
Grooming	• Universal cuff • Built-up handles • Long-handled brush • Lap tray
Feeding	• Universal cuff • Plate guard • Mobile arm support • Built-up utensils
Dressing	• Button hook • Zipper pull • Velcro • Dressing stick • Shoe horn • Sock aid • Elastic shoelaces
Additionally, a hip kit includes: • Sock aid • Dressing stick • Shoe horn • Elastic shoelaces • Reacher • Long-handled bath sponge	

UNIT 3-16 INTERVENTION

EASILY CREATED ADAPTIVE EQUIPMENT

Do-it-yourself adaptive equipment is a cost-effective alternative to help facilitate occupational participation. In addition, do-it-yourself adaptive equipment can be modified to best suit the client's needs.[80]

ADAPTATION	METHOD	EXAMPLES OF USE
Long-handled items	A wooden dowel rod or PVC pipe can be used to add an extension to a handle. Be mindful that the diameter is appropriate for the client's grip.	Brooms, bath sponge
Built-up handles	Dycem, medical tape, wash cloths, pool noodle cutouts, rubber bands, or other available material can be wrapped around handles to increase the diameter for grip.	Makeup applicators, brush, toothbrush, cooking handles, cabinet handles, utensils
	Cut a tennis ball along the seam to create a built-up jar opener.	Opening kitchen jars
Leg lifter	Loop a gait belt around feet to aid in lifting legs.	Bringing legs over the bathtub
Clothing modifications	Sew Velcro onto clothing using whip-stitch techniques to replace buttons, or use Velcro for other clothing modifications.	Dressing
Button hook	Create a button hook for clients who have fine motor difficulties or require one-handed dressing by bending a paperclip and taping it to a plastic spoon or pencil.	Buttoning a shirt

(continued)

UNIT 3-17 INTERVENTION

EASILY CREATED ADAPTIVE EQUIPMENT (CONTINUED)		
ADAPTATION	METHOD	EXAMPLES OF USE
Adding contrast	Colored tape, paint, or paper can be used as an anchor or to make items more visible for individuals with visual impairments.	Colored place mats, contrast on light switches, stairs, cutting board, hot/cold temperature controls
Tactile cues	Puff paint, raised dots, or textured fabrics can be used to aid clients who have visual impairments with finding the location of commonly used buttons or items.	Microwave, dishwasher, washer/dryer start button
Opening via pulling	Tie a piece of rope around handles to increase the ease of opening drawers, cabinets, etc.	Cabinets, drawers, oven door, microwave door, refrigerator
Wrist holder to limit item dropping	Use a piece of ribbon or other material to create an extra hold of item around the wrist so that a dropped item does not fall to the floor each time. This assists individuals with coordination, lack of grip, or other impairments that cause frequent item dropping.	Toothbrush, makeup applicators

UNIT 3-17 INTERVENTION

HOME MODIFICATIONS

Home modification interventions should be driven by home safety assessments, pragmatics, and occupation. It is important for the client to be able to participate in his or her chosen occupations. Some modifications may require hiring a contractor to install the modifications.[81,82]

AREA IN THE HOME	COMMONLY RECOMMENDED MODIFICATIONS[83]
Bathroom	• Grab bars and anchors • Faucet replacement with level handles • Floor-to-ceiling pole in bathroom • Tub bench • Hand-held shower and shower head holder bracket • Shower chair • Toilet frame • Raised toiled seat • Adapted faucets • Anti-slip tape or shower mat
Bedroom	• Stationary beds with clearance for transfers • Mattress height adjusted for wheelchair • Adjusted shelf height for access • Bedside rail • Bedside commode • Carbon monoxide and smoke detector
Kitchen	• Cabinet hardware • Adjusted counter and sink height for access • Adapted faucets • Adaptive kitchen equipment • Front-load dishwasher, washer, and dryer • Side-by-side refrigerator doors • Carbon monoxide and smoke detector

(continued)

HOME MODIFICATIONS (CONTINUED)

AREA IN THE HOME	COMMONLY RECOMMENDED MODIFICATIONS[83]
Stairs	• Round handrails with 2-inch diameter • Handrail height at 34 to 38 inches • Handrails on both sides of stairs • Stair height less than 7 inches and stair depth greater than 11 inches • Anti-slip tape • Color-contrasted tape
Door entry	• Angled entry mat • Remove or cover door thresholds • Ramp at 12:1 ratio. The ramp should be 1 foot in length for every inch of height • Door clearance should be 5 feet x 5 feet for swing-out doors and 3 feet x 5 feet for swing-in doors • Door width between 32 and 34 inches • Adapt door handles for client's hand function • Ensure drive way is level, smooth, and adequately lit
Throughout the home	• Floor lamps, motion-detected lights, or timed lights for safety • Offset door hinges to widen doorways an extra 1.5 to 2 inches • Furniture height should be even with wheelchair height • Hallway width 36 inches • Nonslip floor surfaces • Remove small rugs and secure large rugs • Memory cues • Smoke and carbon monoxide detectors on each level • Strobe door bells may help clients with low hearing • Bump dots may help clients with low vision • Pathways cleared of clutter and furniture rearranged

UNIT 3-18 INTERVENTION

ERGONOMIC MODIFICATIONS	
WORK STATION ERGONOMICS	
Ergonomics is the science of creating an environment that best promotes function in the workplace. A workstation that is designed with good ergonomics reduces injury and increases comfort, health, and safety. Other benefits of ergonomics include increased efficiency, productivity, and quality. Occupational therapy practitioners' training allows them to identify hazardous workplace conditions and make design recommendations to improve ergonomics.[84]	
Ergonomic Recommendations	
Workstation[85]	• Alternate between a sitting and standing workstation. • A standing workstation is best when exerting downward force. • A seated workstation is best to complete fine motor tasks that require minimal reaching and force.
Desk[85]	• Clients should sit with 90-degree angles at the hips, knees, and ankles. • Desk modifications include raising or lowing the chair or desk. surface, or using books or other props under the client's feet. • Clients should minimize time spent looking down and take frequent 30-second breaks to bring the neck back into a neutral position.
Computer use[85]	• Position the head straight and level with the eyes hitting the top third of the screen. • Elbow flexion should be minimized to 90 degrees or less, and wrists should be kept in a neutral position to avoid compression at the carpal tunnel. • Clients using the computer should be advised to take frequent breaks.
Explore more: A computer workstation checklist can be found at https://www.osha.gov/SLTC/etools/computerworkstations/checklist_evaluation.html	

(continued)

UNIT 3-19 INTERVENTION

ERGONOMIC MODIFICATIONS (CONTINUED)

DRIVING ERGONOMICS AND CAR SAFETY TIPS

Occupational therapy practitioners can improve client safety in the car by analyzing the environment and making recommendations based on ergonomics. The car components should all be adjusted to best fit the driver. Adaptive devices are available to improve driving function.[86]

Vehicle Components	Recommendations	Adaptive Devices Available
Steering wheel	• The driver's line of sight should be at least 3 inches above the steering wheel. • There should be at least 10 inches between the driver's breastbone and steering wheel air bag.	• Steering wheel covers increase grip and protect hands from extreme temperatures.
Head restraint	• The head restraint should be positioned less than 3 inches from the center of the back of the driver's head. • The head restraint should not to be too high or too low against the neck.	• The head restraint is not typically adapted. This is an automotive safety feature that limits rearward movement of the occupant's head in the event of a collision.
Brakes	• The driver must be able to press down the brake pedal completely without trouble reaching. • The driver must be able move the foot from the gas to brake pedal without difficulty.	• Hand controls for brake and gas accommodate an inability or inefficiency with using foot pedals. • Pedal extensors position pedals within closer reach of feet.

(continued)

UNIT 3-19 INTERVENTION

ERGONOMIC MODIFICATIONS (CONTINUED)		
Vehicle Components	*Recommendations*	*Adaptive Devices Available*
Seatbelt	• The lap belt should fit low and tight across hips and pelvis, not the stomach. • The shoulder belt should cross over the breastbone and should not be against the neck. • Consider the ease of reaching the seatbelt for buckling and ease of unbuckling.	• Seat belt extenders from vehicle manufacturers increase ease of buckling when the driver's reach or rotation is limited.
Mirrors	• Consider the mirror position and blind spot visibility while seated in the driver's seat.	• Larger/extended/ panoramic mirrors increase view.
Driver	• Consider the driver's ability to transfer into and out of the car. • Consider the driver's ability to turn his or her head to look over the shoulder when checking the blind spot, switching lanes, or reversing. • The driver's sitting position should be comfortable.	• Seat cushions relieve back pain or can improve line of sight. • Seat lifts and swivel seats increase efficiency with getting in and out of the car. • Devices that assist with opening car doors. • Key turner.

Find a CarFit event near your client at https://www.car-fit.org

JOB ACCOMMODATIONS

Occupational therapy practitioners can facilitate participation in work occupations for clients who have disabilities through our knowledge of the client, the task, the environment, and the available resources. A key resource for job accommodations following illness or injury is the Job Accommodation Network.[87] Guidelines for job accommodations upon return to work can be found at askjan.org. Most accommodations are low cost or free.

Simple accommodations to enhance job performance include the following examples[88]:

- Alternate keyboards or voice recognition software can assist someone who has fine motor difficulties.

- Headphones can help limit distractions and enhance performance of an employee with attentional deficits.

- Frequent breaks throughout workday can assist with attentional difficulties or fatigue.

- Flexible work schedules, such as being able to work later in the day or work from home.

- Additional office lighting can aid an employee who has low vision.

DRIVING REHABILITATION AND COMMUNITY MOBILITY

Driving-related interventions can include enhancement of driving performance skills, client and family education, and education regarding community mobility options (eg, bus, train, app-based transportation services).[89] Details on possible interventions are outlined in the following table. Remember to always document any recommendations or referrals.

Education	• Increase client's awareness and self-regulatory behaviors. • The client and practitioner may decide that the client will only drive during daylight hours, on familiar routes, or close to the client's home.
Skills training	• Computer-based skills training to improve processing speed • Hazard perception skills training • Driving simulators, a time-effective and safe alternative to behind-the-wheel driving • Training related to vehicle adaptations
Performance review	• Video the driver's performance to review and analyze with the client. • Give feedback and coaching on simulations and task performance.
Vehicle modification	• Vehicle modification and adaptation • CarFit helps older drivers find a car that best fits them. Information can be found at https://www.car-fit.org Refer to Section One, Unit 3-19 for information for on vehicle modifications.
Psychoeducation	• Provide caregiver support and psychoeducation during transition to driving cessation.
Identify alternatives to driving	• Help the client identify alternative modes of transportation that allow him or her to meet occupational needs. • Address whether the client has the necessary performance skills for alternative modes of transportation. • Locate resources, such as home-delivery services or transportation pick-up services, to help client maintain independence.

References

1. Ross SE, Lin CT. The effects of promoting patient access to medical records: a review. *J Am Med Inform Assoc.* 2003;10(2):129–138. doi:10.1197/jamia.M1147

2. American Occupational Therapy Association. Standards of practice for occupational therapy. *Am J Occup Ther.* 2015;69(suppl 3):6913410057p1-6913410057p6. doi:10.5014/ajot.2015.696S06

3. American Occupational Therapy Association. Occupational therapy practice framework: domain and process (3rd ed). *Am J Occup Ther.* 2017;68(suppl 1):S1-S48. doi:10.5014/ajot.2014.682006

4. Keogh E, Moore DJ, Duggan GB, Payne SJ, Eccleston C. The disruptive effects of pain on complex cognitive performance and executive control. *PLoS ONE.* 2013;8(12):e83272. doi:10.1371/journal.pone.0083272

5. Perry GS, Patil SP, Presley-Cantrell LR. Raising awareness of sleep as a healthy behavior. *Prev Chronic Dis.* 2013;10:E133. doi:10.5888/pcd10.130081

6. Hawker GA, Mian S, Kendzerska T, French M. Measures of adult pain: visual analog scale of pain (VAS pain), numeric rating scale for pain (NRS pain), McGill pain questionnaire (MPQ), short-form McGill pain questionnaire (SF-MPQ), chronic pain grade scale (CPGS), short form-36 bodily pain scale (SF-36 BPS), and measure of intermittent and constant osteoarthritis pain (ICOAP). *Arthritis Care Res (Hoboken).* 2011;63(suppl 11):S240-S252. doi:10.1002/acr.20543

7. Gates DH, Walters LS, Cowley J, Wilken JM, Resnik L. Brief report—range of motion requirements for upper-limb activities of daily living. *Am J Occup Ther.* 2016;70(1):7001350010p1-7001350010p10. doi:10.5014/ajot.2016.015487

8. American Occupational Therapy Association. The role of occupational therapy in wound management. *Am J Occup Ther.* 2013;67(suppl.):S60-S68. doi:10.5014/ajot.2013.67S60

9. Martin DC. The mental status examination. In: Walker HK, Hall WD, Hurst JW, eds. *Clinical Methods: The History, Physical, and Laboratory Examinations.* 3rd ed. Boston, MA: Butterworths; 1990:924-929.

10. Gutman SA. The cranial nerves. In: *Quick Reference Neuroscience for Rehabilitation Professionals: The Essential Neurologic Principles Underlying Rehabilitation Practice.* 3rd ed. Thorofare, NJ: SLACK Incorporated; 2017:68-98.

11. Chou YH, Lin KC. The quick neurological screening test: Psychometric considerations. *Journal of Occupational Therapy Association, R.O.C.* 1998;16:37-51.

12. Conable KA, Rosner AL. A narrative review of manual muscle testing and implications for muscle testing research. *J Chiropr Med.* 2011;10(3);157-165. doi:10.1016/j.jmc.2011.04.001

13. American Occupational Therapy Association. Occupational therapy's role in acute care. American Occupational Therapy Association. https://www.aota.org/~/media/Corporate/Files/AboutOT/Professionals/WhatIsOT/RDP/Facts/Acute-Care.pdf. Published 2017. Accessed April 22, 2019.

14. Centers for Medicare & Medicaid Services. Medicare hospital quality chartbook 2010. https://www.cms.gov/Medicare/Quality-Initiatives-Patient-Assessment-Instruments/HospitalQualityInits/Downloads/HospitalChartBook.pdf. Published September 29, 2010. Accessed April 22, 2019.

15. Centers for Medicare & Medicaid Services. Long-term care hospitals. https://www.medicare.gov/coverage/long-term-care-hospitals.html#1351. Accessed April 22, 2019.

16. Silver B, Lyda-McDonald B, Bachofer H, Gage B. Developing outpatient therapy payment alternatives (DOTPA): 2010 utilization report. Centers for Medicare & Medicaid Services. https://www.cms.gov/Medicare/Billing/TherapyServices/Downloads/2010-DOTPA-Utilization-Report.pdf. Published January 2013. Accessed April 22, 2019.

17. Centers for Medicare & Medicaid Services. Home health services. https://www.medicare.gov/coverage/home-health-services.html. Accessed April 22, 2019.

18. Centers for Medicare & Medicaid Services. Inpatient rehabilitation therapy services: complying with documentation requirements. https://www.cms.gov/Outreach-and-Education/Medicare-Learning-Network-MLN/MLNProducts/downloads/Inpatient_Rehab_Fact_Sheet_ICN905643.pdf. Published 2012. Accessed April 22, 2019.

19. American Occupational Therapy Association. Occupational therapy's role in skilled nursing facilities. American Occupational Therapy Association. https://www.aota.org/~/media/Corporate/Files/AboutOT/Professionals/WhatIsOT/RDP/Facts/FactSheet_SkilledNursingFacilities.pdf. Published 2015. Accessed April 22, 2019.

20. Centers for Medicare & Medicaid Services. Medicare skilled nursing facility (SNF) transparency data (CY2013). CMS.gov. https://www.cms.gov/Newsroom/MediaReleaseDatabase/Fact-sheets/2016-Fact-sheets-items/2016-03-09.html. Published March 9, 2016. Accessed April 22, 2019.

21. American Occupational Therapy Association. Guidelines for documentation of occupational therapy. *Am J Occup Ther.* 2013;67:S32-S38. doi:10.5014/ajot.2013.67S32

22. Sames KM. *Documenting Occupational Therapy Practice.* 3rd ed. Upper Saddle River, NJ: Pearson; 2015.

23. Darragh AR, Campo MA, Frost L, Miller M, Pentico M, Margulis H. Safe-patient-handling equipment in therapy practice: implications for rehabilitation. *Am J Occup Ther.* 2013;67(1):45-53. doi:10.5014/ajot.2013.005389

24. Klyczek JP, Bauer-Yox N, Fiedler RC. The interest checklist: a factor analysis. *Am J Occup Ther.* 1997;51(10):815-823. doi:10.5014/ajot.51.10.815

25. Abu-Awad Y, Unsworth CA, Coulson M, Sarigiannis M. Using the Australian therapy outcome measures for occupational therapy (AusTOMs-OT) to measure client participation outcomes. *Br J Occup Ther.* 2014;77(2):44-49. doi:10.4276/030802214X13916969446958

26. Burnett J, Dyer CB, Naik AD. Convergent validation of the Kohlman Evaluation of Living Skills as a screening tool of older adults' ability to live safely and independently in the community. *Arch Phys Med Rehabil.* 2009;90(11):1948-1952. doi:10.1016/j.apmr.2009.05.021

27. Fisher AG. *Assessment of Motor and Process Skills. Vol 1: Development, Standardization, and Administration Manual.* 6th ed. Fort Collins, CO: Three Star Press; 2006.

28. Fisher AG. *Assessment of Motor and Process Skills. Vol. 2: User Manual.* 6th ed. Fort Collins, CO: Three Star Press; 2006.

29. Williams JH, Drinka TJK, Greenberg JR, Farrell-Holtan J, Euhardy R, Schram M. Development and testing of the assessment of living skills and resources (ALSAR) in elderly community-dwelling veterans. *Gerontologist.* 1991;31(1):84-91. doi:10.1093/geront/31.1.84

30. Kuo J, Fleming J, Dermer B, et al. Reliability of the original and revised versions of the assessment of living skills and resources. *Aust J Occup Ther.* 2007;54(3):194-202. doi:10.1111/j.1440-1630.2006.00625.x

31. Wilby HJ. A description of a functional screening assessment developed for the acute physical setting. *Br J Occup Ther.* 2005;68(1):39-44. doi:10.1177/030802260506800107

32. Haley SM, Andres PL, Coster WJ, Kosinski M, Ni P, Jette AM. Short-form activity measure for post-acute care. *Arch Phys Med Rehabil.* 2004;85(4):649-660.

33. Baum C, Edwards DF. *Activity Card Sort (ACS).* Bethesda, MD: AOTA Press; 2001.

34. Sander AM, Seel RT, Kreutzer JS, Hall KM, High WM, Rosenthal M. Agreement between persons with traumatic brain injury and their relatives regarding psychosocial outcome using the community integration questionnaire. *Arch Phys Med Rehabil.* 1997;78(4):353-357. doi:10.1016/S0003-9993(97)90225-2

35. Whiteneck G, Harrison-Felix C, Mellick D, Brooks C, Charlifue S, Gerhart K. Quantifying environmental factors (a measure of physical, attitudinal, service, productivity, and policy barriers). *Arch Phys Med Rehabil.* 2004;85:1324–1335. doi:10.1016/j.apmr.2003.09.027

36. Heinemann A, Miskovic A, Gray D, et al. Measuring environmental factors: unique and overlapping international classification of functioning, disability and health coverage of 5 instruments. *Arch Phys Med Rehabil.* 2016;97(12):2113-2122. doi:10.1016/j.apmr.2016.05.021

37. Williams A, Fossey E, Harvey C. Sustaining employment in a social firm: use of the work environment impact scale V2.0 to explore views of employees with psychiatric disabilities. *Br J Occup Ther.* 2010;73(11):531-539. doi:10.4276/03080221 0X12892992239279

38. Sandqvist JL, Törnquist KB, Henriksson CM. Assessment of work performance (AWP)—development of an instrument. *Work.* 2006;26(4):379-387.

39. Burns T. *Cognitive Performance Test (CPT).* Pequannock, NJ: Maddak; 2006.

40. Árnadóttir G. *The Brain and Behavior: Assessing Cortical Dysfunction Through Activities of Daily Living.* St. Louis, MO: Mosby; 1990.

41. Katz S, Down TD, Cash HR, Grotz, RC. Progress in the development of the index of ADL. *Gerontologist.* 1970;10(1):20-30.

42. Huang M, Chan K, Zanni J, et al. Functional status score for the ICU: an international clinimetric analysis of validity, responsiveness, and minimal important difference. *Crit Care Med.* 2016;44(12):e1164. doi:10.1097/CCM.0000000000001949.

43. Berney S, Skinner EH, Denehy L, Warrillow S. Development of a physical function outcome measure (PFIT) and a pilot exercise training protocol for use in intensive care. *Crit Care Resusc.* 2009;11(2):110-115.

44. Corner EJ, Wood W, Englebretsen C, et al. The Chelsea critical care physical assessment tool (CPAx): validation of an innovative new tool to measure physical morbidity in the general adult critical care population; an observational proof-of-concept pilot study. *Physiotherapy.* 2003;99(1):33-41. doi:10.1016/j.physio.2012.01.003

45. Hodgson C, Needham D, Haines K, et al. Feasibility and inter-rater reliability of the ICU mobility scale. *Heart Lung.* 2014;43(1)19-24. doi:10.1016/j.hrtlng.2013.11.003

46. Meyer MJ, Stanislaus AB, Lee J, et al. Surgical intensive care unit optimal mobilisation score (SOMS) trial: a protocol for an international, multicentre, randomised controlled trial focused on goal-directed early mobilisation of surgical ICU patients. *BMJ open.* 2013;3(8):e003262. doi:10.1136/bmjopen-2013-003262

47. McWilliams D, Atkins G, Hodson J, Boyers M, Lea T, Snelson C. Feasibility and reliability of the Manchester mobility score as a measure of physical function within the intensive care unit. *Journal of the Association of Chartered Physiotherapists in Respiratory Care.* 2016;48:26-33. http://www.acprc.org.uk/Data/Publication_ Downloads/Journalvol482016(1).pdf. Published 2016. Accessed April 22, 2019.

48. Perme C, Nawa RK, Winkelman C, Masud F. A tool to assess mobility status in critically ill patients: the Perme intensive care unit mobility score. *Methodist Debakey Cardiovasc J.* 2014;10(1):41-49.

49. Law M, Baptiste S, Carswell A, McColl MA, Polatajko H, Pollock N. *The Canadian Occupational Performance Measure.* 3rd ed. Toronto, ON: CAOT; 1998.

50. Colquhoun HL, Letts LJ, Law MC, MacDermid JC, Missiuna CA. Administration of the Canadian occupational performance measure: effect on practice. *Can J Occup Ther.* 2012;79(2)120-1288. doi:10.2182/cjot.2012.79.2.7

51. Coates R, Irvine C, Sutherland C. Development of an aphasia-friendly Canadian Occupational Performance Measure. *BMJ.* 2015;78:196-199. doi:10.1177/0308022614549962

52. Mackintosh S. Functional independence measure. *Aust J Physiother.* 2009;55(1):65. doi:10.1016/S0004-9514(09)70066-2

53. Uniform Data System for Medical Rehabilitation. *The FIM® Instrument: Its Background, Structure, and Usefulness.* www.udsmr.org/Documents/The_FIM_Instrument_Background_Structure_and_Usefulness.pdf. Published 2014. Accessed June 17, 2019.

54. Mahoney FI, Barthel DW. Functional evaluation: the Barthel index. *Md State Med J.* 1965;14:61-65.

55. Baum C, Morrison T, Hahn M, Edwards D. *Executive Function Performance Test: Test Protocol Booklet.* St. Louis, MO: Washington University School of Medicine; 2003.

56. Baum CM, Connor LT, Morrison T, Hahn M, Dromerick AW, Edwards DF. Reliability, validity, and clinical utility of the executive function performance test: a measure of executive function in a sample of people with stroke. *Am J Occup Ther.* 2008;62(4):446-455. doi:10.5014/ajot.62.4.446

57. American Occupational Therapy Association. Home safety and accessibility assessments. https://www.aota.org/Practice/Productive-Aging/Home-Mods/Rebuilding-Together/assessments.aspx. Updated 2018. Accessed April 22, 2019.

58. American Association of Retired Persons. Caregiving checklist. AARP. https://assets.aarp.org/external_sites/caregiving/checklists/checklist_homeSafety.html. Published 2003. Updated 2007. Accessed April 22, 2019.

59. Fisher GS, Ewonishon K. *Cougar Home Safety Assessment-Version 4.0.* Dallas, PA: Misericordia University; 2006. http://www.misericordia.edu/uploaded/documents/academics/ot/ot_research/home_safety/ot_finalcougar07.pdf. Published 2006. Accessed April 22, 2019.

60. Chiu T, Oliver R, Ascott P, et al. *Safety Assessment of Functional and the Environment for Rehabilitation-Health Outcome Measurement and Evaluation (SAFER-HOME), Version 3 Manual.* Toronto, ON: COTA Health: 2006.

61. Gitlin LN, Schinfeld S, Winter L, Corcoran M, Boyce AA, Hauck WW. Evaluating home environments of persons with dementia: interrater reliability and validity of the home environmental assessment protocol (HEAP). *Disabil Rehabil.* 2002;24(1-3):59-71.

62. Stark SL, Sommervill EK, Morris JC. In-home occupational performance evaluation (I-HOPE). *Am J Occup Ther.* 2010;64(4):580-589. doi:10.5014/ajot.2010.08065

63. Clemson L. *Home Fall Hazards.* West Brunswick, Victoria: Co-ordinates Therapy Services; 1997.

64. Sanford JA, Pynoos J, Tejral A, Browne A. Development of a comprehensive assessment for delivery of home modifications. *Phys Occup Ther Geriatr.* 2009;20(2):43-55. doi:10.1080/J148v20n02_03

65. Dickerson AE. Driving assessment tools used by driver rehabilitation specialists: survey of use and implications for practice. *Am J Occup Ther.* 2013;67(5):564-573. doi:10.5014/ajot.2013.007823

66. Dickerson AE. Screening and assessment tools for determining fitness to drive: a review of the literature for the pathways project. *Occup Ther Health Care.* 2014;28(2):82-121. doi:10.3109/07380577.2014.904535

67. Unsworth C. OT-driver off road assessment (OT-DORA). American Occupational Therapy Association. http://www.aota.org/practice/productive-aging/driving/practitioners/screen/ot-dora.aspx. Updated 2016. Accessed April 22, 2019.

68. American Occupational Therapy Association. Driving & community mobility: screening and assessments. https://www.aota.org/Practice/Productive-Aging/Driving/Practitioners/assessments.aspx. Published 2018. Accessed April 22, 2019.

69. Malfetti JL, Winter DJ. Drivers 55 plus: test your own performance. A self-rating form of questions, facts and suggestions for safe driving. https://www.researchgate.net/publication/234637891_Drivers_55_Plus_Test_Your_Own_Performance_A_Self-Rating_Form_of_Questions_Facts_and_Suggestions_for_Safe_Driving. Published January 1986. Accessed April 22, 2019.

70. Wang CC, Kosinski CJ, Schwartzberg JG, Shanklin AV. *Physician's Guide to Assessing and Counseling Older Drivers.* Washington, DC: National Highway Traffic Safety Administration; 2003.

71. Owsley C, Stalvey B, Wells J, Sloane ME. Older drivers and cataract: driving habits and crash risk. *J Gerontol A Biol Med Sci.* 1999;54A:M203-M211.

72. Schmall, V. Dementia and driving fact sheet. Family Caregiver Alliance. 2002. https://www.caregiver.org/dementia-driving. Published 2002. Accessed April 22, 2019.

73. Guariglia S, Smallfield S. The role of occupational therapy in medication management in acute care. *Gerontol Spec Interest Sect Q.* 2015;38(1):1-3.

74. Gibson RW, D'Amico M, Jaffe L, Arbesman M. Occupational therapy interventions for recovery in the areas of community integration and normative life roles for adults with serious mental illness: a systematic review. *Am J Occup Ther.* 2011;65:247-256. doi:10.5014/ajot.2011.001297

75. Hofmeyer MR, Alexander NB, Nyquist LV, Medell JL, Koreishi A. Floor-rise strategy training in older adults. *J Am Geriatr Soc.* 2002;50(10):1702-1706. doi:10.1046/j.1532-5415.2002.50463.x

76. Kraskowsky LH, Finlayson M. Factors affecting older adults' use of adaptive equipment: review of the literature. *Am J Occup Ther.* 2011;55:303-310. doi:10.5014/ajot.55.3.303

77. Centers for Disease Control and Prevention. Adult obesity facts. https://www.cdc.gov/obesity/data/adult.html. Published 2016. Updated March 5, 2018. Accessed April 22, 2019.

78. Seeger MS, Fisher LA. Adaptive equipment used in the rehabilitation of hip arthroplasty patients. *Am J Occup Ther.* 1982;36(8):503-508. doi:10.5014/ajot.36.8.503

79. Parker MG, Thorslund M. The use of technical aids among community-based elderly. *Am J Occup Ther.* 1991;45(8):712-718. doi:10.5014/ajot.45.8.712

80. Therapeutic Recreation Process II. Adapted equipment ideas. State University of New York Cortland. http://colfax.cortland.edu/nysirrc/articles-handouts/SUNY%20Cortland%20TR%20Students%20Adapted%20Equipment%20Book.pdf. Published 2015. Accessed April 22, 2019.

81. DuBroc W, Pickens ND. Becoming "at home" in home modifications: professional reasoning across the expertise continuum. *Occup Ther Health Care.* 2015;29(3):316-329. doi:10.3109/07380577.2015.1010129

82. Hwang E, Cummings L, Sixsmith A, Sixsmith J. Impacts of home modification on aging-in-place. *J Hous Elderly.* 2011;25:246-257. doi:10.1080/02763893.2011.595611

83. American Association of Retired Persons. Home fit guide. https://www.aarp.org/content/dam/aarp/livable-communities/documents-2015/HomeFit2015/AARP%20HomeFit%20Guide%202015.pdf. Published 2015. Accessed April 22, 2019.

84. American Occupational Therapy Association. Ergonomics. www.aota.org/~/media/ Corporate/Files/AboutOT/Professionals/WhatIsOT/WI/Facts/ergonomics.pdf. Revised 2017. Accessed June 17, 2019.

85. Occupational Safety and Health Administration. Computer workstations e-tool. United States Department of Labor. https://www.osha.gov/SLTC/etools/computer-workstations/checklist_evaluation.html. Published 2016. Accessed April 22, 2019.

86. American Society on Aging. CarFit. https://www.flhsmv.gov/ddl/Carfit-Brochure-2009.pdf. Published 2009. Accessed April 22, 2019.

87. Job Accommodation Network. Searchable online accommodation resource. JAN. http://askjan.org/soar/index.htm. Published 2016. Accessed April 22, 2019.

88. Schreuer N, Myhill WN, Aratan-Bergman T, Samant D, Blanck P. Workplace accommodations: Occupational therapists as mediators in the interactive process. *Work.* 2009;34:149-160.

89. Dickerson A, Schold Davis E. Driving and Transportation Alternatives for Older Adults. *AOTA.* https://www.aota.org/About-Occupational-Therapy/Professionals/ PA/Facts/Driving-Transportation-Alternatives.aspx. Published 2012. Accessed April 22, 2019.

SECTION TWO

Central Nervous System

Sit W, Neville M.
Handbook of Occupational Therapy for
Adults With Physical Disabilities (pp 111-219).
© 2020 SLACK Incorporated.

CASE

DIAGNOSIS: STROKE

While working in an inpatient rehabilitation facility, I encountered a woman who had suffered a stroke that left her profoundly impacted and functioning at a low level. She demonstrated extreme difficulty with comprehension and following instructions. Fortunately, she had a very supportive husband. During one of our therapy sessions, I interviewed him about his wife and asked, "What does she like to do?" He informed me that she enjoyed playing the ukulele and traveling with her friends. I asked him to bring their ukulele records to the next session. After that, we played the ukulele albums for her during therapy sessions, and her friends came to visit. Even though my client had low motivation and low function, we were able to identify meaningful activities for her.

Several months after the client was discharged, the inpatient rehabilitation facility held a rehabilitation reunion event around Christmas. Discharged former patients were invited to join us and celebrate. I spotted my client at the reunion, and she was almost unrecognizable. She was wearing a dress, had applied makeup, and had fixed up her hair. She said to me, "William, I wanted to dress up to show you that I am better now." She continued, "Even though I could not speak or understand what was happening, I remember you playing ukulele music for me." Her words have stayed with me as a reminder of the importance of engaging clients in activities that are meaningful to them. Even seemingly insignificant things can have a profoundly positive impact on the client.

STRUCTURES, FUNCTIONS, AND PATHOLOGIES: SKILLS AND FACTORS ASSOCIATED WITH AREAS OF THE BRAIN	
AREA OF BRAIN	**ROLE AND SYMPTOMS INDICATING DAMAGE**
Frontal lobes[1-3]	Functions of the frontal lobes include attention, problem solving, planning, judgment, motivation, expressive language, sequencing, and motor integration. Symptoms of frontal lobe damage include the following: • Difficulty sequencing • Perseveration (repetition of a thought or action) • Personality changes • Inflexible thinking • Difficulty initiating voluntary movements • Difficulty inhibiting inappropriate emotional, social, and sexual behavior • Broca's aphasia (inability to speak fluently without effort): ○ Indicative of left frontal lobe damage *(continued)*

STRUCTURES, FUNCTIONS, AND PATHOLOGIES: SKILLS AND FACTORS ASSOCIATED WITH AREAS OF THE BRAIN (CONTINUED)	
AREA OF BRAIN	ROLE AND SYMPTOMS INDICATING DAMAGE

Parietal lobes[2,3]	Functions of the parietal lobes include tactile perception, spatial awareness, awareness of body parts, object naming, right/left orientation, visual attention, and eye-hand coordination.
	
	Symptoms of parietal lobe damage include the following:
	• Difficulty naming objects
	• Right and left confusion
	• Sensory processing changes
	• Impaired spatial orientation
	• Lack of awareness of body parts
	• Apraxia (inability to perform a motor task)
	• Difficulties with mathematics and astereognosis (inability to identify an object through sense of touch):
	    ○ Indicative of left parietal lobe damage
	• Contralateral (opposite side) neglect and hemi-inattention, and difficulty constructing items:
	    ○ Indicative of right parietal lobe damage
	
	(continued)

UNIT 1-23 NEED TO KNOW

STRUCTURES, FUNCTIONS, AND PATHOLOGIES: SKILLS AND FACTORS ASSOCIATED WITH AREAS OF THE BRAIN (CONTINUED)

AREA OF BRAIN	ROLE AND SYMPTOMS INDICATING DAMAGE
Temporal lobes[2,3]	Functions of the temporal lobes include short-term memory, language comprehension, interpreting music, selective attention, face recognition, and object categorization. Symptoms of temporal lobe damage include the following: • Difficulty understanding spoken language • Short-term memory loss • Increased aggressive behavior • Difficulty identifying and categorizing objects • Difficulty recognizing faces and visually locating objects • Wernicke's aphasia (inability to comprehend speech and produce meaningful speech): ◦ Indicative of left temporal lobe damage • Right temporal lobe (contralateral, or opposite side, neglect and hemi-inattention)
Occipital lobes[3,4]	Functions of the occipital lobes include visual perception, processing, and reading. Symptoms of occipital lobe damage include the following: • Visual field cuts or homonymous hemianopsia (inability to see one-half of the visual field in the side opposite of the lesion) • Difficulty identifying colors • Hallucinations and visual distortions • Alexia and agraphia (difficulty reading and writing) • Cortical blindness

(continued)

STRUCTURES, FUNCTIONS, AND PATHOLOGIES: SKILLS AND FACTORS ASSOCIATED WITH AREAS OF THE BRAIN (CONTINUED)	
AREA OF BRAIN	**ROLE AND SYMPTOMS INDICATING DAMAGE**

Thalamus[3,5]	Functions of the thalamus include processing sensory information with the exception of olfactory processing. Symptoms of thalamus damage include the following:
	• Contralateral (opposite side) limb ataxia (movements that lack smoothness and coordination)
	• Visual neglect, visuospatial deficits, and anosognosia (impairments in self-awareness):
	    ◦ Indicative of right thalamus lesions
	• Aphasia (difficulty producing speech), paraphasia (impaired flow of speech), anomia (difficulty recalling names of objects), dysarthria (slowed or slurred speech), apathy, agitation, and ipsilateral conjugate deviation of eyes (eye deviates on the side of damage):
	    ◦ Indicative of left thalamus lesions
	
	(continued)

STRUCTURES, FUNCTIONS, AND PATHOLOGIES: SKILLS AND FACTORS ASSOCIATED WITH AREAS OF THE BRAIN (CONTINUED)

AREA OF BRAIN	ROLE AND SYMPTOMS INDICATING DAMAGE
Hypothalamus[3,5]	Functions of the hypothalamus are related to maintenance of homeostasis. The hypothalamus regulates body temperature, blood pressure, metabolic rate, water intake, digestion, eating, reproductive behavior, defensive behavior, emotional expression, and sleep-wake cycles. Symptoms of hypothalamus damage include the following: • Refusal of food and malnutrition or weight gain • Hormonal imbalance • Fatigue • Cold intolerance • Amenorrhea (the absence of menstrual cycles) • Loss of libido (the sex drive) • Dizziness • Weakness • Loss of vision • Constipation
Amygdala[3,5]	Functions of the amygdala include emotion, motivation, and interpretation of nonverbal communication. Symptoms of amygdala damage include the following: • Mood changes • Euphoria or indifference • Emotional lability • Decreased social intelligence • Symptoms of depression, including worthlessness, anhedonia (inability to experience pleasure), and suicidal thoughts or behaviors

(continued)

STRUCTURES, FUNCTIONS, AND PATHOLOGIES: SKILLS AND FACTORS ASSOCIATED WITH AREAS OF THE BRAIN (CONTINUED)	
AREA OF BRAIN	ROLE AND SYMPTOMS INDICATING DAMAGE
Hippocampus[3,5]	Functions of the hippocampus include storing declarative memories and learning. Symptoms of hippocampus damage include the following: • Forgetfulness • Learning impairment • Anterograde amnesia (inability to store new memories)
Cerebellum[3,4]	Functions of the cerebellum include coordination of voluntary movement, gross and fine motor coordination, balance and equilibrium, postural control, and eye movement. Symptoms of cerebellum damage include the following: • Ataxia (loss of coordinated movement) • Nystagmus (rapid and uncontrolled eye movements) • Dysmetria (inability to judge scale and distance) • Dysdiadochokinesia (inability to perform alternating and rapid motions) • Dysarthria (slowed speech) • Slurred speech • Dizziness/vertigo • Tremors • Difficulty walking

(continued)

UNIT 1-23 NEED TO KNOW

Structures, Functions, and Pathologies: Skills and Factors Associated With Areas of the Brain (continued)

Area of Brain	Role and Symptoms Indicating Damage
Brainstem[3,4]— Midbrain, pons, and medulla	Functions of the brainstem include control of breathing, heart rate, swallowing, reflexes, digestion, blood pressure, sweating, and temperature. The brainstem regulates consciousness, sleeping, sensing balance, and the level of alertness. Symptoms of brainstem damage include the following: • Dysphagia (impaired swallowing) • Impaired balance • Dizziness/vertigo • Sleep difficulties including insomnia or sleep apnea • Paresis or paralysis • Double vision • Impaired heart rate, blood pressure, or respiration • Locked-in syndrome

Upper Motor Neuron Dysfunction

Upper motor neuron cell bodies originate in the cerebral cortex and brain stem. Symptoms of upper motor neuron lesions include hypertonia, spasticity, hyperreflexia, and abnormal reflexes such as positive pathological reflexes and reduced superficial reflexes.[3]

Pathology	Signs and Symptoms
Amyotrophic lateral sclerosis (ALS)[3]	ALS involves a breakdown of motor neurons in the brain, brainstem, and spinal cord. ALS results in both upper and lower motor neuron impairments. Signs and symptoms of ALS include the following: • Progressive weakness that begins in the hands, feet, or face • Loss of ability to swallow • Loss of respiration • Paralysis • Spasticity and hyperreflexia

(continued)

STRUCTURES, FUNCTIONS, AND PATHOLOGIES: SKILLS AND FACTORS ASSOCIATED WITH AREAS OF THE BRAIN (CONTINUED)

Pathology	Signs and Symptoms
Cerebellar ataxia[3]	Signs and symptoms of cerebellar ataxia include the following: • Lack of coordinated movements, especially in the trunk and extremities • Dysmetria • Dysrhythmia
Cerebrovascular accident (CVA)[3]	Refer to the CVA symptoms table in this unit for more information.
Huntington's chorea[3]	Huntington's chorea is a progressive condition of genetic cause. The onset occurs mid-life and results in the death of neurons in the caudate putamen. Signs and symptoms of Huntington's chorea include the following: • Chorea (involuntary jerking movements) • Ataxia • Changes in personality • Dementia
Multiple sclerosis (MS)[3]	MS is a progressive disorder in which the myelin sheaths of the neurons deteriorate. Signs and symptoms of MS include the following: • Motor weakness and difficulty swallowing • Fatigue • Loss of sensation • Visual impairment • Spasticity • Dysarthria • Intention tremor • Nystagmus • Incontinence • Changes to cognitive and affective systems

(continued)

STRUCTURES, FUNCTIONS, AND PATHOLOGIES: SKILLS AND FACTORS ASSOCIATED WITH AREAS OF THE BRAIN (CONTINUED)

Pathology	Signs and Symptoms
Parkinson's disease[3]	Parkinson's disease is a progressive basal ganglia disorder resulting in the loss of the dopamine neurotransmitter.
	Signs and symptoms of Parkinson's disease include the following:
	• Tremor
	• Bradykinesia
	• Instability of posture
	• Rigidity
Traumatic brain injury (TBI)[3]	TBI refers to damage to the brain resulting from some kind of traumatic event.
	Signs and symptoms of TBI include the following:
	• Changes to or loss of cognitive functions
	• Changes to or loss of sensory and motor functions
	• Impairments to coordination
	• Speech impairments
	• Behavioral changes
	• Swallowing impairments
	• Coma

LOWER MOTOR NEURON DYSFUNCTION

Lower motor neuron cell bodies originate in the spinal cord and in cranial nerve nuclei located in the brainstem. Symptoms of lower motor neuron lesions include muscle atrophy, flaccidity, reduced or absent sensation, and loss of reflexes.[3]

(continued)

STRUCTURES, FUNCTIONS, AND PATHOLOGIES: SKILLS AND FACTORS ASSOCIATED WITH AREAS OF THE BRAIN (CONTINUED)

PATHOLOGY	SIGNS AND SYMPTOMS
ALS[3]	ALS involves a breakdown of motor neurons located in the brain, brainstem, and spinal cord. ALS results in both upper and lower motor neuron impairments. Signs and symptoms of ALS include the following: • Progressive weakness that begins in the hands, feet, or face • Loss of ability to swallow • Loss of respiration • Paralysis • Spasticity and hyperreflexia
Guillain-Barré syndrome[3]	Guillain-Barré syndrome results from dysfunction in the immune system and results in breakdown of myelin sheaths in the peripheral nerves. Signs and symptoms of Guillain-Barré syndrome include the following: • Progressive weakness • Loss of reflexes • Abnormal sensation in the distal extremities
Myasthenia gravis[3]	Myasthenia gravis is a disorder occurring at the post-synaptic membrane of the neuromuscular junction. Signs and symptoms of myasthenia gravis include the following: • Symmetrical weakness affecting the limbs proximally, neck, diaphragm, and eyeballs • Weakness that worsens with repetition • Sensation and reflexes exhibit no impairments

(continued)

STRUCTURES, FUNCTIONS, AND PATHOLOGIES: SKILLS AND FACTORS ASSOCIATED WITH AREAS OF THE BRAIN (CONTINUED)	
Pathology	Signs and Symptoms
Myopathy[3]	Myopathy is presented as muscular weakness. Examples of myopathy disorders include muscular dystrophy, dermatomyositis, and polymyositis. Signs and symptoms of myopathy include the following: • Weakness that is worse proximally • Sensation and reflexes exhibit no impairments
Neuropathy[3]	Neuropathy is a neuron disorder affecting the axons or myelin sheaths Signs and symptoms of neuropathy include the following: • Motor and sensory losses resulting in symptoms of lower motor neuron dysfunction • Neuropathy can be related to diabetes and presents in a stocking/glove distribution
Spinal cord injury (SCI)[3]	Refer to Unit 2-33 in this section for information on SCIs. *(continued)*

STRUCTURES, FUNCTIONS, AND PATHOLOGIES: SKILLS AND FACTORS ASSOCIATED WITH AREAS OF THE BRAIN (CONTINUED)

NEUROTRANSMITTERS

Neurotransmitter	Functions[3]	Link to Disabilities[3]
Serotonin	• General level of arousal • Sleep and appetite regulation • Mood	• Low levels are linked to depression and anxiety • High levels are linked to obsessive compulsive disorder
Norepinephrine	• Attention to sensory information • Increases heart rate and bronchiole dilation • Mood	• High levels are linked to panic disorder, posttraumatic stress disorder, and fear
Acetylcholine	• Selected attention • Contraction of skeletal muscle • Slows heart rate and increases digestion	• Low levels are linked to Myasthenia gravis and Alzheimer's disease
Dopamine	• Motor control • Goal related behavior • Motivation • Pleasurable feelings • Cognition and planning	• Low levels are linked to Parkinson's disease • High levels are linked to schizophrenia and psychosis

(continued)

STRUCTURES, FUNCTIONS, AND PATHOLOGIES: SKILLS AND FACTORS ASSOCIATED WITH AREAS OF THE BRAIN (CONTINUED)

Neurotransmitter	Functions[3]	Link to Disabilities[3]
Glutamate	• Learning and memory	• High levels are linked to seizures and neuronal death
Gamma-aminobutyric acid (GABA)	• Sedation • Inhibition	• Low levels are linked to neural over activity, epilepsy, involuntary muscle contraction, and anxiety
Endorphins	• Decreased perception of pain • Mood • Concentration • Creativity and sensitivity	• Dysregulation is linked to impulsivity, depression, and addiction
Substance P	• Pain sensation and perception • Control of respiratory and cardiovascular systems in central nervous system • Mood regulation in central nervous system	• Complex regional pain syndrome

(continued)

STRUCTURES, FUNCTIONS, AND PATHOLOGIES: SKILLS AND FACTORS ASSOCIATED WITH AREAS OF THE BRAIN (CONTINUED)

COMMON CEREBROVASCULAR ACCIDENT (STROKE) SYMPTOMS

Artery Affected	Signs
Anterior cerebral artery (ACA)[1,3]	The client's contralateral lower limb is more severely affected with an ACA CVA. This may include the loss of sensation and hemiplegia Common symptoms with an ACA CVA include the following: • Apraxia • Perseveration • Behavioral abnormalities • Urinary incontinence • Possibility of transcortical aphasia with a left hemisphere ACA CVA • Possibility of left hemi-inattention with a right hemisphere ACA CVA
Middle cerebral artery (MCA)[3]	The client's contralateral upper limb and face are more severely affected in an MCA CVA. This may include the loss of sensation and hemiparesis. Common symptoms with an MCA CVA include the following: • Homonymous hemianopsia Right hemisphere MCA CVA symptoms include the following: • Hemi-inattention to left side • Difficulty understanding spatial relationships • Constructional apraxia • Impulsiveness • Emotional lability Left hemisphere MCA CVA symptoms include the following: • Aphasia • Frustration • Being overly cautious

(continued)

STRUCTURES, FUNCTIONS, AND PATHOLOGIES: SKILLS AND FACTORS ASSOCIATED WITH AREAS OF THE BRAIN (CONTINUED)	
Artery Affected	*Signs*
Posterior cerebral artery[3,4]	Common symptoms in a posterior cerebral artery CVA include the following: • Contralateral sensory loss and hemiparesis • Homonymous hemianopsia • Cortical blindness • Visual agnosia
Basilar artery[3,4]	Common symptoms in a basilar artery CVA include the following: • Bilateral sensory loss • Tetraplegia and locked in syndrome • Decorticate or decerebrate rigidity • Vertigo, vomiting, nausea, nystagmus • Oculomotor nerve palsy

FAST Warning Signs of a Stroke	
FAST stands for Face drooping, Arm weakness, Speech difficulty, and Time to call 911.[6,7] Practitioners can use the FAST acronym when a stroke is suspected with a client. These warning signs can also be beneficial for occupational therapists to use when educating clients and family members on quick recognition of the signs.	
Face drooping	One side of person's face droops or feels numb. To test for face drooping, ask the person to smile and observe for symmetry.
Arm weakness	One arm is weak or drifts downward when both arms are raised.
Speech difficulty	The person's speech is slurred. He or she will have trouble repeating a short sentence such as "The sky is blue."
Time to call 911	If any of these symptoms are present, immediately call 911.

UNIT 1-24 NEED TO KNOW

NEUROENDOCRINE DYSFUNCTION FOLLOWING BRAIN INJURY

Neuroendocrine dysfunction is common after someone has sustained a brain injury. Dysfunctions may involve the pituitary gland, growth hormone deficiencies, luteinizing and follicle-stimulating hormone deficiencies, and adrenocorticotropic deficiencies.[8,9]

Screening	Neuroendocrine dysfunction can be detected by screening tests of the following hormones: • Thyroid-stimulating hormone • Insulin-like growth factor 1 • Cortisol • Prolactin • Luteinizing hormone • Follicle-stimulating hormone • Testosterone • Estradiol (in nonmenstruating females)
Clinical symptoms	• Weakness and fatigue • Intolerance to cold • Sexual dysfunction • Menstrual abnormalities • Increased body fat • Decreased muscle mass • Diabetes insipidus • Decreased exercise tolerance • Memory impairments • Decreased ability to concentrate
Treatment	Hormone replacement therapy is used as a lifelong treatment to control symptoms of neuroendocrine dysfunction. The client may experience improvements in concentration, attention, processing speed, memory, mood, sleep, weight control, sexual performance, activities of daily living (ADLs), and quality of life.

COMMON ASSESSMENTS ACROSS PRACTICE SETTINGS

ASSESSMENT	ACUTE	INPATIENT	HOME HEALTH	SNF	OUTPATIENT
Common Assessments Across Practice Settings					
Mini-Mental State Examination	✓	✓		✓	✓
St. Louis University Mental Status Examination	✓	✓			✓
Bells Test	✓	✓			
Stroke Impact Scale		✓			✓
Rivermead Behavioral Memory Test		✓			✓
Test of Everyday Attention		✓			✓
Comprehensive Trail-Making Test		✓			✓
Dynamic Loewenstein Occupational Therapy Cognitive Assessment		✓			✓
Arm Motor Ability Test		✓			✓
Wolf Motor Function Test		✓			✓
Berg Balance Scale		✓			✓
Neurobehavioral Cognitive Status Examination (Cognistat)		✓			✓
Clock Drawing Test		✓			✓
					(continued)

UNIT 2-26 EVALUATION

COMMON ASSESSMENTS ACROSS PRACTICE SETTINGS (CONTINUED)

ASSESSMENT	ACUTE	INPATIENT	HOME HEALTH	SNF	OUTPATIENT
Motor-Free Visual Perception Test		✓			✓
Spinal Cord Independence Measure		✓			✓
Confusion Assessment Method for the Intensive Care Unit (ICU)	✓				
Glasgow Coma Scale	✓				
Rancho Los Amigos Level of Cognitive Functioning Scale	✓	✓		✓	
National Institutes of Health Stroke Scale	✓	✓			
Allen Cognitive Levels	✓	✓			
Montreal Cognitive Assessment	✓	✓	✓		
Global Deterioration Scale	✓	✓			✓
American Spinal Injury Association Impairment Scale	✓				
Modified Ashworth Scale	✓	✓	✓	✓	✓
Fugl-Meyer Assessment of Motor Recovery Following a Stroke	✓	✓			✓

SNF: skilled nursing facility.

(continued)

COMMON ASSESSMENTS
ACROSS PRACTICE SETTINGS (CONTINUED)

MINI-MENTAL STATE EXAMINATION[10]

- Purpose: Assesses cognitive performance
- Context: Adult clients with any diagnosis
- Format: Oral questionnaire and paper-and-pencil tasks
- Time to administer: 5 to 10 minutes
- Materials: Questionnaire, watch, writing utensil, and 4 sheets of blank paper
- Cost: $76 and up for manual
- Website: https://www.parinc.com/products/pkey/237

ST. LOUIS UNIVERSITY MENTAL STATUS EXAMINATION[11]

- Purpose: Assesses presence of cognitive deficits and changes in cognition over time
- Context: Older adults, clients with Alzheimer's or dementia
- Format: Pencil-and-paper questionnaire
- Time to administer: 4 to 10 minutes
- Materials: Score sheet and writing utensil
- Cost: Free
- Website: https://www.slu.edu/medicine/internal-medicine/geriatric-medicine/aging-successfully/assessment-tools/mental-status-exam.php

BELLS TEST[12]

- Purpose: Assesses visual neglect
- Context: Clients with stroke, TBI, and other central nervous damage
- Format: Pencil-and-paper object cancellation task
- Time to administer: Less than 5 minutes
- Materials: Test sheet, score sheet, writing utensil, and stopwatch
- Cost: Free
- Website: https://www.strokengine.ca/en/assess/bt

(continued)

UNIT 2-26 EVALUATION

COMMON ASSESSMENTS ACROSS PRACTICE SETTINGS (CONTINUED)

STROKE IMPACT SCALE[13]

- Purpose: Assesses quality of life following a stroke
- Context: Clients with stroke in inpatient or outpatient setting
- Format: Self-report questionnaire
- Time to administer: 15 to 20 minutes
- Materials: Questionnaire form and writing utensil
- Cost: Free
- Website: https://www.strokengine.ca/pdf/sis.pdf

RIVERMEAD BEHAVIORAL MEMORY TEST[14]

- Purpose: Assesses memory abilities and impairments
- Context: Inpatient and outpatient settings
- Format: Performance-based test
- Time to administer: 30 minutes
- Materials: Assessment kit and manual
- Cost: $111 and up for manual
- Website: https://images.pearsonclinical.com/images/assets/RBMT-3/RBMT3MrktCollateral.pdf

TEST OF EVERYDAY ATTENTION[15]

- Purpose: Assesses selective attention, sustained attention, and attention switching
- Context: Clients across diagnoses in inpatient and outpatient settings
- Format: Performance-based test
- Time to administer: 45 to 60 minutes
- Materials: Assessment kit and manual
- Cost: $405
- Website: https://www.pearsonclinical.com/psychology/products/100000182/test-of-everyday-attention-the-tea.html#tab-pricing

(continued)

COMMON ASSESSMENTS
ACROSS PRACTICE SETTINGS (CONTINUED)

COMPREHENSIVE TRAIL-MAKING TEST[16]

- Purpose: Assesses frontal lobe and executive functioning
- Context: Clients with brain injury or stroke in an inpatient or outpatient setting
- Format: Paper-and-pencil test
- Time to administer: 5 to 12 minutes
- Materials: Manual and record booklets
- Cost: $145
- Website: https://www.parinc.com/Products/Pkey/74

DYNAMIC LOEWENSTEIN OCCUPATIONAL THERAPY COGNITIVE ASSESSMENT[17,18]

- Purpose: Assesses neurological deficits to develop cognitive profile
- Context: Clients with brain injury, stroke, progressive neurological conditions, and dementia
- Format: Performance-based test
- Time to administer: 30 to 45 minutes
- Materials: Assessment kit and manual
- Cost: $329
- Website: https://www.therapro.com/Browse-Category/Cognitive-Assessments/DLOTCA.html#

ARM MOTOR ABILITY TEST[19]

- Purpose: Assesses impairments in ADL following a stroke
- Context: Clients with stroke
- Format: Performance-based test
- Time to administer: 15 to 25 minutes
- Materials: Manual and nonstandardized equipment such as a cardigan, shoes with laces, and a spoon
- Cost: Free
- Website: https://www.rehab.research.va.gov/jour/05/42/6/pdf/daly-append2.pdf

(continued)

UNIT 2-26 EVALUATION

COMMON ASSESSMENTS ACROSS PRACTICE SETTINGS (CONTINUED)

WOLF MOTOR FUNCTION TEST[20,21]

- Purpose: Assesses upper extremity motor deficits
- Context: Clients with brain injury and stroke
- Format: Timed, performance-based test
- Time to administer: 6 to 30 minutes
- Materials: Manual, standardized template, and nonstandardized equipment such as index cards, 12-oz beverage in a can, and a box
- Cost: Free
- Website: https://www.uab.edu/citherapy/images/pdf_files/CIT_Training_WMFT_Manual.pdf

BERG BALANCE SCALE[22]

- Purpose: Assesses balance to determine fall risk
- Context: Geriatric clients in inpatient and outpatient settings
- Format: Performance-based scale
- Time to administer: 10 to 15 minutes
- Materials: Manual, chair with armrests, measuring tape, and a step stool
- Cost: Free
- Website: https://www.sralab.org/sites/default/files/2017-07/berg.pdf

  Refer to Section Three, Unit 2-53 for information on the Berg Balance Scale.

NEUROBEHAVIORAL COGNITIVE STATUS EXAMINATION (COGNISTAT)[23]

- Purpose: Assesses cognitive impairment
- Context: Clients with brain injury, stroke, dementia, psychiatric disorders, and substance abuse
- Format: Online or paper test
- Time to administer: 15 to 20 minutes
- Materials: Online system, tokens, and stimulus booklet and a training course
- Cost: $475
- Website: https://www.cognistat.com/cognistat-assessment-system-products-and-pricing

(continued)

COMMON ASSESSMENTS ACROSS PRACTICE SETTINGS (CONTINUED)

CLOCK DRAWING TEST[24]

- Purpose: Assesses for dementia, cognitive impairments, and visual inattention and neglect
- Context: Inpatient and outpatient settings
- Format: Paper-and-pencil test
- Time to administer: Less than 5 minutes
- Materials: Writing utensil and a piece of paper
- Cost: Free
- Website: https://www.sralab.org/sites/default/files/2017-07/Clock%20Drawing%20Test%20Instructions.pdf

MOTOR-FREE VISUAL PERCEPTION TEST[25,26]

- Purpose: Assesses visual perception without influence of motor ability
- Context: Clients across ages and diagnoses and clients with stroke
- Format: Performance-based test
- Time to administer: 10 to 20 minutes
- Materials: Manual and assessment kit
- Cost: $175
- Website: http://www.therapro.com/Browse-Category/Visual-Perception-and-Visual-Skills/Motor-Free-Visual-Perception-Test-4-MVPT-4.html

(continued)

UNIT 2-26 EVALUATION

COMMON ASSESSMENTS ACROSS PRACTICE SETTINGS (CONTINUED)
SPINAL CORD INDEPENDENCE MEASURE[27]
• Purpose: Assesses self-care performance in people with SCIs • Context: Clients with SCIs • Format: Performance-based observation • Time to administer: 30 to 60 minutes • Materials: Rating sheet, writing utensil, and ADL supplies • Cost: Free • Website: https://www.sralab.org/sites/default/files/2017-07/SCIM.pdf
CONFUSION ASSESSMENT METHOD FOR THE ICU[28]
• Purpose: Diagnoses delirium at bedside based on 4 diagnostic criteria: acute onset or fluctuation course, inattention, altered consciousness, and disorganized thinking. • Context: ICU • Format: Screening tool • Time to administer: Less than 5 minutes • Materials: Flowsheet pocket card • Cost: Free • Website: http://www.icudelirium.org/delirium/monitoring.html

GLASGOW COMA SCALE

SUMMARY

- Purpose: Describes level of consciousness (LOC) in clients with newly acquired brain injury or head trauma
- Context: Clients with potential brain injuries, trauma, and coma
- Format: Observation and rating scale
- Time to administer: Quick
- Materials: None
- Cost: Free
- Website: www.glasgowcomascale.org

The Glasgow Coma Scale (GCS) is a method for assessing a person's level of consciousness at the time of initial assessment and reassessment.[29,30] The GCS is typically used with clients who have sustained a brain injury. The therapist presents specific stimuli and records the client's basic motor, verbal, and eye response. A score of 1 in each category indicates no response.[29,30]

SCORING

The GCS is the total of the 3 scores. Higher scores indicate a higher conscious state.

Scoring Interpretation

- GCS total 3 to 8: Severe
- GCS total 9 to 12: Moderate
- GCS total 13 to 15: Mild

A score of 8 or below indicates that the client is in a coma or is comatose. A score above 8 indicates that the client is emerging from a coma. Half of patients with a score of less than 8 at 6 hours do not survive.

(continued)

UNIT 2-27 EVALUATION

UNIT 2-27   EVALUATION

GLASGOW COMA SCALE (CONTINUED)

BASIC MOTOR RESPONSE	VERBAL RESPONSE	EYE OPENING
The therapist should deliver a 2-step command. Ask the client to squeeze your hand while opening his or her mouth and sticking out his or her tongue (Note: in the case of an SCI, ask the client to stick out his or her tongue only). • **Score of 6:** Client obeys the command Record the client's motor response to a pain or pressure stimulus by pinching the trapezius on one side. Repeat on the other side. • **Score of 5:** Localized response—client attempts to remove the pain stimulus • **Score of 4:** Arm flexion • **Score of 3:** Arm extension • **Score of 2:** Generalized response • **Score of 1:** No response ○ If the sides differ, record the response on the better side.	Record verbal response by asking the client to tell you what his or her name is or what month it is. • **Score of 5:** Conversational and oriented—client responds with correct answers • **Score of 4:** Confused—client can speak in phrases or sentences but cannot give correct answers • **Score of 3:** Single or nonsense words • **Score of 2:** Sounds such as groans • **Score of 1:** No response or sounds Record "Not testable" if factors such as an endotracheal tube prevent a verbal response.	Record eye response by observing when the client opens his or her eyes. • **Score of 4:** Spontaneous eye opening • **Score of 3:** Eyes open to speech or shouting • **Score of 2:** Eyes open to pressure or pain stimuli (applied to nail tip for up to 10 seconds) • **Score of 1:** No eye opening Record "Not testable" if local factors such as swelling prevent opening.

RANCHO LOS AMIGOS LEVEL OF COGNITIVE FUNCTIONING SCALE

SUMMARY

- Purpose: Describes the client's cognition and behavior following brain injury
- Context: Clients with brain injury and consciousness disorders
- Format: Observation with rating scale
- Time to administer: Less than 15 minutes
- Materials: None
- Cost: Free
- Website: www.neuroskills.com/resources/rancho-los-amigos-revised.php

Rancho Los Amigos Levels of Cognitive Functioning Scale describes the client's LOC, behavior, and impairments following a TBI. The scale has 8 or 10 sequential levels that clients typically progress through after injury.[31,32] The length of time spent in each level varies per person, and a client may stop progressing at any stage. Understanding the level of your client will assist with treatment planning.

(continued)

UNIT 2-28 EVALUATION

RANCHO LOS AMIGOS LEVEL OF COGNITIVE FUNCTIONING SCALE (CONTINUED)

LEVEL	DESCRIPTION	SUPPORT NEEDED
Level 1: No response	Client is unconscious and unresponsive.	• Prevent contractures using passive range of motion (ROM). • Introduce familiar stimuli, including the client's favorite music, reading aloud to them from their favorite book, playing a TV show, or using scents. • **Client requires total assistance.**
Level 2: Generalized response	Client demonstrates nonspecific and inconsistent reactions to stimuli. Client demonstrates a reflex response to pain.	• Responses may be significantly delayed. • Continue presenting familiar auditory, tactile, visual, vestibular, olfactory, and gustatory stimuli. • **Client requires total assistance.**
Level 3: Localized response	Client demonstrates localized responses to stimuli (ie, client turns toward or away from auditory stimuli, blinks in response to strong light, or follows a moving object in their visual field). Client responds inconsistently to simple commands, such as "Squeeze my hand."	• Continue presenting familiar stimuli. • Ask client to perform simple commands, such as, "close your eyes," "squeeze my hand," raise your hand." Provide tactile cues as needed. • **Client requires total assistance.**

(continued)

RANCHO LOS AMIGOS LEVEL OF COGNITIVE FUNCTIONING SCALE (CONTINUED)

LEVEL	DESCRIPTION	SUPPORT NEEDED
Level 4: Confused, agitated	Client's behavior may be aggressive. Client may attempt to remove restraints or tubes, and client may cry or scream disproportionately to stimuli even after it is removed.	• Create a quiet and calming environment with minimal distractions. • Engage client in automatic gross motor movements such as walking. • **Client requires maximum assistance.**
Level 5: Confused, inappropriate, nonagitated	Client may wander. Client may demonstrate severely impaired recent memory, may be unable to learn new information, and may exhibit socially inappropriate behavior.	• A vail bed may be used to minimize flight risk. • Provide a structured schedule and environment. • Involve client in self-care. • Reduce distractions. • Use cognitive retraining interventions. • **Client requires maximum assistance.**
Level 6: Confused, appropriate	Client no longer wanders. Client's verbal expressions are appropriate, and his or her memory of the past is improved. Client can sustain attention for 30 minutes with familiar tasks in a nondistracting environment with moderate redirection.	• Provide a structured schedule and environment to establish routines. • Client can be supervised for self-care. • Cognitive retraining interventions can be used. • Improve client's self-awareness, as the client may be unaware of his or her impairments and safety risks. • **Client requires moderate assistance.**

(continued)

UNIT 2-28 EVALUATION

RANCHO LOS AMIGOS LEVEL OF COGNITIVE FUNCTIONING SCALE (CONTINUED)		
LEVEL	**DESCRIPTION**	**SUPPORT NEEDED**
Level 7: Automatic, appropriate	Client lacks safety judgment, executive and higher-level problem-solving skills, and is extremely inflexible to changes in scheduling and environment. Client demonstrates a carry-over of new learning, but may overestimate his or her abilities.	• Cognitive retraining interventions may be used. • Community reintegration is beneficial. • Work-related skills training may be appropriate. • **Client requires minimum or standby assistance or is modified independent, depending on task complexity.**
Level 8: Purposeful, appropriate	Client is aware of how impairments interfere with task completion, but still requires assistance for corrective action. Client requires no assistance once the task is learned. Client thinks about consequences with minimum assistance. Client can sustain attention with familiar tasks for 1 hour in distracting environments. Client may show signs of depression and overestimates or underestimates his or her abilities.	• Vocational Rehabilitation may be appropriate. • Instrumental activities of daily living (IADL) training and participation in leisure activities is appropriate. • Client may use assistive memory devices for his or her daily schedule, to-do lists, and important information. • **Client requires minimum or standby assistance or is modified independent, depending on task complexity.**

(continued)

RANCHO LOS AMIGOS LEVEL OF
COGNITIVE FUNCTIONING SCALE (CONTINUED)

LEVEL	DESCRIPTION	SUPPORT NEEDED
Level 9: Purposeful, appropriate	Client is aware of how impairments interfere with task completion and can take corrective action, but standby assistance may be needed to anticipate and prevent problems.	• Client uses assistive memory devices. • Client can carry out familiar ADLs, IADLs, work, and leisure tasks independently. Minimum assistance may be required for unfamiliar tasks when requested. • Client needs cues to anticipate problems. • **Client may require standby assistance on request. Client requires minimum or standby assistance or is modified independent, depending on task complexity**
Level 10: Purposeful, appropriate	Client can complete multiple tasks simultaneously with more time, breaks, or with use of compensatory strategies.	• Client is independent with use of extra time, periodic breaks, assistive memory devices, and compensatory strategies. • **Client is modified independent.**

Reprinted with permission from Rancho Los Amigos.

Resources available for families about each Rancho level, developed by the Rancho Los Amigos National Rehabilitation Center, can be accessed at http://file.lacounty.gov/SDSInter/dhs/218115_RLOCFOriginalFamilyGuide-English.pdf

References:

Davis, A.E., & Gimenez, A. Cognitive-behavioral recovery in comatose patients following auditory sensory stimulation. *J Neurosci Nurs.* 2003;35(4):202-214.

Hart, T., Kozlowski, A. J., Whyte, J., Poulsen, I., Kristensen, K., Nordenbo, A., & Heinemann, A. W. Functional recovery after severe traumatic brain injury: an individual growth curve approach. *Arch Phys Med Rehabil.* 2014;95:2103-2110.

Landa-Gonzalez, B. Multicontextual occupational therapy intervention: a case study of traumatic brain injury. *Occup Ther Int.* 2001;8(1):49-62.

UNIT 2-28 EVALUATION

NATIONAL INSTITUTES OF HEALTH STROKE SCALE

SUMMARY

- Purpose: Assesses severity of impairments following stroke and helps identify client's long-term needs
- Context: Clients with stroke
- Format: Observation with rating scale
- Time to administer: Less than 10 minutes
- Materials: Pin for sensory test, and paper with a list of words
- Cost: Free
- Website: https://stroke.nih.gov/resources/scale.htm

The National Institutes of Health Stroke Scale consists of 15 items to aid the practitioner in determining stroke severity. The test considers the client's LOC; gaze; visual field; muscle strength in the face, arms, and legs; motor and sensory function; language; speech clarity; and attention.[33]

SCORING

Add the totals of each category. Higher scores indicate more severe deficits.

- Below 5: Mild impairment
- 5 to 14: Moderate impairment
- 15 to 25: Severe impairment

(continued)

NATIONAL INSTITUTES OF HEALTH STROKE SCALE (CONTINUED)

ITEM	DESCRIPTION	SCORE
1a. LOC	Rate the client's responsiveness.	0: Alert 1: Drowsy 2: Stuporous 3: Coma
1b. LOC questions	Ask the client what month it is and how old he or she is.	0: Age and month are correct 1: Only one is correct 2: Both are incorrect
1c. LOC commands	Instruct the client to open and close his or her eyes. Ask the client to make a fist with his or her unaffected hand and then release the fist.	0: Client performed both correctly 1: Client performed one correctly 2: Client did not follow instructions
2. Best gaze	Observe the client's horizontal eye movements as he or she tracks you, or instruct the client to follow your finger with his or her eyes.	0: Normal eye movements 1: Partial gaze palsy 2: Forced deviation
3. Visual	Assess for hemianopia by introducing objects into the client's visual field quadrants.	0: No visual loss 1: Partial hemianopia 2: Complete hemianopia 3: Bilateral hemianopia
4. Facial palsy	Look for symmetry and ask the client to perform the following actions: • Show teeth • Raise eyebrows • Close and open eyes	0: Normal symmetry 1: Minor facial palsy 2: Partial facial palsy 3: Complete facial palsy

(continued)

UNIT 2-29 EVALUATION

NATIONAL INSTITUTES OF HEALTH STROKE SCALE (CONTINUED)

ITEM	DESCRIPTION	SCORE
5a. Motor arm (left)	Instruct the client to elevate his or her left arm to 90 degrees if the client is seated (45 degrees if supine) and observe the amount of movement or drift that occurs in 10 seconds.	0: No drift 1: Drift 2: Unable to resist gravity 3: No movement against gravity 4: No movement at all 0: Amputation or joint fusion
5b. Motor arm (right)	Instruct the client to elevate his or her right arm to 90 degrees if the client is seated (45 degrees if supine) and observe the amount of movement or drift that occurs in 10 seconds.	0: No drift 1: Drift 2: Unable to resist gravity 3: No movement against gravity 4: No movement at all 0: Amputation or joint fusion
6a. Motor leg (left)	Instruct the client to elevate his or her left leg, while in supine, to 30 degrees. Observe the amount of movement or drift that occurs in 5 seconds.	0: No drift 1: Drift 2: Unable to resist gravity 3: No movement against gravity 4: No movement at all 0: Amputation or joint fusion
6b. Motor leg (right)	Instruct the client to elevate his or her right leg, while in supine, to 30 degrees. Observe the amount of movement or drift that occurs in 5 seconds.	0: No drift 1: Drift 2: Unable to resist gravity 3: No movement against gravity 4: No movement at all 0: Amputation or joint fusion

(continued)

NATIONAL INSTITUTES OF HEALTH STROKE SCALE (CONTINUED)

ITEM	DESCRIPTION	SCORE
7. Limb ataxia	Instruct the client to touch a finger to his or her nose. Perform the heel-to-shin test with the client in supine by asking the client to place one heel on the opposite shin, and then to slide the heel down the shin toward his or her feet. Observe for smoothness of movement.	0: Ataxia is absent 1: Ataxia is present in one limb 2: Ataxia is present in 2 limbs 0: Amputation or joint fusion
8. Sensory	Administer a pinprick test to the client's face, trunk, arms, and legs, and compare the response on each side of the body. If the client's consciousness is altered, watch for a grimace or asymmetrical withdrawal.	0: Normal 1: Partial sensory loss 2: Severe sensory loss
9. Best language	Ask the client to name items in the room, to describe an image, or to read a sentence.	0: No aphasia 1: Mild to moderate aphasia 2: Severe aphasia 3: Mute

(continued)

UNIT 2-29 EVALUATION

NATIONAL INSTITUTES OF HEALTH STROKE SCALE (CONTINUED)		
ITEM	DESCRIPTION	SCORE
10. Dysarthria	Ask the client to read words from a list. Assess the clarity of speech.	0: Articulation is normal 1: Mild to moderate dysarthria 2: Near to intelligible 0: Intubated or other barrier
11. Extinction and inattention (formerly referred to as *neglect*)	Identify neglect by using the information from previous tests, or present dual stimuli at once.	0: No neglect 1: Partial neglect 2: Complete neglect

ALLEN COGNITIVE LEVELS

SUMMARY

- Purpose: Describes cognitive function
- Context: Individuals suspected to have cognitive deficits
- Format: Observation of performance
- Time to administer: 20 minutes
- Materials:
  - ○ 3 and 3/4 x 4 and 3/4 inch punched leather rectangle board
  - ○ 1 instruction manual
  - ○ 1 blunt sewing needle
  - ○ 1 hank of waxed linen thread
  - ○ 2 Perma-Lok lacing needles (Tandy Leather)
  - ○ 1 hank of leather lacing
- Cost: $199 for the complete screening assessment and materials. Portions of the assessment and replacement tools may also be purchased for a cost.
- Website: www.allen-cognitive-levels.com

Allen Cognitive Levels are used to describe cognitive functioning in individuals based on their motor response, attention, assistance required, and functional activities.[34]

(continued)

UNIT 2-30 EVALUATION

UNIT 2-30 EVALUATION

ALLEN COGNITIVE LEVELS (CONTINUED)

LEVEL	MOTOR ACTION	ATTENTION SPAN	ASSIST LEVEL	OCCUPATIONAL THERAPY FUNCTIONAL ACTIVITIES	FUNCTIONAL MILESTONES
1	Automatic reactions and reflexive responses	Seconds	Total assistance	Sensory stimulation	1.0: Client is conscious. Client withdraws from noxious stimuli. 1.4: Client swallows. 1.8: Client raises body parts. Client can pivot transfer.
2	Postural reactions	Minutes	Maximum assistance	Gross motor activities, including games and dance	2.2: Client stands. 2.4: Client walks aimlessly. Client displays one-word communication. 2.8: Client uses grab bars for support.
3	Manual actions	30 minutes	Moderate assistance	Simple, repetitive activities and familiar ADLs, such as face-washing	3.0: Client grasps objects. 3.2: Client can distinguish between objects and speaks in short phrases. 3.6: Client understands cause and effect.

(continued)

ALLEN COGNITIVE LEVELS (CONTINUED)

LEVEL	MOTOR ACTION	ATTENTION SPAN	ASSIST LEVEL	OCCUPATIONAL THERAPY FUNCTIONAL ACTIVITIES	FUNCTIONAL MILESTONES
4	Goal-directed actions	Hours	Minimum assistance	Multistep tasks and simple crafts, but client has difficulties with new learning or generalization	4.0: Client is independent with self-care. Client can sequence to prepare snacks or make small purchases. 4.2: Client walks to familiar places in the neighborhood and can follow a simple and familiar bus route. 4.6: Client scans the environment. Client can live alone with daily assistance for safety and reminders for household chores. 4.8: Supportive employment with a job coach is possible.

(continued)

UNIT 2-30   EVALUATION

UNIT 2-30 EVALUATION

ALLEN COGNITIVE LEVELS (CONTINUED)

LEVEL	MOTOR ACTION	ATTENTION SPAN	ASSIST LEVEL	OCCUPATIONAL THERAPY FUNCTIONAL ACTIVITIES	FUNCTIONAL MILESTONES
5	Exploratory actions (trial and error)	Weeks	Standby assistance	Standby assistance	5.0: Client demonstrates intonation (ie, rise and fall) in speech. 5.6: Client demonstrates social bonding, anticipates safety, and is capable of driving and of caring for a child.
6	Planned actions (absence of cognitive disability)	Can attend to past and future	Independent	Follows multistep and complex verbal or written cues	6.0: Client can engage in premeditated activities.

(continued)

ALLEN COGNITIVE LEVELS (CONTINUED)

TITLES OF 6 LEVELS AND 27 MODES OF PERFORMANCE FOR ALLEN COGNITIVE SCALE'S HIERARCHY OF FUNCTIONAL COGNITION

Titles of Cognitive Levels	*Titles of Modes*				
	.0	.2	.4	.6	.8
(Pre-Conscious State prior to Level 1)	Coma				Generalized reflexive actions
Level 1: Automatic actions	1.0 Withdrawing from noxious stimuli	1.2 Responding to stimuli in 1 sensory system	1.4 Locating stimuli	1.6 Rolling body in bed	1.8 Raising body part
Level 2: Postural actions	2.0 Overcoming gravity for sitting	2.2 Using righting reactions for standing	2.4 Walking	2.6 Walking to a location	2.8 Grasping for stabilizing
Level 3: Manual actions	3.0 Grasping objects	3.2 Distinguishing objects	3.4 Sustaining actions on objects	3.6 Noting effects of actions on objects	3.8 Using all objects

(continued)

UNIT 2–30 EVALUATION

ALLEN COGNITIVE LEVELS (CONTINUED)

Titles of Cognitive Levels	Titles of Modes				
	.0	.2	.4	.6	.8
Level 4: Goal-directed actions	4.0 Sequencing familiar actions	4.2 Differentiating features of objects	4.4 Completing a goal	4.6 Personalizing features of objects	4.8 Learning by rote memorization
Level 5: Exploratory actions	5.0 Comparing and varying actions and objects	5.2 Discriminating sets of actions and objects	5.4 Self-directing learning	5.6 Considering social standards	5.8 Consulting with others
Level 6: Planned actions	6.0 Planning actions				

Sources. Developed as an educational handout by D. B McCraith and C. A. Earhart. Copyright © 2016, 2017, 2018, 2019 by ACLS and LACLS Committee, Camarillo, CA. Permission required to reproduce this handout.

(continued)

ALLEN COGNITIVE LEVELS (CONTINUED)

ALLEN COGNITIVE LEVEL SCREENING

Allen Cognitive Level screening is used for Allen levels 3.0 through 5.8. Individuals at lower levels do not work with objects, and those at higher levels are concerned with symbolic cues.

Allen Cognitive Level Screening Kit Materials

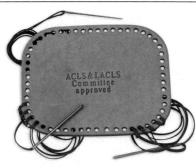

- 3 and 3/4 x 4 and 3/4 inch punched leather rectangle board
- 1 instruction manual
- 1 blunt sewing needle
- 1 hank of waxed linen thread
- 2 Perma-Lok lacing needles
- 1 hank of leather lacing

Allen Cognitive Level Screening Tips

- Set up the tasks.
- Review the instructions well enough to combine verbal instructions with demonstrations.
- Administer the screening in an environment with minimal distractions.
- Always start with the running stitch.
- If a person has visual impairments, hand tremors, or hemiplegia, you may need to use a leather board with larger holes.
- You may hold the leather board for support if someone has use of only one hand.
- You may give encouragements during the screening, such as "Take your time," "I appreciate your efforts," and "You are doing fine."
- If a person has done a lot of lacing in the past, the score may be higher than his or her actual ability to function because it is not measuring new problem-solving abilities.

Information regarding Allen Cognitive Level screening can be found at http://www.allen-cognitive-levels.com/acls.htm

(continued)

UNIT 2-30 EVALUATION

ALLEN COGNITIVE LEVELS (CONTINUED)

RUNNING STITCH

Instructions

- Say, "I am interested in seeing how you follow directions and concentrate. I will show you how to do a stitch now, so watch carefully what I do."
- Say, "Take the needle and push it down through the next hole and pull the thread through the hole. Push the needle up through the next hole. Pull the needle through the hole and tighten it. Do not skip any holes. Now you do it."

Error Correction

- Ask, "Is yours like mine?"
- If "No," Ask, "How is it different?" "Can you fix it?"
- If "Yes," Say, "You have a mistake. Can you find it? Show me where it is."
  - ○ If the client does not identify the error, say, "Your mistake is right here. I want you to make yours look just like mine."
  - ○ If the client does not fix the error, say, "Would you like me to show you again?" Or switch to a larger board if needed.

Scoring

- 3.0: Client grasps the leather or pushes it away. Client may not attempt to grasp the lacing, or client may grasp the lacing once it is handed to him or her, and move lacing in a random manner.
- 3.2: Client pushes the needle through at least one hole, which can be the wrong location. Client may skip holes.
- 3.4: Client completes at least 3 running stitches with no more than 2 demonstrations. Client does not skip holes.

(continued)

ALLEN COGNITIVE LEVELS (CONTINUED)

WHIPSTITCH

Instructions

- Say, "See how the leather lacing has a dark, smooth side and a light, rough side."
- Say, "Always keep the smooth, dark side up as you do each stitch, being careful not to twist the lacing. Now I will show you another stitch. Watch me carefully. Take the lacing and bring it around to the front, over the edge of the leather. Push the needle through the hole and tighten it. Be sure the lacing isn't twisted. Do not skip any holes. Now you do 3 stitches."
- If the client does not make any errors by crossing in the back or by twisting the lacing spontaneously, the administrator takes the board and introduces errors.
- Say, "I am going to make a mistake to see if you can correct it." Ask, "Can you show me my mistake? Can you fix it?" "I made another mistake. Can you show me my mistake? Can you fix it?"
- If the client tries to take the stitch out to correct the twist, say, "Can you do it without taking the lacing out of the hole?"

Error Correction

Same process as running stitch error correction.

Scoring

- 3.6: Client does at least one whipstitch in the correct location with no skipped holes.
- 3.8: Client does not recognize twist or cross errors in the back when cued. Client does recognize a running stitch error, but is unconcerned about the error. Client may continue until he or she is out of space. Client may ask, "Am I done?"
- 4.0: Client does recognize twists or the cross in back as an error when it is pointed out. Client does not attempt to correct twist or cross errors. Client corrects running stitch errors on the back when pointed out.
- 4.2: Client corrects twists by redoing the last stitch. Client does not untwist while the lacing is still in the hole. Client corrects cross errors in the back.
- 4.4: Client can untwist at least 1 whipstitch without pulling it out. Client stops after 3 stitches.

(continued)

UNIT 2-30 EVALUATION

UNIT 2-30 EVALUATION

ALLEN COGNITIVE LEVELS (CONTINUED)

SINGLE CORDOVAN STITCH

Instructions

- Hand the leather to the person and point to this stitch. Ask, "Can you do this stitch by yourself?"
- If the client demonstrates a response of frustration, panic, or refusal:
    - Ask, "Would you like to be shown how?"
    - If so, continue: "Watch me carefully. Bring the needle to the front of the leather. Push the needle through the next hole toward the back of the leather. Do not pull the lacing tight, but leave a small loop in it. Bring the lacing to the front of the leather. This time put the needle through the loop you have made. Keep the needle to the left of the lacing. (Show the insertion of the needle.) Pull the lacing through the loop toward the back of the leather. Tighten the lacing from the back hole, then tighten the long lacing end. Make sure the lacing is not twisted. Now you do 3 stitches."
- Only 2 demonstrations may be scored.

Error Correction

Same process as running stitch error correction.

Scoring

- 5.8: Client completes 3 single cordovan stitches without a demonstration or a verbal cue by examining the sample stitches and using trial and error.
- 5.6: Client completes 3 single cordovan stitches without a demonstration but requires a cue (a verbal cue or pointing to location of error) to do the stitch correctly.
- 5.4: One (but only one) demonstration is given. Client corrects errors in directionality, tangled lacing, or tightening in sequence without a second demonstration by altering actions 2 or more times.

(continued)

ALLEN COGNITIVE LEVELS (CONTINUED)

Scoring

If 2 demonstrations were given:

- 5.2: Client corrects errors in directionality, tangled lacing, or tightening in sequence with a second demonstration. The loops are tightened in sequence. The tension may be a little loose, but no other errors remain.

- 5.0: Client corrects errors in directionality, tangled lacing, or tightening in sequence but cannot replicate solutions. A little improvement or alteration occurs with a second demonstration, but errors remain.

- 4.8: Client does not tighten the lacing in sequence, only pulls on the needle, and may or may not recognize errors. Little to no improvement is noted with the first or second demonstration.

- 4.6: Client's right and left orientation of the lacing and needle are incorrect when going through the loop. Little to no improvement is noted with the first or second demonstration.

- 4.4: Client goes from the front to back through the hole (like the whipstitch) but inserts the needle through the loop from the back as if it were one step (ie, the lacing is under the loop but does not wrap around it). Or, directionality goes from the front to the back through the hole but back to front through the loop or vice versa. Client does not benefit from first or second demonstration.

- 4.2: Client repeats the whipstitch or does the whipstitch followed by an attempt to do a second unrelated step. Client does not benefit from first or second demonstration.

MONTREAL COGNITIVE ASSESSMENT

SUMMARY

- Purpose: Detects mild cognitive dysfunction
- Context: Clients with Alzheimer's disease, brain tumor, dementia, Huntington's disease, Parkinson's disease, stroke, and temporal dementia
- Format: Interview-based observation
- Time to administer: 10 minutes
- Materials: Montreal Cognitive Assessment (MoCA) testing score sheet form (3 versions available at http://www.mocatest.org to reduce reassessment practice effects) pencil, and stopwatch
- Cost: Free
- Website: http://www.mocatest.org

The MoCA is a rapid screen used to detect mild cognitive dysfunction. The MoCA assesses 16 items in 11 categories.[35]

SCORING

A score of 26 or more out of 30 is considered normal. One point is added to the raw score for individuals who have 12 or fewer years of formal education.

(continued)

MONTREAL COGNITIVE ASSESSMENT (CONTINUED)

ADMINISTRATION INSTRUCTIONS EXAMPLE

Task	Examiner Instructions	Scoring
Visuospatial/Executive (5 Points)		
1. Alternating trail making	"Please draw a line, going from a number to a letter in ascending order. Begin here [point to (1)] and draw a line from 1 to A then to 2 and so on. End here [point to (E)]."	The client should score 1 point for drawing the following pattern: 1-A-2-B-3-C-4-D-5-E, without drawing any lines that cross. Any error that is not immediately self-corrected earns a score of 0.
2. Visuoconstructional skills (cube)	While pointing to the cube: "Copy this drawing of a cube, as accurately as you can, in the space below."	The client should score 1 point for a correct drawing that includes the following: • 3-dimensional • All lines are drawn • No line is added • Lines are relatively parallel and their length is similar (rectangular prisms are accepted)

(continued)

UNIT 2-31 EVALUATION

MONTREAL COGNITIVE ASSESSMENT (CONTINUED)

Task	Examiner Instructions	Scoring
3. Visuoconstructional skills (clock)	"Draw a clock. Put in all the numbers and set the time to 10 after 11."	• Contour (1 point): The clock face must be a circle with only minor distortion acceptable (eg, slight imperfection on closing the circle). • Numbers (1 point): All clock numbers must be present with no additional numbers. Numbers must be in the correct order and placed in the approximate quadrants on the clock face. Roman numerals are acceptable. Numbers can be placed outside the circle contour. • Hands (1 point): There must be 2 hands jointly indicating the correct time. The hour hand must be clearly shorter than the minute hand. Hands must be centered within the clock face with their junction close to the clock center.
Naming (3 Points)		
4. Naming 3 animals	Beginning on the left, point to each figure and say: "Tell me the name of this animal."	The client should score 1 point for each correct response (up to 3 points; eg, camel, lion, rhino). *(continued)*

MONTREAL COGNITIVE ASSESSMENT (CONTINUED)

Task	Examiner Instructions	Scoring
Memory (No Points Given Yet)		
5. Memory	Read a list of 5 words at a rate of 1 word per second, giving the following instructions: "This is a memory test. I am going to read a list of words that you will have to remember now and later on. Listen carefully. When I am through, tell me as many words as you can remember. It does not matter in what order you say them." Trial 1: Mark a check for each word the subject recalls. Read the list a second time with the following instructions: "I am going to read the same list for a second time. Try to remember and tell me as many words as you can, including the words you said the first time." Trial 2: Put a check in the allocated space for each word the subject recalls after the second reading. At the end of the second trial, inform the subject, "I will ask you to recall those words again at the end of the test."	No points are given yet.

(continued)

UNIT 2-31 EVALUATION

MONTREAL COGNITIVE ASSESSMENT (CONTINUED)

Task	Examiner Instructions	Scoring
Attention (6 Points)		
6. Forward digit span	"I am going to say some numbers, and when I am through, repeat them to me exactly as I said them." Read the 5-number sequence at a rate of 1 digit per second.	The client should score 1 point for a correctly repeated sequence.
7. Backward digit span	"Now I am going to say some more numbers, but when I am through, you must repeat them to me in backward order." Read the 3-number sequence at a rate of 1 digit per second.	The client should score 1 point for a correctly repeated backward sequence.
8. Vigilance	Read the list of letters at a rate of 1 letter per second, after giving the following instruction: "I am going to read a sequence of letters. Every time I say the letter A, tap your hand once. If I say a different letter, do not tap your hand."	The client should score 1 point if there are zero to one errors (an error is a tap on a wrong letter or a failure to tap on the letter A).

(continued)

MONTREAL COGNITIVE ASSESSMENT (CONTINUED)

Task	Examiner Instructions	Scoring
9. Serial 7s	"Now, I will ask you to count by subtracting 7 from 100, and then, keep subtracting 7 from your answer until I tell you to stop." Give this instruction twice if necessary.	The client should score 0 points for no correct subtraction.
		The client should score 1 point for 1 correct subtraction.
		The client should score 2 points for 2 or 3 correct subtractions.
		The client should score 3 points for 4 or 5 correct subtractions.
		Each subtraction is evaluated independently. If the participant responds with an incorrect number but continues to correctly subtract 7 from it, give 1 point for each correct subtraction. For example, a participant may respond "92, 85, 78, 71, 64" where the "92" is incorrect, but all subsequent numbers are subtracted correctly. This is one error, and the item would be given a score of 3 because the subject has made 4 correct subtractions.

(continued)

UNIT 2-31 EVALUATION

UNIT 2-31 EVALUATION

MONTREAL COGNITIVE ASSESSMENT (CONTINUED)

Task	Examiner Instructions	Scoring
Language (3 Points)		
10. Sentence repetition	"I am going to read you a sentence. Repeat it after me, exactly as I say it [pause]: 'I only know that John is the one to help today.'" Following the response, say: "Now I am going to read you another sentence. Repeat it after me, exactly as I say it [pause]: 'The cat always hid under the couch when dogs were in the room.'"	The client should score 1 point for correctly repeating the first sentence and 1 point for correctly repeating the second sentence. Repetition must be exact. Be alert for errors that are omissions (eg, omitting "only" or "always") and substitutions or additions (eg, "John is the one who helped today," substituting "hides" for "hid", or altering plurals).
11. Verbal fluency	"Tell me as many words as you can think of that begin with a certain letter of the alphabet that I will tell you in a moment. You can say any kind of word you want, except for proper nouns (like Bob or Boston), numbers, or words that begin with the same sound but have a different suffix, for example, love, lover, loving. I will tell you to stop after one minute. Are you ready? [pause] Now, tell me as many words as you can think of that begin with the letter F. [time for 60 seconds] Stop." Record the subject's response in the bottom or side margins.	The client should score 1 point for generating 11 words or more in 60 seconds.

(continued)

Montreal Cognitive Assessment (CONTINUED)

Task	Examiner Instructions	Scoring
Abstraction (2 Points)		
12. Abstraction	Ask the subject to explain what each pair of words has in common, starting with the example: "Tell me how an orange and a banana are alike." If the subject answers in a concrete manner, then say only one additional time: "Tell me another way in which those items are alike." If the subject does not give the appropriate response (fruit), say, "Yes, and they are also both fruit." Do not give any additional instructions or clarification. After the practice trial, say: "Now, tell me how a train and a bicycle are alike." Following the response, administer the second trial, saying: "Now tell me how a ruler and a watch are alike." Do not give any additional instructions or prompts.	Only the last 2 item pairs are scored. The client should score 1 point for a correct response to the train-to-bicycle comparison. Correct responses include means of transportation, means of traveling, and you can take trips in both. The client should score 0 points for a response that indicates that they both have wheels. The client should score 1 point for a correct response to the ruler-to-watch comparison. Correct responses include measuring instruments, and both are used to measure. The client should score 0 points for a response that indicates they both have numbers

(continued)

UNIT 2-31 EVALUATION

UNIT 2-31 EVALUATION

MONTREAL COGNITIVE ASSESSMENT (CONTINUED)

Task	Examiner Instructions	Scoring
Delayed Recall (5 Points)		
13. Delayed recall	"Earlier, I read you some words, which I asked you to remember. Tell me as many of those words as you can remember." Make a check mark in the allocated space for each of the words correctly recalled spontaneously without any cues. An optional section uses cues for recall but is not scored.	The client should score 1 point for each word (up to 5) recalled freely without any cues.
Orientation (6 Points)		
14. Orientation	"Tell me the date today." If the subject does not give a complete answer, then prompt accordingly by saying: "Tell me the [year, month, exact date, and day of the week]." Then say, "Now, tell me the name of this place, and which city it is in."	The client should score 1 point for each correct answer (up to 6). The correct answer is the exact date and place (eg, name of hospital, clinic, or office). No points are allocated if the subject makes an error of 1 day for the day and date.

GLOBAL DETERIORATION SCALE

SUMMARY

- Purpose: Describes cognitive function in clients who have or may develop dementia. It is also used to describe stages of impairment.
- Context: Adults with memory impairments, dementia, and Alzheimer's disease
- Format: Observation
- Time to administer: Quick
- Materials: None
- Cost: None
- Website: https://www.fhca.org/members/qi/clinadmin/global.pdf

The Global Deterioration Scale (GDS) is a popular method that describes stages of dementia and cognitive function in adults with memory impairments. Level 1 on the GDS indicates no cognitive decline or memory impairments while level 7 indicates severe cognitive decline and late stage dementia.[36] The scale can be used to determine the level of care required by the client. Refer to Unit 3-42 in this section for interventions for altered mental status and dementia.

LEVEL	CATEGORY	DESCRIPTION OF IMPAIRMENTS
1	No cognitive decline	The client has no complaints of memory impairments.
2	Very mild cognitive decline	The client experiences forgetfulness regarding placement of familiar objects or memory of names, but there is no objective evidence of memory deficits.
3	Mild cognitive decline	The client's performance in a demanding employment setting is decreased. Denial may be present. For example, the client may have difficulty remembering what he or she just read.
4	Moderate cognitive decline	The client has deficits in remembering current or recent events, difficulty handling finances, problems remembering his or her past history, and/or difficulty performing complex tasks.

(continued)

GLOBAL DETERIORATION SCALE (CONTINUED)		
LEVEL	CATEGORY	DESCRIPTION OF IMPAIRMENTS
5	Moderately severe cognitive decline or early dementia	The client requires assistance to survive. The client may be unable to remember his or her phone number, address, names of grandchildren, or name of high school. The client experiences disorientation to time or place, and may need assistance with choosing proper clothing.
6	Severe cognitive decline or middle dementia	The client may forget his or her spouse's name. The client may also be incontinent, require assistance for dressing and bathing and have personality and emotional changes, such as delusional behavior or obsessive symptoms.
7	Very severe cognitive decline or late dementia	The client is incontinent and requires assistance for toileting and feeding. The client has lost speech, the ability to walk, smile, sit up, and hold his or her head up.

Reisberg B, Ferris SH, de Leon, MJ, et. al.,. The global deterioration scale for assessment of primary degenerative dementia. *Am J Psychiatry*. 1982;139:1136-1139. Copyright © 1983 Barry Reisberg, MD. Reproduced with permission.

UNIT 2-32 EVALUATION

AMERICAN SPINAL INJURY
ASSOCIATION IMPAIRMENT SCALE

SUMMARY

- Purpose: Documents the severity of an SCI based on sensory and motor impairments
- Context: Clients with an SCI
- Format: Neurologic exam
- Time to administer: Varies
- Materials: Assessment sheet and pin to test sensory level
- Cost: Free to download
- Website: http://asia-spinalinjury.org/information/downloads

The American Spinal Injury Association (ASIA) Impairment Scale measures the severity of an SCI by testing major muscle movements and key dermatomes and helps identify the level of spinal injury.[37,38]

STEP 1: DETERMINE SENSORY LEVELS FOR RIGHT AND LEFT SIDES

Sensory test points

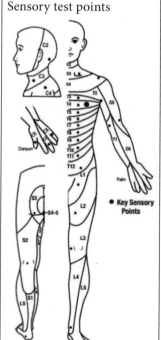

Test the client's sensation on the right and left sides using pin prick and light touch at each sensory test point.

Score:

- 0: Sensation is absent
- 1: Sensation is impaired
- 2: Sensation is normal
- NT: Not testable

Pin-prick score total: Add up the right and left sides. The total is out of 112.

Light-touch score total: Add up the right and left sides. The total is out of 112.

Does the client have any anal sensation? Yes or no

The sensory level is the most caudal and intact dermatome for both pin-prick and light-touch sensation.

(continued)

American Spinal Injury Association Impairment Scale (continued)

Step 2: Determine Motor Levels for Right and Left Sides

Motor test points:

- C5: Elbow flexors
- C6: Wrist extensors
- C7: Elbow extensors
- C8: Finger flexors (the distal phalanx of middle finger)
- T1: Finger abductors (the little finger)
- L2: Hip flexors
- L3: Knee extensors
- L4: Ankle dorsiflexors
- L5: Long toe extensors
- S1: Ankle plantar flexors

Test the client's muscle function for each motor test point on the right and left sides.

Score right and left:

- 0: Total paralysis of muscles
- 1: Palpable or visible muscle contraction
- 2: Active movement in a gravity eliminated position
- 3: Active movement against gravity
- 4: Active movement against some resistance
- 5: Active movement against full resistance
- NT: Not testable

Total motor score: Add up right and left side. The total is out of 100.

Does the client have voluntary anal contraction (VAC)?
Yes or No

The motor level is the lowest level of muscle function with a grade of at least 3 when the client is tested supine. The levels above the motor level must be intact with a grade of 5.

If there is no myotome to test, then the motor level is presumed to be the same as the sensory level if the testable motor function above that level is also normal.

(continued)

UNIT 2-33 EVALUATION

AMERICAN SPINAL INJURY
ASSOCIATION IMPAIRMENT SCALE (CONTINUED)

STEP 3: DETERMINE THE NEUROLOGICAL LEVEL OF INJURY

Compare the scores for the sensory and motor level. The neurological level of injury (NLI) is the most caudal segment of the cord with intact sensation and antigravity (a muscle grade of 3 or greater) muscle function strength. Both sensation and muscle function must be normal above the NLI. For example, if the sensory level is C7 and motor level is C5, then the NLI is C5.

STEP 4: DETERMINE IF THE INJURY IS COMPLETE OR INCOMPLETE

A complete or incomplete SCI is defined as the absence or presence of sacral sparing.

An SCI is complete when the following criteria are all met:
- The client has no VAC.
- The S4 to S5 sensory scores are 0.
- The client has no deep anal pressure sensation.

If all 3 of the above criteria are not met, then the injury is incomplete.

STEP 5: DETERMINE THE ASIA IMPAIRMENT SCALE GRADE

Is the injury complete?

Yes → The ASIA Impairment Scale grade is A. Document the zone of partial preservation as the lowest dermatome or myotome on each side with some preservation.

No → Continue grading below.

Is the injury Motor Complete?

Yes → The ASIA Impairment Scale grade is B.

No → The injury is not motor complete if there is VAC or if motor function exists more than 3 levels below the motor level on a given side. Continue grading below.

Note: When differentiating between ASIA Impairment Scale B and ASIA Impairment Scale C, nonkey muscle functions more than 3 levels below the motor level on each side should be tested.

(continued)

UNIT 2-33 EVALUATION

| AMERICAN SPINAL INJURY |
| ASSOCIATION IMPAIRMENT SCALE (CONTINUED) |

Muscle functions:
- C5: Shoulder flexion, extension, abduction, adduction, internal rotation, external rotation; elbow supination
- C6: Elbow pronation; wrist flexion
- C7: Finger flexion at proximal joint, extension; thumb flexion, extension, abduction in plane of thumb
- C8: Finger flexion at metacarpophalangeal joint; thumb opposition, abduction, adduction perpendicular to palm
- T1: Abduction of index finger
- L2: Hip adduction
- L3: Hip external rotation
- L4: Hip extension, abduction, internal rotation; knee flexion; ankle inversion and eversion; toe metatarsophalangeal and interphalangeal extension
- L5: Hallux and toe distal interphalangeal and proximal interphalangeal flexion and abduction
- S1: Hallux adduction

Are at least half (or more) of the key muscles below the NLI graded 3 or better?

No → The ASIA Impairment Scale grade is C.

Yes → The ASIA Impairment Scale grade is D.

Are sensation and motor functions normal in all segments?

Yes → The ASIA Impairment Scale grade is E.

Note: The ASIA Impairment Scale E grade is used in follow-up testing when an individual with a documented SCI has recovered normal function. If no deficits are found at initial testing, then the individual is neurologically intact. The ASIA Impairment Scale does not apply in this instance.

(continued)

UNIT 2-33 EVALUATION

AMERICAN SPINAL INJURY
ASSOCIATION IMPAIRMENT SCALE (CONTINUED)

ASIA SCALE GRADE DESCRIPTIONS

A = Complete

- No sensory or motor function is preserved in the sacral segments S4 to S5.

B = Sensory Incomplete

- Sensory but not motor function is preserved below the neurological level and includes the sacral segments S4 to S5 (light touch or pin prick sensations are present at S4 to S5, or deep anal pressure is present).
- No motor function is preserved more than 3 levels below the motor level on either side of the body.

C = Motor Incomplete

- Motor function is preserved at the most caudal sacral segments for VAC or the patient meets the criteria for sensory incomplete status (sensory function is preserved at the most caudal sacral segments of S4 to S5 by light touch, pin prick, or deep anal pressure).
- The client has some sparing of motor function more than 3 levels below the ipsilateral (same side) motor level on either side of the body. This includes key or nonkey muscle functions to determine motor incomplete status.
- Less than half of the key muscle functions below the single NLI have a muscle grade of 3 or greater.

D = Motor Incomplete

- The same criteria as above, but at least half (or more) of the key muscle functions below the single NLI have a muscle grade of 3 or greater.

E = Normal

- A client with prior deficits has sensation, and motor function grade is normal in all segments as tested with the International Standards for Neurological Classification of Spinal Cord Injuries.
- Someone without an initial SCI does not receive an ASIA Impairment Scale grade.

An ASIA Impairment Scale form can be found courtesy of the American Spinal Injury Association at http://asia-spinalinjury.org/wp-content/uploads/2016/02/International_Stds_Diagram_Worksheet.pdf

Reprinted with permission from the American Spinal Injury Association. (2011). *International standards for neurological classification of spinal cord injury*. Atlanta, GA: American Spinal Injury Association.

(continued)

UNIT 2-33 EVALUATION

AMERICAN SPINAL INJURY ASSOCIATION IMPAIRMENT SCALE (CONTINUED)	
COMMON INCOMPLETE SPINAL CORD INJURIES[3]	
Central cord syndrome	Central cord syndrome is usually present in the cervical region of the spinal column. It presents as a greater loss of motor control and sensation in the upper extremities as compared to the lower extremities.
Anterior cord syndrome	Anterior cord syndrome presents as a loss of motor control, loss of pain sensation, and loss of temperature sensation. The client can feel touch, vibration, and proprioception.
Brown-Sequard syndrome	Brown-Sequard syndrome describes the area of damage that occurs on one half of the spinal cord. Brown-Sequard syndrome presents as a loss of voluntary movement on the side of damage and loss of pain and temperature sensation on the opposite side.
Conus medullaris syndrome	Conus medullaris syndrome presents as a flaccid bowel and bladder with sexual dysfunction and lower limbs affected.
Cauda equina syndrome	Cauda equina syndrome presents as a flaccid bowel and bladder with sexual dysfunction and the lower limbs affected.

MODIFIED ASHWORTH SCALE

SUMMARY

- Purpose: Measures spasticity by assessing resistance during passive muscle stretch
- Context: Clients with central nervous system disorders, including MS, cerebral palsy, TBI, and stroke
- Format: Observation and hierarchical rating scale
- Time to administer: Very quick
- Materials: None
- Cost: Free
- Website: https://www.sralab.org/rehabilitation-measures/ ashworth-scale-modified-ashworth-scale

The Modified Ashworth Scale is a quick and easy way to assess muscle tone in clients recovering from central nervous system disorders.[39,40]

INSTRUCTIONS FOR GRADING MUSCLE TONE

1. Position the client in supine. Instruct the client to relax.
2. To test a muscle that acts as a flexor, place the joint in a maximally flexed position, and move the joint to a position of maximal extension in a 1-second period.
3. To test a muscle that acts as an extensor, place the joint in a maximally extended position, and move the joint to a position of maximal flexion in a 1-second period.

Note: Testing should be completed prior to measuring ROM to obtain the most accurate grading of muscle tone.

(continued)

UNIT 2-34 EVALUATION

MODIFIED ASHWORTH SCALE (CONTINUED)

SCORING

- 0: There is no increase in muscle tone (note: this may indicate normal tone or muscle flaccidity).
- 1: There is a slight increase in muscle tone. You may feel a catch and release or minimal resistance when the joint is moved at end range.
- 1+: There is a slight increase in muscle tone. You may feel a catch followed by minimal resistance. The tone affects less than half of the joint's ROM.
- 2: There is an increase in muscle tone through most of the range, but the joint can still be moved easily.
- 3: There is considerable increase in muscle tone. Passive movement of the joint is difficult.
- 4: There is rigidity in flexion or extension (note: this may indicate high spasticity or contracture).

FUGL-MEYER ASSESSMENT OF MOTOR RECOVERY FOLLOWING A STROKE

SUMMARY

- Purpose: Assesses sensorimotor impairment and recovery in clients who have hemiplegia following a stroke
- Context: Clients with stroke, suspected motor deficits, or hemiplegia
- Format: Performance-based observation and rating scale
- Time to administer: Varies. It should take 20 minutes to administer the motor segment only; 30 minutes to administer the total Fugl-Meyer; and 60 to 90 minutes to administer all subscales.
- Materials: Assessment sheet, tennis ball, spherical cone, and knee hammer
- Cost: Free
- Website:
  - Upper Extremity: www.gu.se/digitalAssets/1328/1328946_fma-ue-english.pdf
  - Lower Extremity: https://neurophys.gu.se/digitalAssets/1520/1520603_fma-ue-protocol-english-updated-20150311.pdf

The Fugl-Meyer Assessment of Sensorimotor Recovery is designed for use with clients who have hemiplegia following a stroke. Domains assessed by the Fugl-Meyer include motor function, sensory function, balance, joint ROM, and joint pain.[41,42] Practitioners commonly elect to assess each domain separately. The motor segment has score sheets to test the upper extremity as well as the lower extremity.

SCORING

Higher scores indicate better sensorimotor function.

- Score of 0 on an item indicates the client cannot perform the task, a reflex is absent, or anesthesia (lack of sensation) is present.
- Score of 1 on an item indicates the client performed part of the task or demonstrated hyperesthesia or dysesthesia.
- Score of 2 on an item indicates that the client can perform the task, a reflex is present, and sensation is normal.

(continued)

UNIT 2-35 EVALUATION

FUGL-MEYER ASSESSMENT OF MOTOR RECOVERY FOLLOWING A STROKE (CONTINUED)

Maximum Scores

- 226 points for the full assessment. The maximum score indicates full sensorimotor recovery.
- 66 points for the upper extremity motor domain.
- 34 points for the lower extremity motor domain.
- 24 points for the sensory domain.
- 14 points for the balance domain.
- 44 points for the joint ROM domain.
- 44 points for the joint pain domain.

COMMON INTERVENTIONS ACROSS PRACTICE SETTINGS

INTERVENTION	ACUTE	INPATIENT	HOME HEALTH	SNF	OUTPATIENT
Pain Management Strategies	✓	✓	✓	✓	✓
Bed Positioning With Hemiplegia	✓	✓		✓	
Motor Control/Motor Learning					
Basal Ganglia–Related Treatment Guidelines	✓	✓	✓	✓	✓
Cognitive Rehabilitation Strategies	✓	✓	✓	✓	
Allen Cognitive Level Guidelines	✓	✓	✓	✓	
Altered Mental Status and Dementia Intervention Strategies	✓	✓	✓	✓	
Functions Associated With Spinal Cord Injury Levels and Preserving Upper Extremity Function After a Spinal Cord Injury	✓	✓		✓	
Splinting for Spinal Cord Injuries	✓	✓			✓
Central Nervous System Precautions and Contraindications	✓	✓	✓	✓	✓

UNIT 3-36 INTERVENTION

Pain Management Strategies[43]

Occupational therapy clients can manage their pain through the application of modalities, education, prescribed exercises, home programs, or biofeedback. The following table includes ideas for each of these pain management strategies.

Treatment Mechanism	Treatment Examples
Modalities	• Ice • Heat • Massage balls • Swiss balls • Peanut balls • Thera Cane • Still point inducer for neck pain • Foam rollers • Yoga-based stretching • Paraffin • Alpha stimulation • Transcutaneous electrical nerve stimulation • Galvanic stimulation • Kinesio taping • Sport taping • Manual therapy as needed • Desensitization devices • Splinting as needed
Education	• Stress management • Nutrition • Benefits of exercise • Sleep hygiene habits • Abdominal breathing • Posture • Positive communication

(continued)

PAIN MANAGEMENT STRATEGIES[43] (CONTINUED)	
TREATMENT MECHANISM	TREATMENT EXAMPLES
Exercises	• Functional activities using heavy and light weight lifting to meet goals related to returning to work, changing jobs, or improving the client's quality of life
Home programs	• Surgical scar management and desensitization • Osteoporosis training for maintaining function • Weightbearing and walking programs for complex regional pain syndrome and lower extremity injuries • Consistent stretching and icing • Keeping a pain journal to track the dates and time of pain flare-ups and what activities may increase the pain
Biofeedback	• Measures muscle tension with electromyogram • Relaxation techniques • Reduce neck and back pain

BED POSITIONING WITH HEMIPLEGIA

Positioning of an individual with hemiplegia, such as those who have had a stroke, is an important factor for comfort, health, and safety. Always remember to ask the client if the position is comfortable, and help the client move to a more comfortable position if necessary. Be sure that the client's position changes every 2 to 4 hours to prevent skin breakdown. The following are tips for safe positioning of a person with hemiplegia.[44-46]

CLIENT POSITION	RECOMMENDATIONS
Client is lying on the unaffected side.	• Pillows can be used to support the client's head. • Place the affected shoulder forward with the scapula protracted, and support the affected arm with pillows. • Bring the unaffected leg forward with the knee in flexion, and support the affected leg extended backward or slightly flexed. • Place a pillow behind the client's back for additional support to prevent him or her from rolling backward.
Client is lying on the affected side.	• Make sure that this position does not impact the client's ability to breathe. • Pillows can be used to support the client's head and protract the affected scapula. • Support the affected arm with the wrist and fingers extended and the palm up. • Position the affected leg in line with the trunk or slightly flexed forward. • Bring the client's unaffected leg forward with the knee in flexion, and use pillows to keep the legs separated. • Place a pillow behind the client's back for additional support to prevent him or her from rolling backward.

(continued)

UNIT 3-38 INTERVENTION

BED POSITIONING WITH HEMIPLEGIA (CONTINUED)

CLIENT POSITION	RECOMMENDATIONS
Client is lying supine.	• Pillows can be used to support the client's shoulders and arms. • Be sure to keep the affected arm supported with pillows.
Client is seated.	• Support the client's affected arm with a pillow. • Keep both of the client's feet positioned on the footrests of a wheelchair or flat on the floor.
Client is transferring.	• If the affected arm cannot be directly supported against gravity, support the affected arm with a sling to reduce pain and subluxation. • Once the transfer is completed, the sling can be removed and pillows or another supportive surface may be used to support the affected arm.

UNIT 3-38 INTERVENTION

MOTOR CONTROL/MOTOR LEARNING

BASAL GANGLIA–RELATED TREATMENT GUIDELINES

Basal ganglia impairments may be present in clients who have Parkinson's disease, MS, Huntington's disease, stroke, tumors, TBI, infection, multiple system atrophy, Wilson's disease, progressive supranuclear palsy, and dystonia. Common symptoms include tremor, bradykinesia, and gait freezing. Intervention guidelines are outlined below.[47-49]

Impairment	Intervention Guidelines
Tremor[47]	Interventions for a client with tremors include weighted utensils, wrist cuffs, compensatory strategies, and adaptive devices.
	Weighted utensils and wrist cuffs may be more effective for some clients than for others. They may not be effective long-term due to habituation. Evidence suggests that weighted cuffs may be more effective at reducing tremor for clients with MS or cerebellar lesions rather than basal ganglia-related disorders such as Parkinson's.[47]
	Compensatory strategies and adaptive devices that can help improve occupational functioning in individuals with basal ganglia disorders include the following ideas:
	• Drinking from a cup with a lid to avoid spills
	• Use of a plate guard, rocker knife, and specialized self-stabilizing utensil
	• Utilizing a buttonhook, or replacing buttons with another type of fastener
	• Minimizing the degrees of freedom by stabilizing the client's elbow on the table
	• Stabilizing objects by using nonslip materials
	(continued)

UNIT 3–39 INTERVENTION

MOTOR CONTROL/MOTOR LEARNING (CONTINUED)	
Impairment	*Intervention Guidelines*
Bradykinesia and gait freezing[48,49]	Interventions for a client with bradykinesia and gait freezing include high amplitude and high intensity movements and external cues. High amplitude and high intensity movements may include programs such as the LSVT BIG programs, but they require a certification. External cues to improve movement efficiency include the following ideas: • Auditory cues including music or a metronome • Visual cues including lines on the floor, a walker with laser lights, or use of a mirror • Cognitive cues including rehearsal of movement • Tactile cues

UNIT 3-39 INTERVENTION

COGNITIVE REHABILITATION STRATEGIES

Cognitive rehabilitation following stroke or brain injury is based on neuroplasticity (ie, the ability of the brain to change). Components that enhance neuroplasticity include repetition, particularly repetition of meaningful tasks, and the ability to promote generalization, such as performing the same task or strategy in multiple environments and contexts.[50]

Task-specific training leads to client-centered occupational outcomes and is supported by evidence. For example, teaching a client scanning strategies by using letter cancellation activities may not generalize to the ability to read a book. The general method for task-specific training involves identification and performance of the intended task, then gradually fading cues out as learning takes place.[50]

Cognitive rehabilitation is often categorized into 2 main approaches: remediation and adaptation. A combination of the 2 approaches is an effective intervention method.[50]

REMEDIATION APPROACH	ADAPTATION APPROACH
Method: Improves cognitive function by targeting underlying deficits	**Method:** Increases participation in functional occupations through modifications and adaptations to compensate for deficits
Examples: Cancellation tasks, design copying, and tabletop cognitive exercises	**Examples:** Compensatory strategies (eg, the lighthouse scanning strategy, using memory devices) and environmental modifications
Client must be able to generalize the intervention to functional activities. The client must be capable of far or very far transfers of learning.	

(continued)

COGNITIVE REHABILITATION STRATEGIES (CONTINUED)

THERAPY STRATEGIES DURING COGNITIVE REHABILITATION

Targeted Function	Intervention Strategies
Awareness[51,52]	• Educate the client and client's family about the client's condition and cognitive difficulties that he or she may face.
	• Apply a metacognitive strategy by asking the client to consider and anticipate performance difficulties he or she may encounter prior to and during the task. Ask the client to reflect on his or her performance and think about future methods of problem solving.
	• Provide verbal feedback through general prompts to cue error correction and follow with specific prompts if necessary. Video feedback of the client's performance and the use of a mirror during therapy may be beneficial.
	• Teach the client scanning strategies for visual neglect and limb activation cueing for motor neglect.
	• Monitor the client for potential signs of depression or anxiety as the awareness of deficits increases.
Attention[51,52]	• Modify the environment to reduce distractions, and/or instruct the client to wear earplugs.
	• The client may use checklists for daily activities.

(continued)

COGNITIVE REHABILITATION STRATEGIES (CONTINUED)

Targeted Function	Intervention Strategies

Apraxia[52]	• First, determine the cause of apraxia:
	  ◦ Ideational/conceptual apraxia (eg, the client may use a toothbrush to comb hair, or may place a sock over a shoe)
	  ◦ Ideomotor apraxia (eg, the client may have clumsy movements, difficulty crossing midline, or difficulty sequencing movements)
	• Educate caregivers and family members on apraxia and the importance of avoiding over-assistance.
	• Apply cueing strategies including gestures, tactile cues, visual cues, or auditory cues.
	• Teach by chaining information and repetition.
	• Apply an errorless learning technique to prevent the client from learning errors during task performance.
	• For ideomotor apraxia, decrease the degrees of freedom during tasks. For example, instruct the client to rest his or her elbow on the table.

Agnosia[52]	• Utilize additional senses. Touching or tracing can help a client with visual agnosia identify objects. Individuals with prosopagnosia (difficulty with face recognition) can identify others by their voice or distinguishing features. • Describe known pieces to assist with identification, such as the color, shape, and location of the object.

(continued)

COGNITIVE REHABILITATION STRATEGIES (CONTINUED)	
Targeted Function	*Intervention Strategies*
Memory[51,52]	• Utilize memory aids such as checklists, calendars, alarms, labels, and mnemonics. • Use repetition to promote overlearning. • Errorless learning: instead of trial and error, reduce the potential for clients to remember mistakes more than the therapist's correction by preventing errors as the client is performing the activity.
Problem solving[51,52]	• Encourage the client to define the problem and break it down into manageable steps. • Think of alternative solutions to the problem. • Focus on important areas. For example, safety and emergencies, community and transportation, medication, and stating one's rights. • Use simulated scenarios to practice problem solving.
Executive function[51,52]	• Promote self regulation strategies, including verbal self instruction. • Internalize self monitoring. • May require structuring the environment to support the client. Options include cue cards, feedback, and role modeling.
Perception vs cognition[51,52]	• Use scanning strategies and environmental cues.

UNIT 3-40 INTERVENTION

ALLEN COGNITIVE LEVEL GUIDELINES

Understanding Allen Cognitive Levels can help practitioners plan appropriate treatments for clients with dementia.[53]

LEVEL	OCCUPATIONAL THERAPY FOCUS AND GUIDELINES
1	• Use sensory stimulation to promote arousal.
2	• Client responds to proprioceptive cues such as hand-over-hand guidance. This can aid retrieval of procedural memory. • The client's ability to imitate movements is approximate or partial. • Therapy activities to stimulate cognitive function may include postural movements and gross motor activities, such as hitting a balloon or dancing.
3	• Client can imitate demonstrated manual actions. Tactile cues are useful for stimulating self-care tasks stored in procedural memory. • Clients can perform some self-care independently. • No new learning is present. • Clients can manipulate objects, such as simple craft projects, and perform repetitive tasks. • Task supplies should be stored within client's reach. • Demonstrate steps one at a time during tasks and activities. • Clients need frequent cues to continue tasks, as clients are not goal oriented. • Activities should last up to 30 minutes. • Clients should not be left alone. Caregivers should child-proof the environment.

(continued)

ALLEN COGNITIVE LEVEL GUIDELINES (CONTINUED)	
LEVEL	OCCUPATIONAL THERAPY FOCUS AND GUIDELINES
4	• Client can perform ADLs independently. • Visual cues are helpful. For example, provide a sample of a completed craft project so the client can work toward a goal. • The therapist can demonstrate several steps at a time. • Activities can last up to 1 hour. • Reduce distractions by removing clutter and presenting only the items needed for the task in the client's visual field. • In group activities, each client should have his or her own set of supplies. • Keep dangerous or harmful items out of sight. Clients should not use machinery or electrical appliances if their cognitive level is below 4.6. • Client can be left alone for periods of time at level 4.6 with daily supervision or assistance.
5	• Client may be viewed as accident prone due to a trial-and-error approach. • Goals for intervention include safety and abstract planning. • Written instructions or diagrams can be beneficial reminders for clients during task performance and may prevent errors from occurring. • Clients enjoy trying new activities and approaches rather than following one set of instructions. Allow clients the freedom to make choices rather than create an exact replica. • Clients can engage in ongoing projects that last more than one session. The learning carries over into later sessions. • Clients may not anticipate problems. Activities should encourage the client's ability to anticipate, plan, and make decisions and judgments. For example, menu planning, weekly scheduling, budgeting, and packing for trips encourage the client to plan. Asking the client cause-and-effect questions, such as "what will happen if you do 'X'," is beneficial.
6	• Clients perform trial and error covertly through visualization and anticipate potential problems. • Clients can read and follow written instructions.

UNIT 3-41 INTERVENTION

ALTERED MENTAL STATUS AND DEMENTIA INTERVENTION STRATEGIES

ALTERED MENTAL STATUS

Altered mental status (AMS) can result in symptoms that overlap across 2 or more causes, such as impaired ability to follow directions, fatigue, decreased concentration, confusion, and agitation. Recognizing the cause of AMS is important in order to provide proper treatment services.[54]

Delirium

Delirium is a sudden and acute change in mental status with onset over hours to days. The incidence of delirium in ICU settings is reported between 45% and 87%.[55] Delirium indicates a medical emergency but is reversible with treatment. Causes of delirium may include infection such as a urinary tract infection, toxins, certain drugs, endocrine or metabolic imbalances, or trauma. Cognitive symptoms often fluctuate as hyperactive or hypoactive.

Management of Delirium

Management is a multidisciplinary process. Effective ways to manage delirium include[56]:

- Orienting the client to time and place
- Providing calming sensory input and preventing sensory overload (eg, reduce lighting or play soft music)
- Creating a familiar environment
- Engaging the client in ADLs and meaningful activities
- Providing cognitively stimulating activities
- Ensuring early mobilization

Dementia

Dementia is a progressive and irreversible decline in mental function with onset over months to years.

Discussed in more detail later.

Depression

Depression is a mood disorder, with symptoms such as sadness, anhedonia (ie, inability to feel pleasure), fatigue, irritability, and anxiety, that persist for weeks. Depression is usually reversible with treatment.

(continued)

UNIT 3-42 INTERVENTION

ALTERED MENTAL STATUS AND
DEMENTIA INTERVENTION STRATEGIES (CONTINUED)

Communication Techniques

Effective communication techniques for individuals with AMS include:

- Introduce yourself each time you enter the client's room.
- Do not argue with the client. If the client becomes agitated or upset, distract or change the topic or task if necessary.
- Speak in a soothing voice, and use a low pitch when speaking.
- Reduce environmental distractions. For example, turn off the TV or radio, and provide one part of a project at a time.
- Provide short, clear instructions.

(continued)

ALTERED MENTAL STATUS AND
DEMENTIA INTERVENTION STRATEGIES (CONTINUED)

DEMENTIA INTERVENTION STRATEGIES

Dementia encompasses a variety of diseases, but general intervention strategies for broad dementia stages are outlined in this table.

Early Stages of Dementia
(Global Deterioration Scale Stage 1 to 3)[36,57]

In early stages of dementia, the client's difficulties with higher-level executive skills may affect job performance and driving. Assist the client with staying active in meaningful occupations and health management. The client may wish to develop a life legacy project as a meaningful activity. At GDS stage 3, the client may have difficulties with new learning. Be sure to provide the client with increased repetition, modeling, or hand-over-hand assistance when teaching a new task or home exercise program.

Middle Stages of Dementia
(Global Deterioration Scale Stage 4 to 5)[36,57]

In the middle stages of dementia, the client requires assistance with complex IADLs. The client can perform manual actions such as stacking and folding towels. Engage the client in reminiscence activities as meaningful engagement. The client may also enjoy dolls and soft toys.

At GDS stage 5, the client is unable to live alone due to safety concerns with performing ADLs. Home modifications may be beneficial. These include labeling drawers and cabinets, removing clutter, modifying the front door to prevent wandering, and adapting methods for medication management. Adaptive devices such as extended handles and grab bars can serve as safety cues, while other devices such as buttonhooks may cause confusion rather than being beneficial.

Late Stages of Dementia
(Global Deterioration Scale Stage 6 to 7)[36,57]

In the late stages of dementia, the client needs increasing assistance with ADLs. Comforting activities for the client may include singing, rocking, nonverbal communication, and sensory stimulation. The therapist may focus on caregiver education for safe transfers, skin protection, and avoiding contractures. The caregiver may also benefit from resources to obtain respite care or otherwise decrease the burden.

UNIT 3-42 INTERVENTION

FUNCTIONS ASSOCIATED WITH SCI LEVELS AND PRESERVING UPPER EXTREMITY FUNCTION AFTER AN SCI

FUNCTIONS ASSOCIATED WITH SCI LEVELS

For individuals with an SCI in rehabilitation settings, spending more time on ADL training is associated with higher functional outcomes on measurements, such as the Functional Independence Measure.[58] Functional outcomes may differ depending on the client's age and other medical conditions, including factors such as obesity.[59] Functional outcomes are also dependent on the presence or absence of SCI-related complications.[58]

It is important to provide education on prevention of pressure sores, regular skin checks, monitoring for autonomic dysreflexia, bowel and bladder care, and other methods of self-management. ADL training should be graded or adapted as needed with a progression toward modified independence with the fewest adaptive devices.[58] For example, dressing training may begin with the client in bed and may progress toward dressing while seated in a chair, or transfer training may initially include use of a transfer board but may be possible without the use of a sliding board after the client gains upper extremity strength.

Summary of Interventions for Clients With Spinal Cord Injuries

- ADL training
- Education on skin checks and prevention of pressure sores
- Education and training on bowel and bladder care
- Adaptive devices, although these should be graded so that the client uses fewest adaptive devices possible

The following table outlines the functional muscles and movements, necessary equipment, and expected outcomes for each level of SCI. The level indicates the last segment with a muscle grade of 3 or greater.[60]

(continued)

UNIT 3-43 INTERVENTION

UNIT 3-43   INTERVENTION

FUNCTIONS ASSOCIATED WITH SCI LEVELS AND PRESERVING UPPER EXTREMITY FUNCTION AFTER AN SCI (CONTINUED)

Level	Functional Muscles Innervated	Equipment Needs	Expected Functional Outcomes
C1 to C3	• Sternocleidomastoid • Cervical paraspinal • Neck accessories The muscles innervated at this level are necessary for neck flexion, extension, and rotation.	• Ventilator • Suction equipment • Communication devices • Power wheelchair operated with head or pneumatic control • Trendelenburg bed • Hoyer lift or transfer board • Mouth stick • Electronic aid for daily living devices	A person with an injury at this level is expected to require total assistance with ADLs and a full-time caregiver. Expected functional abilities include the following: • Propelling a power wheelchair • Using a communication device • Instructing others in his or her care • Talking, chewing, sipping, and blowing
C4	• Upper trapezius • Diaphragm • Cervical paraspinal The muscles innervated at this level are necessary for neck flexion, extension, and rotation; scapular elevation; and inspiration.	• May need ventilator due to low respiratory reserve • Power wheelchair operated with head or pneumatic control • Trendelenburg bed • Hoyer lift or transfer board • Mouth stick • Electronic aid for daily living devices	A person with an injury at this level is expected to require total assistance with ADLs and a full-time caregiver. Expected functional abilities include the following: • Shrugging his or her shoulders to control devices • Inability to cough

(continued)

FUNCTIONS ASSOCIATED WITH SCI LEVELS AND PRESERVING UPPER EXTREMITY FUNCTION AFTER AN SCI (CONTINUED)

Level	Functional Muscles Innervated	Equipment Needs	Expected Functional Outcomes
C5	• Biceps, brachialis, brachioradialis • Rhomboids • Deltoid • Serratus anterior (partial) The muscles innervated at this level are necessary for shoulder flexion, abduction, and extension; elbow flexion and supination; and scapular adduction and abduction.	• Long opponens splint • Wheelchair pressure relief cushion • Power recline and/or tilt wheelchair • Trendelenburg bed • Transfer board • Adaptive devices	A person with an injury at this level is expected to require a part- or full-time caregiver. The client will need assistance for approximately 10 hours daily for personal care and 6 hours daily for home care. Expected functional abilities include the following: • Eating, light hygiene, and driving with adaptive equipment and help with setup

(continued)

UNIT 3-43 INTERVENTION

FUNCTIONS ASSOCIATED WITH SCI LEVELS AND PRESERVING UPPER EXTREMITY FUNCTION AFTER AN SCI (CONTINUED)

Level	Functional Muscles Innervated	Equipment Needs	Expected Functional Outcomes
C6	• Extensor carpi radialis longus and brevis • Supinator • Clavicular pectoralis • Serratus anterior • Latissimus dorsi The muscles innervated at this level are necessary for scapular protraction, partial horizontal adduction, forearm supination, and radial wrist extension.	• Tenodesis splint • Adaptive devices • Universal cuff • Manual or power wheelchair • Hydraulic standing frame • Padded tub bench • Transfer board	A person with an injury at this level is expected to require a part-time caregiver. The client will need assistance for approximately 6 hours daily for personal care and 4 hours daily for home care. Expected functional abilities include the following: • Tenodesis grasp for self-feeding, personal hygiene, grooming, and upper extremity dressing • May require some assistance with light meal preparation *(continued)*

FUNCTIONS ASSOCIATED WITH SCI LEVELS AND PRESERVING UPPER EXTREMITY FUNCTION AFTER AN SCI (CONTINUED)

Level	Functional Muscles Innervated	Equipment Needs	Expected Functional Outcomes
C7 to C8	• Triceps • Flexor carpi radialis • Pronator quadratus • Extensor carpi ulnaris • Flexor digitorum superficialis and profundus • Partial lumbricals • Latissimus dorsi • Sternal pectoralis • Extensor communis • Pronator/flexor/extensor/abductor pollicis The muscles innervated at this level are necessary for elbow extension; wrist flexion; finger flexion and extension; and thumb flexion, extension, and abduction.	• Padded tub bench • Adaptive devices • Transfer board • Manual rigid or folding wheelchair • Hydraulic or standard standing frame	The client will need assistance for approximately 6 hours daily for personal care and 2 hours daily for home care. Expected functional abilities include the following: • Modified independence with eating, grooming, dressing, and bathing • Extension of elbows for sliding board transfers • Modified independence with light meal preparation and homemaking

(continued)

UNIT 3-43 INTERVENTION

FUNCTIONS ASSOCIATED WITH SCI LEVELS AND PRESERVING UPPER EXTREMITY FUNCTION AFTER AN SCI (CONTINUED)

Level	Functional Muscles Innervated	Equipment Needs	Expected Functional Outcomes
T1 to T9	• Intrinsic muscles of hand, including thumbs (lumbricals) • Internal and external intercostals • Erector spinae The muscles innervated at this level are necessary for finger adduction and abduction and full upper extremity use.	• Elevated padded toilet seat • Manual rigid or folding lightweight wheelchair • Transfer board • Standing frame	A person with an injury at this level is expected to be modified independent with self-care. The client will need assistance for approximately 3 hours daily for home care. Expected functional abilities include the following: • Independence with complex meal preparation and light housecleaning *(continued)*

FUNCTIONS ASSOCIATED WITH SCI LEVELS AND PRESERVING UPPER EXTREMITY FUNCTION AFTER AN SCI (CONTINUED)

Level	Functional Muscles Innervated	Equipment Needs	Expected Functional Outcomes
T10 to L1	• Intercostals • External obliques • Rectus abdominis The muscles innervated at this level are necessary for trunk stability.	• Padded toilet seat • Manual rigid or folding lightweight wheelchair • Standing frame • Forearm crutches or walker • Knee-ankle-foot orthosis • Vehicle hand controls	The client will need home care assistance for approximately 2 hours each day a helper is available. Expected functional abilities include the following: • Independence or requiring some assistance with functional ambulation
L2 to S5	• Fully intact abdominals and trunk muscles • Partial hip flexors, extensors, abductors, adductors, knee flexors, extensors, ankle dorsiflexors, plantar flexors	• Padded toilet seat and tub bench • Manual rigid or folding lightweight wheelchair • Standing frame • Forearm crutches or cane as indicated • Knee-ankle-foot or ankle-foot orthosis • Vehicle hand controls	The client will need homemaking assistance for approximately 1 hour or less each day there is a helper available. Expected functional abilities include the following: • Independence or requiring some assistance with functional ambulation

(continued)

UNIT 3-43 INTERVENTION

FUNCTIONS ASSOCIATED WITH SCI LEVELS AND PRESERVING UPPER EXTREMITY FUNCTION AFTER AN SCI (CONTINUED)

PRESERVING UPPER EXTREMITY FUNCTION AFTER A SPINAL CORD INJURY[61]

Wheelchair Recommendations

- Provide manual wheelchair users with a fully customized wheelchair that is as light as possible.
- Adjust the wheelchair's rear axle as far forward as possible without compromising stability.
- When the user's hand is placed on the top center of the pushrim, there should be a 100- to 120-degree angle between the upper arm and the forearm. If there is not, adjust the rear axle.
- Educate the client to use long, smooth strokes and to drift his or her hand down naturally below the pushrim when not in contact with it.

Additional Upper Extremity Recommendations

- Educate clients with an SCI about the risk of upper limb pain and injury, prevention and fitness, and various treatment options.
- Assess the client for proper transfer technique.
- Minimize the frequency of repetitive upper limb tasks.
- Minimize the force required to complete upper limb tasks.
- Minimize the extreme positions of joints.

UNIT 3-43 INTERVENTION

SPLINTING FOR SPINAL CORD INJURIES

Hand splinting is common for clients with C5, C6, C7, or C8 level injuries. One purpose for hand splinting is to prevent contractures, which can develop quickly due to muscle paralysis and from effects of edema below the lesion level following an SCI.[62]

Primary purposes of hand splinting include the following.[62]

- Maintain ROM
- Prevent contractures
- Encourage functional use of the hands for daily activities

Resting hand splints are commonly worn at night, while splints that promote functional movement are commonly worn during the day. Functional splints promote tenodesis and include wrist–cock-up splints, short opponens splints, and long opponens splints.[62]

RESTING HAND SPLINTS	FUNCTIONAL SPLINTS
• Resting hand splints typically promote a wrist position that ranges from neutral to 30 degrees of extension. • Metacarpophalangeal joints are in flexion. • Interphalangeal joints may be slightly flexed, and the thumb is midway to opposition.	• Wrist–cock-up splints promote wrist extension with a universal cuff, and a short or long opponens splint. • Long opponens splints are used for clients with quadriplegia, who have zero to poor wrist extension, to keep the thumb in opposition. • Short opponens splints are used for clients with quadriplegia, who have fair to good wrist extension, to keep the thumb in opposition.

In acute stages of rehabilitation, the client's splint may be designed to prevent overstretching of extensors. A boxing glove splint is a wrist–cock-up splint with a palmar pad. The splint is bandaged to the client's hand and provides compression in order to prevent edema. For a C6-level injury, a hand roll may be placed to support the fingers in a flexed position to prevent overstretching.[62]

(continued)

UNIT 3-44 INTERVENTION

SPLINTING FOR SPINAL CORD INJURIES (CONTINUED)	
MOST USED STATIC SPLINTS	
A survey of occupational therapists ranked the most common static splints used with each level in order from highest to lowest percentage.[62]	
Level of Injury	*Ranking of Splints*
C5	The most commonly used static splint is a resting hand splint, followed by long opponens, dorsal wrist splint, and wrist–cock-up splint.
C6	The most commonly used static splint is a resting hand splint, followed by short opponens, wrist–cock-up splint, dorsal wrist splint, and long opponens splint.
C7	The most commonly used static splint is a short opponens splint, followed by a resting hand splint, wrist–cock-up splint, dorsal wrist splint, and long opponens splint.
Dynamic splints (eg, wrist-drive splints for prehension that are useful when eating, writing, or completing grooming tasks) are most commonly used in clients with C6- or C7-level injuries.	
	(continued)

UNIT 3–44 INTERVENTION

SPLINTING FOR SPINAL CORD INJURIES (CONTINUED)

MOST USED DYNAMIC SPLINTS

A survey of occupational therapists ranked the most common dynamic splints used with each level in order from highest to lowest percentage.[62]

Level of Injury	Ranking of Splints
C5	The most commonly used dynamic splint is a ratchet splint, followed by an external powered wrist splint, wrist flexor hinge, and a Rehabilitation Institute of Chicago (RIC) tenodesis splint.
C6	The most commonly used dynamic splint is a wrist flexor hinge splint, followed by an RIC tenodesis splint, and a ratchet splint.
C7	The most commonly used dynamic splint is a wrist flexor hinge splint, followed by an RIC tenodesis splint.
C8	Dynamic splints are rarely used.

Functional task-specific splints may also be used. Writing splints are used to hold a pen for handwriting or to hold a stylus for phone or tablet use. Typing splints assist to stabilize a finger for use with a keyboard. Universal cuffs are another functional splint with a variety of uses, as are adapted utensils to help clients dine with dignity.

Central Nervous System Precautions and Contraindications

Understanding common precautions and contraindications is imperative for keeping clients with central nervous system involvement safe. Precautions and contraindications may be related to medication that the client is taking, blood pressure, intracranial pressure (ICP), skin integrity, swallowing, musculoskeletal functioning, or circulation.

Blood Pressure Following Stroke[63]

Tissue plasminogen activator (tPA) is commonly used to break down clots. If tPA is used in treatment, then the client must wait 24 hours prior to any activity that requires moving out of the bed. For clients who had an ischemic stroke, the normal blood pressure ranges for holding therapy differ, depending on if the client was treated using tPA, as follows:

Normal blood pressure range for a client who was not treated with tPA:

- Systolic: 120 to 220 mm Hg
- Diastolic: 60 to 120 mm Hg

Normal blood pressure range for a client who was treated with tPA:

- Systolic: 120 to 185 mm Hg
- Diastolic: 60 to 110 mm Hg

(continued)

CENTRAL NERVOUS SYSTEM
PRECAUTIONS AND CONTRAINDICATIONS (CONTINUED)

BLOOD PRESSURE FOLLOWING STROKE[63]

Condition	Description of Precautions
Orthostatic hypotension[64]	• Orthostatic hypotension is a sudden drop in blood pressure that may occur when the client moves from supine to sitting. • Monitor for orthostatic hypotension by measuring the client's blood pressure in supine, after raising the head of the bed, and when the client is seated at the edge of the bed. • Ask the client about symptoms of dizziness or lightheadedness while moving to a seated position at the edge of the bed. • If the client indicates dizziness or the blood pressure suggests orthostatic hypotension, move the client to a supine position. Raise his or her legs if needed.
SCI[65]	• Clients with SCIs may have a lower resting blood pressure. • Strategies to manage blood pressure for clients with SCIs include compression stockings, sequential compression devices, and an abdominal binder.

(continued)

UNIT 3-45 INTERVENTION

CENTRAL NERVOUS SYSTEM PRECAUTIONS AND CONTRAINDICATIONS (CONTINUED)

BLOOD PRESSURE FOLLOWING STROKE[63]

Condition	Description of Precautions

Autonomic dysreflexia[65]	• Autonomic dysreflexia is a sudden increase in blood pressure that may occur in clients with a T6 or higher SCI.
	• Signs of autonomic dysreflexia include the following:
	  ◦ A pounding headache
	  ◦ Sweating above the level of injury
	  ◦ Nausea
	  ◦ Slow heart rate
	• If the client is experiencing suspected autonomic dysreflexia, take the following precautions:
	  ◦ Raise the client's head and lower his or her legs.
	  ◦ Check if the client needs to empty his or her bladder.
	  ◦ Loosen any tight clothing.
	  ◦ Check for any pressure sores, ingrown nails, or an overly full bowel.
	• If the cause of autonomic dysreflexia cannot be identified, seek immediate medical attention.
	
	(continued)

UNIT 3–45 INTERVENTION

CENTRAL NERVOUS SYSTEM
PRECAUTIONS AND CONTRAINDICATIONS (CONTINUED)

INTRACRANIAL PRESSURE[66]

Following a TBI, the client's ICP may be managed by elevating the head of the bed to 30 degrees.

- Do not lower the head of the bed if there is an open ventricular drain to relieve pressure.

Factors that can increase ICP include the following:

- Turning the head while in supine
- Loud noises
- Suctioning
- Elevated blood pressure

Always check the client's target ranges for ICP before holding therapy:

- The ICP should be less than 20 at maximum in order to hold therapy.

SKIN INTEGRITY AND SENSATION[67]

Condition	Description of Precautions
Loss of sensation	• Clients with loss of sensation are at increased risk of injury or burns from heat. • Always check the client's skin for areas of redness or bruising. • Be cautious of water temperatures and the client's ability to sense heat from heat packs or hot pans from the oven.
Skin breakdown and pressure sores	• In order to prevent skin breakdown and pressure sores, change the bed position at least once every 2 hours. • Instruct clients with SCIs to conduct pressure relief at least 1 minute every hour and to check their skin often using mirrors. • When performing serial recasting, recast about every 2 days and check the skin during these times.

(continued)

UNIT 3-45 INTERVENTION

CENTRAL NERVOUS SYSTEM PRECAUTIONS AND CONTRAINDICATIONS (CONTINUED)	
RANGE OF MOTION AND MOVEMENT OF THE AFFECTED EXTREMITY	
Condition	Description of Precautions
Hemiplegia[44]	• Do not pull on a hemiplegic arm during transfers or exercises. Avoid aggressive ROM and stretching. • Maintain the scapulohumeral rhythm if the client is completing overhead shoulder ranges. • If necessary, manually mobilize the scapula with upward rotation past 90 degrees to prevent impingement. • Avoid overhead pulley exercises to decrease pain.
Heterotopic ossification[68]	• Heterotopic ossification is the presence of abnormal bone growths and is commonly found in the hips, knees, elbows, or shoulders. • Signs of heterotopic ossification include decreased ROM, swelling or warmth over the joint, and a fever. • Heterotopic ossification after an SCI most commonly occurs 3 to 12 weeks after the injury.[68]
Shoulder subluxation[44]	• Support the affected shoulder by using a sling during transfers, taping, or when sitting against gravity. • Maintain the shoulder position by using pillows when sitting or supine in bed.
Contractures[46]	• Prevent contractures through splinting and use of pillows during bed positioning.

(continued)

CENTRAL NERVOUS SYSTEM
PRECAUTIONS AND CONTRAINDICATIONS (CONTINUED)

DEEP VEIN THROMBOSIS[69]

Deep vein thrombosis (DVT) is a blood clot that may occur in either leg and, less commonly, in the arms. Signs of DVT include the following:

- Swelling
- Warmth or coolness
- Discoloration
- Tenderness
- Fever and chills

The client may use compression stockings or sequential compression devices to prevent DVT. If a DVT is identified, check with nursing staff prior to initiating ROM or out-of-bed activities.

UNIT 3-45 INTERVENTION

REFERENCES

1. Roca M, Parr A, Thompson R, et al. Executive function and fluid intelligence after frontal lobe lesions. *Brain.* 2010;133(1):234-247. doi:10.1093/brain/awp269

2. Poldrack RA. Mapping mental function to brain structure: how can cognitive neuroimaging succeed? *Perspect Psychol Sci.* 2010;5(6):753-761. doi:10.1177/1745691610388777

3. Lundy-Ekman L. *Neuroscience: Fundamentals for Rehabilitation.* 4th ed. St. Louis, Mo: Elsevier Saunders; 2013.

4. Demel SL, Broderick JP. Basilar occlusion syndromes: an update. *Neurohospitalist.* 2015;5(3):142-150. doi:10.1177/1941874415583147

5. Gutman S. *Quick Reference Neuroscience for Rehabilitation Professionals: The Essential Neurologic Principles Underlying Rehabilitation Practice.* 3rd ed. Thorofare, NJ: SLACK Incorporated; 2017.

6. Cleveland Clinic. Think FAST when it comes to stroke: knowing the warning signs and how to react can make the difference between life and death. *Heart Advis.* 2013;16(4):1.

7. Robinson TG, Reid A, Haunton VJ, Wilson A, Naylor AR. The face arm speech test: does it encourage rapid recognition of important stroke warning symptoms? *Emerg Med J.* 2013;30(6):467-471. doi:10.1136/emermed-2012-201471

8. Munoz A, Urban R. Neuroendocrine consequences of traumatic brain injury. *Curr Opin Endocrinol Diabetes Obes.* 2013;20(4):354-358. doi:10.1097/MED.0b013e32836318ba

9. Behan LA, Phillips J, Thompson CJ, Agha A. Neuroendocrine disorders after traumatic brain injury. *J Neurol Neurosurg Psychiatry.* 2008;79(7):753-759. doi:10.1136/jnnp.2007.132837

10. Folstein MF, Folstein SE. "Mini mental state". A practical method for grading the cognitive state of patients for clinician. *J Psychiatr Res.* 1975;12:189-198. doi:10.1016/0022-3956(75)90026-6

11. Tariq SH, Tumosa N, Chibnall JT, Perry MH 3rd, Morley JE. Comparison of the Saint Louis University mental status examination and the mini-mental state examination for detecting dementia and mild neurocognitive disorder—a pilot study. *Am J Geriatr Psychiatry.* 2006;14(11):900-1000. doi:10.1097/01.JPG.0000221510.33817.86

12. Gauthier L, Dehaut F, Joanette Y. The Bells test: a quantitative and qualitative test for visual assessment. *International Journal of Clinical Neuropsychology.* 1989;11:49-54.

13. Mulder M, Nijland R. Stroke impact scale. *J Physiother.* 2016;62(2):117. doi:10.1016/j.jphys.2016.02.002

14. Wilson B, Cockburn J, Baddeley A. *The Rivermead Behavioral Memory Test.* Reading, England: Thames Valley Test Company; 1985.

15. Robertson IH, Ward T, Ridgeway V, Nimmo-Smith I. *The Test of Everyday Attention Manual.* Reading, England: Tames Valley Test Company; 1994.

16. Moses J, James A. Test review-comprehensive trail making test (CTMT). *Arch Clin Neuropsychol.* 2004;19(5):703.

17. Itzkovich M, Averbuch S, Elazar B, Katz N. *Loewenstein Occupational Therapy Cognitive Assessment (LOTCA) Battery.* 2nd ed. Pequannock, NJ: Maddak; 2000.

18. Katz N, Itzhovich M, Averbuch S. The Loewenstein occupational therapy cognitive assessment. *Arch Phys Med Rehabil.* 2002;83(8):1179.

19. O'Dell MW, Kim G, Finnen LR, Polistena C. Clinical implications of using the arm motor ability test in stroke rehabilitation. *Phys Med Rehabil.* 2011;92(5):830-836. doi:10.1016/j.apmr.2010.09.020

20. Morris DM, Uswatte G, Crago JE, Cook EW, Taub E. The reliability of the wolf motor function test for assessing upper extremity function after stroke. *Phys Med Rehabil.* 2001;82(6):750-755. doi:10.1053/apmr.2001.23183

21. Wolf SL, Lecraw DE, Barton LA, Jann BB. Forced use of hemiplegic upper extremities to reverse the effect of learned nonuse among chronic stroke and head-injured patients. *Exp Neurol.* 1989;104:125-132.

22. Berg K, Wood-Dauphinee S, Williams JI, Maki B. Measuring balance in the elderly: validation of an instrument. *Can J Public Health.* 1992;83(suppl 2):S7-S11.

23. Mueller J, Kierman R, Langston JW. *Cognistat Manual.* Fairfax, CA: The Northern California Neurobehavioral Group; 2007.

24. Freedman M, Leach L, Kaplan E, Winocur G, Shulman K, Delis DC. *Clock Drawing: A Neuropsychological Analysis.* New York, NY: Oxford University Press; 1994.

25. Colarusso RP, Hammill DD. *Motor-Free Visual Perception Test.* Novato, CA: Academic Therapy Publications; 1972.

26. Brown GT, Rodger S, Davis A. Motor-free visual perception test—revised: an overview and critique. *Br J Occup Ther.* 2003;66(4):159-167. doi:10.1177/030802260306600405

27. Ackerman P, Morrison SA, McDowell S, Vazquez L. Using the spinal cord independence measure III to measure functional recovery in a post-acute spinal cord injury program. *Spinal Cord.* 2010;48(5):380-387. doi:10.1038/sc.2009.140

28. Ely EW, Margolin R, Francis J, et al. Evaluation of delirium in critically ill patients: validation of the confusion assessment method for the intensive care unit (CAM-ICU). *Crit Care Med.* 2001;29:1370-1379.

29. Teasdale G. The Glasgow structured approach to assessment of the Glasgow coma scale. Glasgow Coma Scale. http://www.glasgowcomascale.org. Published 2014. Accessed April 25, 2019.

30. Barlow P. A practical review of the Glasgow coma scale and score. *Surgeon.* 2012;10(2):114-119. doi:10.1016/j.surge.2011.12.003

31. Hagen C, Malkmus D, Durham P. *Levels of Cognitive Functioning.* Downey, CA: Rancho Los Amigos Hospital; 1972.

32. Stenberg M, Godbolt AK, Nygren De Boussard C, Levi R, Stålnacke BM. Cognitive impairment after severe traumatic brain injury, clinical course and impact on outcome: a Swedish-Icelandic study. *Behav Neurol.* 2015;2015. doi:10.1155/2015/680308

33. Kwah LK, Diong J. National Institutes of Health Stroke Scale (NIHSS). *J Physiother.* 2014;60(1):61. doi:10.1016/j.jphys.2013.12.012

34. Allen CA, Austin S, Davis S, Earhart C, McCraith DB, Riska-Williams L. *Manual for the Allen Cognitive Level Screen-5 (ACLS-5) and Large Allen Cognitive Level Screen-5 (LACLS-5).* Camarillo, CA: ACLS and LACLS Committee; 2007.

35. Nasreddine ZS, Phillips NA, Bédirian V, et al. The Montreal cognitive assessment, MoCA: a brief screening tool for mild cognitive impairment. *J Am Geriatr Soc.* 2005;53:695-699. doi:10.1111/j.1532-5415.2005.53221.x

36. Reisberg B, Ferris SH, de Leon MJ, Crook T. The global deterioration scale for assessment of primary degenerative dementia. *Am J Psychiatry.* 1982;139(9):1136-1139. doi:10.1176/ajp.139.9.1136

37. Vissarionov SV, Baindurashvili AG, Kryukova IA. International standards for neurological classification of spinal cord injuries (ASIA/ISNCSCI scale, revised 2015). *Pediatr Traumatol, Orthop and Reconstr Surg.* 2016;4(2):67-72. doi:10.17816/PTORS4267-72

38. Marino RJ, Barros T, Biering-Sorensen F, et al. International standards for neurological classification of spinal cord injury. *J Spinal Cord Med.* 2016;26(suppl 1): S50-S56. doi:10.1080/10790268.2003.11754575

39. Gregson JM, Leathley M, Moore AP, Sharma AK, Smith TL, Watkins CL. Reliability of the tone assessment scale and the modified Ashworth scale as clinical tools for assessing poststroke spasticity. *Arch Phys Med Rehabil.* 1999;80(9):1013-1016. doi:10.1016/S0003-9993(99)90053-9

40. Bohannon RW, Smith MB. Interrater reliability of a modified Ashworth scale of muscle spasticity. *Phys Ther.* 1987;67(2):206-207. doi:10.1093/ptj/67.2.206

41. Fugl-Meyer AR, Jääsko L, Leyman I, Olsson S, Steglind S. The post-stroke hemiplegic patient. *Scand J Rehabil Med.* 1975;7(1):13-31.

42. Lee YY, Hsieh YW, Wu CY, Lin KC, Chen CK. Proximal Fugl-Meyer assessment scores predict clinically important upper limb improvement after 3 Stroke rehabilitative interventions. *Arch Phys Med Rehabil.* 2015;96(12):2137-2144. doi:10.1016/j.apmr.2015.07.019

43. McCormack GL. Pain management by occupational therapists. *Am J Occup Ther.* 1988;42:582-590. doi:10.5014/ajot.42.9.582

44. Smith M. Management of hemiplegic shoulder pain following stroke. *Nurs Stand.* 2012;26(44):35-44. doi:10.7748/ns.26.44.35.s48

45. Liepert J. How evidence based is the positioning of patients with neurological illness? *Dtsch Arztebl Int.* 2015;112(3):33. doi:10.3238/arztebl.2015.0033

46. de Jong LD, Nieuwboer A, Aufdemkampe G. Contracture preventive positioning of the hemiplegic arm in subacute stroke patients: a pilot randomized controlled trial. *Clin Rehabil.* 2006;20(8):656-667. doi:10.1191/0269215506cre1007oa

47. O'Connor RJ, Kini MU. Non-pharmacological and non-surgical interventions for tremor: a systematic review. *Parkinsonism Relat Disord.* 2011;17(7):509-515. doi:10.1016/j.parkreldis.2010.12.016

48. Moroz A, Edgley SR, Lew HL, et al. Rehabilitation interventions in Parkinson disease. *Phys Med Rehabil.* 2009;1(3):S48. doi:10.1016/j.pmrj.2009.01.018

49. Donovan S, Lim C, Diaz N, et al. Laserlight cues for gait freezing in Parkinson's disease: an open-label study. *Parkinsonism Relat Disord.* 2011;17(4):240. doi:10.1016/j.parkreldis.2010.08.010

50. Gillen G. *Cognitive and Perceptual Rehabilitation: Optimizing Function.* St. Louis, MO: Elsevier Mosby; 2009.

51. Cicerone KD, Dahlberg C, Kalmar K, et al. Evidence-based cognitive rehabilitation: recommendations for clinical practice. *Arch Phys Med Rehabil.* 2000;81(12):1596-1615. doi:10.1053/apmr.2000.19240

52. Barman A, Chatterjee A, Bhide R. Cognitive impairment and rehabilitation strategies after traumatic brain injury. *Indian J Psychol Med.* 2016;38(3):172-181. doi:10.4103/0253-7176.183086

53. Cole MB, Tufano R. *Applied Theories in Occupational Therapy: A Practical Approach.* Thorofare, NJ: SLACK Incorporated; 2008.

54. Hamby JR. Appendix E: altered mental status. In: Smith-Gabai H, Holm SE, eds. *Occupational Therapy in Acute Care.* Bethesda, MD: AOTA Press; 2011:589-603.

55. Álvarez EA, Garrido MA, Tobar EA, et al. Occupational therapy for delirium management in elderly patients without mechanical ventilation in an intensive care unit. A pilot randomized clinical trial. *J Crit Care.* 2016;37:85-90. doi:10.1016/j.jcrc.2016.09.002

56. Aguirre E. Delirium and hospitalized older adults: a review of nonpharmacologic treatment. *J Contin Educ Nurs.* 2010;41(4):151-152. doi:10.3928/00220124-20100326-09

57. Smallfield S. Dementia and the role of occupational therapy. American Occupational Therapy Association. www.aota.org/About-Occupational-Therapy/Professionals/PA/Facts/Dementia.aspx. Published 2017. Accessed May 14, 2019.

58. Ozelie R, Gassaway J, Buchman E, et al. Relationship of occupational therapy inpatient rehabilitation interventions and patient characteristics to outcomes following spinal cord injury: the SCIRehab project. *J Spin Cord Med.* 2012;35(6):527-546. doi:10 .1179/2045772312Y.0000000062

59. Yoshimura O, Takayanagi K, Kobayashi R, et al. Possibility of independence in ADL (activities of daily living) for patients with cervical spinal cord injuries – an evaluation based on the Zancolli classification of residual arm functions. *Hiroshima J Med Sci.* 1998;47(2):57.

60. Atkins MS. Spinal cord injury. In: Radomski MV, Latham CAT, eds. *Occupational Therapy for Physical Dysfunction.* 7th ed. Philadelphia, PA: Lippincott Williams & Wilkins; 2014:1168-1214.

61. Paralyzed Veterans of America Consortium for Spinal Cord Medicine. Preservation of upper limb function following spinal cord injury: a clinical practice guideline for health-care professionals. *J Spin Cord Med.* 2005;28(5):433-470.

62. Krajnik SR, Bridle MJ. Hand splinting in quadriplegia: current practice. *Am J Occup Ther.* 1992;46(2):149-156. doi:10.5014/ajot.46.2.149

63. Cumbler E, Glasheen J. Management of blood pressure after acute ischemic stroke: an evidence-based guide for the hospitalist. *J Hosp Med.* 2007;2(4):261-268. doi:10.1002/jhm.165

64. Chhabra L, Spodick DH. Orthostatic hypertension: recognizing an underappreciated clinical condition. *Indian Heart J.* 2013;65(4):454-456. doi:10.1016/j.ihj.2013.06.023

65. Krassioukov A, Claydon VE. The clinical problems in cardiovascular control following spinal cord injury: an overview. *Prog Brain Res.* 2006;152:223-229.

66. Brimioulle S, Moraine JJ, Norrenberg D, Kahn RJ. Effects of positioning and exercise on intracranial pressure in a neurosurgical intensive care unit. *Phys Ther.* 1997;77(12):1682-1689.

67. Regan MA, Teasell RW, Wolfe DL, Keast D, Mortenson WB, Aubut JA. A systematic review of therapeutic interventions for pressure ulcers following spinal cord injury. *Arch Phys Med Rehabil.* 2009;90(2):213-231. doi:10.1016/j.apmr.2008.08.212

68. Craig Hospital. Heterotopic ossification. https://craighospital.org/resources/heterotopic-ossification. Updated January 2015. Accessed April 25, 2019.

69. Centers for Disease Control and Prevention. Venous thromboembolism (blood clots). https://www.cdc.gov/ncbddd/dvt/facts.html. Updated April 18, 2018. Accessed April 25, 2019.

SECTION THREE

Sensory System, Cranial Nerves, and Peripheral Nervous System

Sit W, Neville M.
*Handbook of Occupational Therapy for
Adults With Physical Disabilities* (pp 221-281).
© 2020 SLACK Incorporated.

CASE

DIAGNOSIS: STROKE WITH CRANIAL NERVE IMPLICATIONS

Once, a colleague was working in a rehabilitation facility with a male client who had suffered a stroke. Located in his brainstem, the stroke thus affected the function of his cranial nerves. He experienced difficulties with swallowing and using his facial muscles, resulting in the loss of speech due to his inability to properly utilize his tongue or jaw to form words. He could, however, produce sounds from his throat.

My colleague described the client as a precious man, of whom she was quite fond. One day during therapy, the client—through the use of his letter board—informed my colleague that he was going to write a book. Knowing the client was an author, my colleague asked him, "What will you write a book about?" In answer, he pointed to her, indicating that he wanted to write a book about my colleague and about therapy. He used the letter board to begin spelling "T... H... E... R... A... P... I... S... T..." My colleague exclaimed, "The rapist?!", appalled at what she could possibly have done. The client burst into loud, guttural laughter at the misunderstanding. Indeed, it is rather unfortunate that the word "therapist" can be broken apart that way, but at the very least, it was much to the delight of the client that day.

Dizziness

While most causes of dizziness are peripheral and readily treatable by skilled clinicians specially trained in vestibular rehabilitation, other causes of dizziness can be related to the central nervous system, cardiopulmonary system, endocrine system, or medications—all of which may warrant immediate emergent care for management, dependent upon the client's history.[1]

Understand that the term *dizziness* is more of a general term that must be differentiated among unsteadiness, light-headedness, and vertigo:

- Unsteadiness is the presentation of physical imbalance with mobility that can stem from musculoskeletal and other neuromuscular disorders.
- Light-headedness tends to be related to orthostatic abnormalities where a sudden shift in blood flow may trigger postural sway or imbalance.
- Vertigo pertains to the perception of spinning, either the client spinning or the room around the client spinning, and is related to miscommunication of sensory systems (visual, vestibular, and somatosensory) within the brain.[1,2]

Central Versus Peripheral Dizziness

	Central	Peripheral
Dizziness Description[2]	• Symptoms tend to be constant. • Client may have sensation of vertigo. • Client often experiences a sense of light-headedness. • There is usually a history of loss of consciousness, brain injury, or trauma (if no pertinent history with presentation, then red-flag for referral to doctor/emergency room).	• Symptoms tend to fluctuate. • Client reports a "spinning" or "whirling" feeling. • Client may perceive they or their surroundings are moving in a circular fashion. • The feeling usually only lasts seconds to minutes depending on the cause of dysfunction.

(continued)

DIZZINESS (CONTINUED)

	Central	Peripheral
Effect of Changing Position[2]	• Symptoms are continuous and not dependent on position.	• Symptoms are positional and can fluctuate. • Symptoms may decrease while staying still. • Client is sensitive to motion.
Effect of Closing Eyes[2]	• Dizziness continues.	• Symptoms are reduced.
Nystagmus[2]	• Vertical nonfatiguing nystagmus occurs with position changes. • Nystagmus is direction changing. • Nystagmus increases with fixation.	• Nystagmus has a delayed presentation after the client's position changes. • Nystagmus occurs in direction of vestibular dysfunction. • Falls occur toward the direction of the affected ear.
Hearing Symptoms[2]	• Client may have unexplained sensorineural hearing loss.	• Client reports reduced hearing, pain or fullness in the ear, or ringing (tinnitus).
Visual Symptoms[2]	• Vision loss may occur. • Abnormal saccades may occur. • Abnormal smooth pursuits may occur. • Diplopia may occur. • Oscillopsia may occur.	• Blurry vision may occur. • Oscillopsia (only if bilateral peripheral loss occurs) may be present.
Nausea[2]	• Moderate nausea may be present.	• Nausea may be present, and it is often severe with vomiting.
Presence of Headache[2]	• Headache is common.	• Headache is uncommon.

(continued)

DIZZINESS (CONTINUED)		
	Central	*Peripheral*

Potential Causes[2,3] (If known lesions/ infections. This is not an all-inclusive list.)	• Cerebrovascular accident/transient ischemic attack
	• Brain tumors/traumatic brain injury
	• Migraines
	• Aging, trauma, or psychogenic
	• Vascular insufficiencies (eg, stenosis, occlusion)
	• Cardiac insufficiencies (eg, low-ejection fracture)
	• Abnormal lab values
	• Medications
	• Infection
	• Cerebellar lesion
	• Brainstem lesion
	• Degenerative diseases
	• Epilepsy
		• Otitis
		• Cranial nerve VIII lesion
		• Meniere's syndrome
		   o Presents as fluctuating hearing loss and ringing, and pressure and fullness in the ear.
		• Benign paroxysmal positioning vertigo (BPPV)
		   o Stones in the ear canal may result from prolonged bed rest, trauma, or a viral infection.
		• Vestibular neuritis
		• Ototoxic drugs
		   o Damage to the inner ear may be caused by medications or antibiotics.
		• Mastoid infection
		• Cholesteatoma
		• Local trauma to ear
		• Foreign body
		• Impacted cerumen
		• Otosclerosis
		• Motion sickness
		• Psychogenic

(continued)

DIZZINESS (CONTINUED)	

CEREBELLAR CAUSES OF DIZZINESS

While it is unlikely that an entry-level therapist will need to further distinguish cerebellar causes of dizziness, it may be helpful to understand the subtle differences that occur in symptoms for cerebellar lesions at different locations. The following charts will assist with identifying whether the client's signs align with unilateral, bilateral, or midline cerebellar syndrome.[4]

Unilateral Cerebellar Syndrome[4]

Speech	• Cerebellar speech that presents as jerky and loud
Face	• Cranial nerves: Cranial nerve III palsy in Benedikt's syndrome • Nystagmus present in the direction of gaze • Presence of yellow fat deposit on or near eyelid (xanthelasma)
Upper limbs	• Cerebellar signs include dysdiadochokinesia, dyschronometria, and dysmetria with intention tremor • Assess client's tone for cogwheel and lead-pipe rigidity • Screen for pronator drift
Lower limbs	• Dysdiadochokinesia during a foot tapping test • Dysmetria and intention tremor during toe-to-finger test • Dyssynergia during a heel-shin test
Sitting	• Assess for pendular jerks and the ability to sit up with hands folded
Gait	• Appears broad based and veers towards the side of the lesion
Causes	• Isolated stroke or a tumor in the posterior fossa • Ataxic hemiparesis due to lacunar stroke • Benedikt's syndrome • Cerebellopontine angle tumor and/or neurofibromatosis • Jugular foramen (Arnold-Chiari or Dandy-Walker malformation) • Lateral medullary syndrome • Demyelinating condition such as multiple sclerosis • Parkinsonism in multiple system atrophy

(continued)

DIZZINESS (CONTINUED)	
Bilateral Cerebellar Syndrome[4]	
Speech	• Cerebellar speech and hoarseness of voice
Face	• Gaze-evoked nystagmus • Thyroid swelling (Goitre) • Enlargement of the tongue (macroglossia)
Upper limbs	• Dupuytren's contracture • Dysmetria, dysdiadochokinesia, or dyschronometria • Parkinsonism • Neurofibromatosis features
Lower limbs	• Cerebellar signs • Clawing of toes (Friedreich's ataxia)
Sitting	• Truncal ataxia and pendular jerks
Gait	• Cerebellar ataxia
Causes	• Acquired infection, such as Lyme disease, tabes dorsalis, toxoplasmosis, Creutzfeldt-Jakob disease, HIV, or enteroviruses • Metabolic causes including hypothyroidism or Wilson's disease • Drugs including alcohol, thiamine deficiency, lithium, phenytoin, and carbamazepine • Bilateral strokes • Multiple system atrophy • Neurofibromatosis type 2 with bilateral cerebellopontine angle tumor • Paraneoplastic (cancer of the lung or ovary) • Hereditary causes including ataxia telangiectasia or Friedreich's ataxia
Midline Cerebellar Syndrome (Cerebellar Vermis)[4]	
Speech	• Cerebellar speech
Lower limbs	• Abnormal heel-toe walk test
Sitting	• Truncal ataxia
Causes	• Paraneoplastic (midline tumor)

PUPIL SCALE

Pupil reaction is controlled by the oculomotor cranial nerve, and the pupil scale records the size of the pupil in mm.[5] In a typical client, pupil size and shape are symmetrical, and the average pupil size is between 2 mm and 5 mm.[6] Abnormal pupil size, symmetry, and responsiveness to light may indicate conditions including intracranial pressure, cerebral damage, or compression of the third cranial nerve.[5]

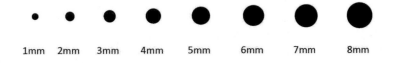

| 1mm | 2mm | 3mm | 4mm | 5mm | 6mm | 7mm | 8mm |

PAIN

Pain is the number one reason that people seek medical attention.[7] The International Association for the Study of Pain defines pain as "an unpleasant sensory and emotional experience associated with actual or potential tissue damage or described in terms of such damage."[8] Thus, pain serves as a protective mechanism to indicate something is wrong.

Sources of pain include nociceptive pain, non-nociceptive (neuropathic) pain, and psychogenic pain.[7]

- Nociceptor pain results from tissue damage.
- Non-nociceptive (neuropathic) pain is caused by direct injury to structures of the nervous system.
- Psychogenic pain shows little or no physical evidence of organic disease or identified injury.

Pain is subjective, individual, and a complex mechanism that includes physical, emotional, and cognitive components. Occupational therapy practitioners should always be aware and mindful of the client's experience of pain when working with the client.

DEFINITIONS

Acute pain[7]	• Has rapid, sudden onset • Acts as a signal to withdraw from potential harm • Described as sharp and localized • Activates sympathetic nervous system, causing diaphoresis (sweating), increased respiratory and pulse rates, and elevated blood pressure
Chronic pain[7]	• Considered pain of long duration with slow and gradual onset • Described as dull, diffuse, and poorly localized • True cause of chronic pain not known or understood • Affects 1 in 5 Americans
Referred pain[7]	• Perceived in an area other than its source • Occurs at a different site from the source of injury or disease • Also known as *trigger points*

(continued)

PAIN (CONTINUED)	
SYNDROMES	
Reflex sympathetic dystrophy[9]	A generic term used to describe posttraumatic pain accompanied by inappropriate autonomic activity and impaired extremity function
Complex regional pain syndrome (CRPS)[9]	CRPS I occurs without an identifiable peripheral nerve injury. CRPS II (formerly known as *causalgia*) is clinical reflex sympathetic dystrophy with a peripheral nerve abnormality. Symptoms of CRPS include the following: • Incapacitating pain and functional compromise • Physiologic changes (trophic, vascular) • Stiffness • Edema • Changes in hair growth, nails, and/or skin (discoloration) • Diagnostic testing may include x-ray and bone scans
Phantom limb pain/residual limb pain[9]	Phantom pain described as stabbing or pins and needles is experienced in 80% of amputees. Residual limb pain is felt as pain in the remaining limb and is reported by 60% of amputees. Neuroma is a common cause of residual limb pain.

UNIT 1–49 NEED TO KNOW

DERMATOMES AND KEY TEST POINTS

Dermatomes refer to areas on the skin with sensory nerves that arise by a shared spinal nerve root. Certain pathologies that originate in a spinal nerve root may present with symptoms, such as a rash or pain, along the dermatome. Additionally, dermatomes are helpful when determining the level of injury for clients with spinal cord injury.[10]

KEY DERMATOME TEST POINTS[11]

- C2: 1 cm lateral to the occipital protuberance
- C3: Supraclavicular fossa at the midclavicle
- C4: Over the acromioclavicular joint
- C5: Lateral antecubital fossa, proximal to the elbow crease
- C6: Dorsal surface of the thumb
- C7: Dorsal surface of the middle finger
- C8: Dorsal surface of the fifth finger
- T1: Medial antecubital fossa, proximal to the medial epicondyle
- T2: Apex of the axilla
- L1: Upper anterior thigh
- L2: Midanterior thigh
- L3: Medial femoral condyle, above the knee
- L4: Medial malleolus
- L5: Dorsum of third metatarsophalangeal joint
- S1: Lateral calcaneus
- S2: Popliteal fossa
- S3: Ischial tuberosity
- S4: Perianal area

(continued)

DERMATOMES AND KEY TEST POINTS (CONTINUED)

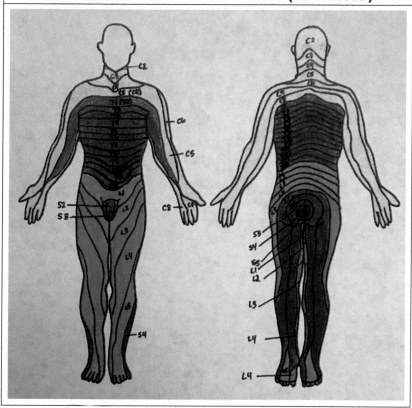

UNIT 2-51 EVALUATION

COMMON ASSESSMENTS ACROSS PRACTICE SETTINGS

ASSESSMENT	ACUTE	INPATIENT	HOME HEALTH	SNF	OUTPATIENT
Common Assessments Across Practice Settings					
Stereognosis (Nottingham Sensory Assessment)	✓	✓		✓	✓
Moberg Pick-Up Test		✓			✓
Cranial Nerve Screening	✓	✓			✓
Vestibular Evaluation					
Vestibular assessments		✓			
Romberg Test					
Berg Balance Scale					
Activities-Specific Balance Confidence Scale					
Functional Gate Assessment					
Dynamic Gate Index					
Modified Clinical Test of Sensory Interaction on Balance (mCTSIB)					
Vision Screening and Assessments					
Brain Injury Visual Assessment Battery for Adults	✓	✓	✓		✓
Pain Evaluation					
McGill Pain Assessment	✓	✓	✓	✓	✓
Shoulder Pain and Disability Index					

(continued)

COMMON ASSESSMENTS ACROSS PRACTICE SETTINGS (CONTINUED)

ASSESSMENT	ACUTE	INPATIENT	HOME HEALTH	SNF	OUTPATIENT
Sensory Tests					
Semmes-Weinstein monofilament test	✓	✓			✓
Static 2-point discrimination					
Moving 2-point discrimination					
Provocative Peripheral Nerve Tests					
Spurling's Neck Compression Test	✓	✓			✓
Shoulder abduction (relief) rest					
Neck distraction test					
Upper limb tension test					
Valsalva maneuver					
Roos Test					
Adson's test					
Straight leg raise test					
Elbow flexion test					
Pressure provocation test					
Tinel's sign (cubital)					
Median nerve compression test/pressure provocation test					
Phalen's test					
Tinel's sign (carpal)					
Froment's sign					
Wartenberg's sign					

SNF: skilled nursing facility.

(continued)

UNIT 2-51 EVALUATION

COMMON ASSESSMENTS
ACROSS PRACTICE SETTINGS (CONTINUED)

STEREOGNOSIS (NOTTINGHAM SENSORY ASSESSMENT)[12]

- Purpose: Assesses ability to identify objects through touch
- Context: Clients with cognitive impairments and sensory deficits in hands
- Format: Performance-based test
- Time to administer: 15 minutes
- Materials: 2 different coins, pen, pencil, comb, scissors, sponge, flannel cloth, cup, glass, and something to occlude vision
- Cost: Free
- Website: https://www.nottingham.ac.uk/medicine/documents/ publishedassessments/nsainstructionsrevised.pdf

MOBERG PICK-UP TEST[13]

- Purpose: Assesses hand functionality
- Context: Clients across diagnoses in inpatient or outpatient settings
- Format: Performance-based test
- Time to administer: 10 to 20 minutes
- Materials: Small objects, container for objects, stopwatch, and something to occlude vision
- Cost: Free
- Website: http://www.danmicglobal.com/517457.aspx

CRANIAL NERVE SCREENING

The 12 pairs of cranial nerves are responsible for an assortment of sensory, motor, or both sensory and motor functions. A cranial nerve screening can provide information about the location of a potential lesion. Information regarding the cranial nerves, their functions, and quick functional tests follows.[14,15]

(continued)

UNIT 2-52 EVALUATION

CRANIAL NERVE SCREENING (CONTINUED)

CRANIAL NERVE	FUNCTION	ASSESSMENT
I: Olfactory nerve	Sensory	Smell	To test the olfactory nerve: • Ask the client to close his or her eyes and obstruct one nostril. • Then ask the client to identify a familiar smell, such as coffee or an orange peel. A lesion to the olfactory nerve may result in the loss of smell (anosmia).
II: Optic nerve	Sensory	Vision	To test the optic nerve, you can do any of the following (use the client's current eyewear if he or she has known visual acuity deficits): • Assess visual acuity with a Snellen chart. • Perform a visual field test. • Obtain results from a funduscopic exam by an ophthalmologist. A lesion to the optic nerve may result in blindness.

(continued)

CRANIAL NERVE SCREENING (CONTINUED)

CRANIAL NERVE	FUNCTION	ASSESSMENT
III: Oculomotor nerve	Motor	Movement of eye up, down, medially, and laterally	To test the oculomotor nerves: • Occlude one eye. • Instruct the client to maintain his or her head in a forward position while scanning a moving stimulus with the eyes. • Move an item, such as a pen, in the shape of an H. • Do not allow client to turn his or her head; do not bring the object too close to the client's face or move the object too quickly. A lesion to the oculomotor nerve may result in an outwardly turned eye (lateral strabismus), double vision (diplopia), drooping eyelid (ptosis), or a shaky eye (nystagmus). To test the pupillary reflex: • Shine a light into the client's eye and observe for pupil constriction.
IV: Trochlear nerve	Motor	Movement of the eye downward and laterally by innervating the superior oblique muscles	The trochlear nerve is tested simultaneously with the oculomotor nerve. A lesion to the trochlear nerve may result in an eye that is turned upward and inward (vertical or medial strabismus), vertical diplopia at near and far distances, nystagmus, difficulty moving the eye downward and laterally, or difficulty walking down steps.

(continued)

UNIT 2-52 EVALUATION

UNIT 2-52 EVALUATION

CRANIAL NERVE SCREENING (CONTINUED)

CRANIAL NERVE	FUNCTION	ASSESSMENT
V: Trigeminal nerve	Sensorimotor	Facial sensation and chewing	To test the sensory function of the trigeminal nerve:

CRANIAL NERVE	FUNCTION	ASSESSMENT
V: Trigeminal nerve	Sensorimotor	Facial sensation and chewing

To test the sensory function of the trigeminal nerve:

- Occlude the client's vision.
- Brush a cotton swab against the affected and unaffected side of the client's cheeks.

To test the motor function of the trigeminal nerve:

- Occlude the client's vision.
- Check for jaw deviation by asking the client to open his or her mouth and move the jaw from side to side.
- Check jaw strength on both sides by asking the client to bite down on a tongue depressor while the therapist tries to pull it out.

A lesion to the trigeminal nerve may result in the loss of facial sensation on the side of the lesion (trigeminal neuralgia), or difficulty chewing with observed jaw deviation toward the affected side.

(continued)

CRANIAL NERVE SCREENING (CONTINUED)

CRANIAL NERVE	FUNCTION	ASSESSMENT
VI: Abducens nerve	Motor	Innervates the lateral rectus muscle to abduct the eye, allowing the client to look laterally	The abducens nerve is tested at the same time as the oculomotor and trochlear nerve. A lesion to the abducens nerve may result in the eyeball turning inward (medial strabismus), diplopia, or nystagmus.
VII: Facial nerve	Sensorimotor	Taste, facial expressions, tears, salivation, and closing the eyes	To test the sensory function of the facial nerve: • Present sweet, salty, and sour stimuli to the outer and lateral portions of the anterior tongue. To test the motor function of the facial nerve: • Ask the client to elevate the eyebrows and forehead, smile, frown, pucker the lips, and blow up the cheeks with air. • Observe the client for facial muscle strength and symmetry. A lesion to the facial nerve may result in decreased taste on the anterior tongue, decreased corneal reflex, or Bell's palsy if the lesion is from a lower motor neuron (affecting both the forehead and lower facial muscles).

(continued)

UNIT 2-52 EVALUATION

CRANIAL NERVE SCREENING (CONTINUED)

CRANIAL NERVE	FUNCTION	ASSESSMENT
VIII: Vestibulocochlear nerve	Sensory	Hearing, balance, and the sensation of head positioning with movement	To test the vestibulocochlear nerve: • Check for nystagmus when tracking an object moved in an H or X pattern. • Conduct a Romberg test by assessing the client's balance when standing with his or her eyes closed. A lesion to the vestibulocochlear nerve may result in deafness, ringing of the ears (tinnitus), nystagmus, vertigo, or deficits in balance.

(continued)

CRANIAL NERVE SCREENING (CONTINUED)

CRANIAL NERVE	FUNCTION	ASSESSMENT
IX: Glossopharyngeal nerve	Sensorimotor	Taste, salivation, and swallowing	The glossopharyngeal nerve is assessed with the vagus nerve. To test the sensory function of the glossopharyngeal nerve: • Present sweet, salty, and sour stimuli to the posterior aspect of the tongue. • Ask the client to chew on a lemon rind to test the sensation of bitter tastes. To test the motor function of the glossopharyngeal nerve: • Use a tongue depressor or cotton swab to elicit a gag reflex. • Observe the client's ability to swallow solid food, pureed food, thick liquids, and thin liquids. A lesion to the glossopharyngeal nerve may result in the loss of bitter taste sensation, loss of gag and swallowing reflexes, or difficulty swallowing (dysphagia). *(continued)*

UNIT 2-52 EVALUATION

CRANIAL NERVE SCREENING (CONTINUED)

CRANIAL NERVE	FUNCTION	ASSESSMENT
X: Vagus nerve	Sensorimotor	Swallowing, taste, speech, and parasympathetic regulation	The vagus nerve is assessed with the glossopharyngeal nerve. To test the vagus nerve: • Observe if the client is speaking clearly as opposed to slurring his or her words, speaking with decreased phonal volume, or if the client's voice sounds hoarse. A lesion to the vagus nerve may result in an irregularly rapid heartbeat, difficulty breathing (dyspnea), oxygen deficiency due to trouble breathing (asphyxia), hoarse voice (dysphonia), dysphagia, or slurred speech (dysarthria).

(continued)

CRANIAL NERVE SCREENING (CONTINUED)

CRANIAL NERVE	FUNCTION	ASSESSMENT
XI: Accessory nerve	Motor	Elevates the larynx during swallowing, innervates the sternocleidomastoid for contralateral head rotation, and innervates the upper trapezius for shoulder elevation and shoulder flexion above 90 degrees	To test the accessory nerve: • Ask the client to swallow while you place your index and middle finger over the client's Adam's apple to assess laryngeal muscles. • Compare the client's ability to flex his or her neck laterally and forward, turn the head, and shrug the shoulders on both sides. A lesion to the accessory nerve may result in dysphagia; weakness with head rotation, flexion, and extension; shrugging the shoulder; or flexing the arm above 90 degrees.
XII: Hypoglossal nerve	Motor	Movement of the tongue	To test the hypoglossal nerve: • Ask the client to stick out his or her tongue while you check for deviation to one side. • Ask the client to move his or her tongue side to side, and check for asymmetry or weakness. • Ask the client to use his or her tongue to push against the cheeks and apply resistance. A lesion to the hypoglossal nerve may result in dysarthria, deviation of the tongue toward the side of the lesion, or dysphagia.

UNIT 2-52 EVALUATION

VESTIBULAR EVALUATION

The vestibular evaluation should include a chart review, thorough client interview, visual screening, functional mobility screen, hearing screen, psychological screen, and activities of daily living (ADL) assessment.[1] As part of the vestibular evaluation, identify if the effects on the vestibular system are of cerebellar origin, which occur in the central nervous system, or if they are sensory-related and occur in the peripheral nervous system. Refer to Section Three, Unit 1-47, for information on effects on the vestibular system.

EVALUATION COMPONENT[1]	DESCRIPTION
Chart review	• Review the client's medical chart for past medical history, consults, lab values, radiology reports, and medications that may cause dizziness. • Specifically, be aware of any head trauma or brain injury, acute infections, or recent changes in medications.
Symptoms and fall history	• What is the client's fall history? • Are there certain times of day or certain activities that seem to exacerbate symptoms? • Describe the dizzy spell without using the word dizzy or dizziness. ◦ Key phrases such as "the room is spinning", "words swim on a page when I read," or "I am whirling when I move my head" are major cues into a suspected vestibular dysfunction. • Consider using a client questionnaire such as the Dizziness Handicap Inventory.[16]
Visual screening	• Observe extraocular movements, saccades, smooth pursuits, convergence, and divergence. Look for signs of spontaneous and gaze nystagmus and oscillopsia. These could be potential indicators of vestibular dysfunction.

(continued)

VESTIBULAR EVALUATION (CONTINUED)

EVALUATION COMPONENT[1]	DESCRIPTION
Functional mobility	• Assess the client's body and posture as well as neck range of motion. • Look for speech, face, upper limb, and lower limb signs of cerebellar syndromes (see the following tables). • Screen for dysdiadochokinesis to assess coordination. • Observe the client's gait, static balance, and dynamic balance.
Psychological screening	• Is the client experiencing anxiety or depression? • Identify any recent major life changes.
Environment	• Assess the environment for hazards, such as rugs, uneven pathways, or cluttered walkways.

(continued)

UNIT 2-53 EVALUATION

VESTIBULAR EVALUATION (CONTINUED)

VESTIBULAR ASSESSMENTS

Assessment Name	Description
Romberg Test[17]	• The client stands with feet together and arms either at the side or crossed. • Assess the client's balance with his or her eyes opened first, and then with his or her eyes closed. • The client should be able to sustain this stance for at least 10 seconds without sway with eyes open or closed.

Berg Balance Scale[18]	• The client is asked to perform movements that require balance and weight shifting, such as moving from sitting to standing, standing with his or her eyes closed, standing on one leg, and turning 360 degrees.
	• Equipment required a stopwatch, yardstick, footstool, chair with armrests, chair without armrests, and 15 feet of walking space.
	• The client's total score can be compared to categories that indicate the client's level of fall risk:
	  ○ 41 to 56: Low fall risk. The client can be considered independent with ambulation.
	  ○ 21 to 40: Medium fall risk. The client should ambulate with assistance.
	  ○ 0 to 20: High fall risk. The client likely uses a wheelchair.

Activities-Specific Balance Confidence Scale[19]	• The client is asked to rate perceived confidence to perform ambulatory tasks without falling or experiencing unsteadiness on a scale from 0% to 100% (no confidence to complete confidence). • Equipment required is the survey and a pen or pencil. • The scale has 16 items (score of 0 to 1600 possible). The score is recorded as a percentage, with 100% the highest level of confidence. Maximum score of 1600 divided by 16 items = 100%. • Scores of less than 67% indicate a risk for falling.

(continued)

VESTIBULAR EVALUATION (CONTINUED)

Assessment Name	Description
Functional Gait Assessment[20]	• Designed to assess postural stability with different walking tasks. • Equipment required includes a clear 20-foot long by 12-inch wide walking path, a stopwatch, an obstacle of 9-inch height (2 stacked shoe boxes), and a set of steps with railing. • Scored on performance of each task (0, or severe impairment, to 3, or no impairment) for a total possible score of 30. • Scores of less than 22 indicate an increased risk for falling.
Dynamic Gait Index[21]	• Assesses the ability to adapt balance in the presence of external demands. • Equipment required includes a 20-foot pathway, a shoebox, 2 obstacles of the same size, and stairs. • Scored on performance of each task (0, or severe impairment, to 3, or no impairment) for total possible score of 24. • Scores of less than 19 indicate an increased risk for falling.
mCTSIB[21]	• Assesses sensory contributions to postural control and involves the observation of a patient's attempt to maintain balance. • Equipment required is a stopwatch and medium-density foam pad. • Perform 3 trials for each condition: standing with feet together on firm surface with eyes open then with eyes closed, and on foam surface with eyes open then with eyes closed. • Maximum time to sustain under all conditions is 30 seconds.

UNIT 2-53 EVALUATION

VISION SCREENING AND ASSESSMENTS

A client is considered to have low vision when his or her acuity is 20/70 or less in the better-seeing eye and with best correction. A client is considered legally blind when his or her acuity is 20/200 or less in the better-seeing eye with best correction, or his or her visual field is 20 degrees or less in the better eye.[22]

When conducting a low vision screening, ask the client about the following:

- The onset and duration of the client's visual problems
- The date of the client's last visual examination
- The client's understanding of the diagnosis, prognosis, and effects on occupational performance
- Any optical or nonoptical devices that have been prescribed or are used
- The client's goals related to eyesight and occupational performance

Make sure that the client's eye doctor knows of any significant changes to the client's vision.

(continued)

VISION SCREENING AND ASSESSMENTS (CONTINUED)

VISUAL ASSESSMENT

The client should wear his or her usual glasses during the visual assessment. The client's visual acuity threshold, contrast sensitivity, central and peripheral visual field loss, and oculomotor function should all be included in the assessment.[23]

ASSESSMENT	DESCRIPTION
Visual acuity threshold[24]	The client should attempt to read newspaper-size print from a distance of 40 cm (16 inches): • Moderate impairment is indicated if the client cannot read the print even with eyeglasses. • Moderate impairment is the minimum criteria for Medicare and Medicaid reimbursable rehabilitation. Standardized screening tests for visual acuity include the Minnesota Low-Vision Reading Test (MNREAD) or Smith-Kettlewell Reading Test (SKREAD) near acuity test, or the LEA numbers booklet if it is suspected that the client has very low vision.[25,26]
Contrast sensitivity[24]	The LEA symbol low-contrast test is a standardized screening test for contrast sensitivity.

Central visual field loss[24]	Use the clock face technique:
	• Draw a clock with numbers using a black marker and a star drawn in the center.
	• Place the clock 16 to 18 inches away from the client, or farther if a small scotoma is suspected.
	• Ask the client to look at the clock:
	  ○ If the star is missing or appears unclear compared to the numbers, then a scotoma with central fixation is suspected.
	  ○ If the client sees the star, then ask if any numbers have disappeared. This indicates a scotoma with habitual eccentric viewing.

(continued)

UNIT 2-54 EVALUATION

VISION SCREENING AND ASSESSMENTS (CONTINUED)

ASSESSMENT	DESCRIPTION
Confrontation field testing for peripheral visual field[25,27]	To administer confrontation field testing for the peripheral visual field: • Sit facing the client. • Instruct the client to look at your eyes. • Use your fingers, a pen, or a confrontation testing wand to move from the side toward client's peripheral visual field. • Instruct the client to signal when he or she can see the object.
Oculomotor function	Refer to Unit 2-52 in this section for information on cranial nerve screening.

BRAIN INJURY VISUAL ASSESSMENT BATTERY FOR ADULTS[28]

- Purpose: Assesses visual processing functions including visual acuity, contrast sensitivity, visual field, oculomotor function, visual attention, etc
- Context: Traumatic brain injury, cerebrovascular accident, brain tumor, anoxic brain injury, multiple sclerosis, encephalopathy, eye trauma, macular degeneration, diabetes
- Format: Standardized performance-based assessment
- Time to administer: Subtests can be administered within minutes while the entire battery will take longer.
- Materials: Book containing subtests
- Cost: $495
- Website: http://www.visabilities.com/bivaba.html

PAIN EVALUATION

A pain assessment requires the practitioner to obtain the clients history with pain.[7] This includes investigating the following areas:

- Location: Where is the pain?
- Intensity: What is the level of pain on a scale of 0 to 10?
- Quality: Can you describe the feeling?
- Chronology: When did it start? How long does it last?
- Precipitating factors: What triggers the pain to start?
- Alleviating factors: What lessens or relieves the pain?

   Pain scales are commonly used as a way to describe pain. The pain scale is from 0 to 10.[7]

- 0: No Pain
- 2: Pain that is mild or annoying
- 4: Pain that is moderate or uncomfortable
- 6: Dreadful or severe pain
- 8: Horrible or very severe pain
- 10: Unbearable pain/the worst pain possible

   The following 2 tests can be used to assess pain.

MCGILL PAIN ASSESSMENT[7,29,30]

- Purpose: Assesses subjective pain intensity and quality
- Context: Clients who experience pain
- Format: Self-report
- Time to administer: Up to 30 minutes
- Materials: Paper, pencil, and the form
- Cost: Free
- Website: https://www.sralab.org/sites/default/files/2017-07/McGill%20Pain%20Questionnaire%20%281%29.pdf

SHOULDER PAIN AND DISABILITY INDEX[31]

- Purpose: Assesses pain related to shoulders
- Context: Musculoskeletal systems
- Format: Patient-reported questionnaire
- Time to administer: 5 to 10 minutes
- Materials: Paper, pencil, and the form
- Cost: Free
- Website: https://www.sralab.org/sites/default/files/2017-06/form_spadi.pdf

UNIT 2-56 EVALUATION

SENSORY TESTS

The following tests can be used to evaluate the client's sensation. This table provides a summary of each tool along with instructions for use.

TOOL	SUMMARY	INSTRUCTIONS
Semmes-Weinstein monofilament test[32]	• Purpose: Assesses touch threshold to detect loss of light touch, protective sensation, and deep pressure • Context: Clients with nerve entrapment or nerve injury, including carpal tunnel, cubital tunnel, and ulnar tunnel syndromes • Format: Sensory test • Time to administer: Quick • Materials: Semmes-Weinstein monofilament set and record sheet • Cost: Varies depending on vendor where monofilaments are purchased • Website: https://www.ncmedical.com/item_1278.html	• The client begins seated at a table with his or her vision occluded. • Beginning with larger Semmes-Weinstein monofilaments (color-coded), the examiner applies monofilaments to the client's skin until the skin blanches, often accompanied by monofilament bending. • Instruct the client to indicate when he or she has felt a touch. • Record the results according to assessment hand mapping. Follow the manual for result indications for decreased sensation.

(continued)

SENSORY TESTS (CONTINUED)

TOOL	SUMMARY	INSTRUCTIONS
Static 2-point discrimination[33]	• Purpose: Assesses touch sensation and receptor density. Used to test nerve regeneration • Context: Clients with nerve lacerations • Format: Sensory test • Time to administer: Quick • Materials: Disk-Criminator • Cost: $100 • Website: https://www.ncmedical.com/item_1283.html	• The client begins seated at a table with their vision occluded and palm facing up. • Using the Disk-Criminator, the examiner touches the client's skin with either 1 or 2 points just until the skin blanches. • Begin with more widely spaced points and work toward closer points. • Ask the client to identify how many points were felt on each trial. • The client should be able to correctly identify the number of points on at least 7 of 10 trials. Normal sensation is being able to distinguish 2 points that are less than 6 mm apart. *(continued)*

UNIT 2-56 EVALUATION

SENSORY TESTS (CONTINUED)

TOOL	SUMMARY	INSTRUCTIONS
Moving 2-point discrimination[33]	• Purpose: Assesses touch sensation and receptor density; used to test nerve regeneration • Context: Clients with nerve compression or laceration • Format: Sensory test • Time to administer: Quick • Materials: Disk-Criminator • Cost: $100 • Website: https://www.ncmedical.com/item_1283.html	• The client begins seated at a table with his or her vision occluded and palm facing up. • Using the Disk-Criminator, the examiner touches the client's skin with either 1 or 2 points just until the skin blanches. The examiner moves the Disk-Criminator from proximal to distal on the distal phalanx. • Ask the client to identify how many points were felt on each trial. • The client should be able to correctly identify the number of points on at least 7 of 10 trials. Normal sensation is being able to distinguish 2 points that are less than 5 mm apart. Note: Moving 2-point discrimination returns before static 2-point discrimination does.

PROVOCATIVE PERIPHERAL NERVE TESTS

Peripheral nerve testing can involve provoking symptoms to guide diagnosis and treatment. The following table describes tests for the neck, back, and upper extremities; instructions for administering the test; and potential diagnoses.

Note: The use of any single test for diagnosis cannot be recommended at this time. Combinations of tests may be more accurate. Occupational therapists are not licensed to diagnose pathologies, but the results of these tests may provide a greater understanding of a client's potential peripheral nerve injury.

NAME OF TEST	ADMINISTRATION	POSITIVE TEST MAY INDICATE
Spine		
Cervical[34]		
Spurling's Neck Compression Test[35]	• The client begins seated with his or her neck in neutral alignment. • Instruct the client to laterally flex his or her neck toward the side experiencing symptoms. • If there are no symptoms, then the examiner applies a downward force with combined side flexion. The test is positive if pain is present in the same-side upper extremity with or without the application of the downward force.	Cervical radiculopathy
Shoulder abduction (relief) test[36]	• The client begins seated. • Instruct the client to actively abduct his or her arm and place his or her hand on top of his or her head with the palm facing down. The test is positive if the client's pain is reduced.	Cervical radiculopathy

(continued)

UNIT 2-57 EVALUATION

UNIT 2-57 EVALUATION

PROVOCATIVE PERIPHERAL NERVE TESTS (CONTINUED)

NAME OF TEST	ADMINISTRATION	POSITIVE TEST MAY INDICATE
Neck distraction test[37]	• The client begins lying supine, and the examiner begins seated behind the client's head. • The examiner grasps the back of the client's head with one hand (at the occipital condyles) and cradles the other hand around the client's chin. • A traction force is applied, gently pulling the client's head toward the examiner's body. The test is positive if the client's pain is reduced.	Cervical radiculopathy
Upper limb tension test[38]	• The client begins lying supine, and the examiner stabilizes the scapula by blocking the shoulder. • If there is no pain, then the examiner abducts the client's arm to approximately 110 degrees with the elbow in slight flexion. • Next, the examiner supinates the client's arm while extending the wrist and fingers. The test is positive if pain is present.	Various dysfunctions

(continued)

Provocative Peripheral Nerve Tests (continued)

Name of Test	Administration	Positive Test May Indicate
Valsalva maneuver[34]	• The client begins seated. • Instruct the client to hold his or her breath and "bear" down, as if toileting. The test is positive if pain is present.	Cervical radiculopathy
Thoracic		
Roos Test[39]	• The client begins seated with both arms abducted to 90 degrees and elbows flexed to 90 degrees. • The arms are externally rotated (similar to a goal post position). • Instruct the client to rapidly open and close both hands for 60 seconds. The test is positive if the client's symptoms are reproduced while performing the test.	Thoracic outlet syndrome
Adson's test[39]	• The client begins seated with both arms in approximately 15 degrees of abduction. • Palpate the client's radial pulse. • Instruct the client to inhale, hold his or her breath, tilt his or her head back, and rotate his or her head toward the involved side. The test is positive if there is a change in the client's radial pulse while performing the test or if the client reports paresthesia.	Thoracic outlet syndrome

(continued)

UNIT 2-57 EVALUATION

UNIT 2-57 EVALUATION

PROVOCATIVE PERIPHERAL NERVE TESTS (CONTINUED)

NAME OF TEST	ADMINISTRATION	POSITIVE TEST MAY INDICATE
Lumbar		
Straight leg raise test[40]	• The client begins lying supine with his or her head and neck in neutral alignment. • Support the client's leg at the heel with his or her knee in extension. The ankle is in neutral dorsiflexion. • Raise the leg until the client reports symptoms. Avoid rotating the client's trunk or leg, and do not adduct or abduct the hip. The test is positive if symptoms are present.	Lumbar radiculopathy
Elbow and Forearm		
Elbow flexion test[41]	• The client begins seated with his or her arms in the anatomical position. • Instruct the client to flex both elbows to end range (but not forcibly). The wrists are in extension. • Have the client hold the position for 3 minutes. The test is positive if pain or paresthesias is present along the ulnar nerve distribution (the fourth and/or fifth digits).	Cubital tunnel syndrome

(continued)

PROVOCATIVE PERIPHERAL NERVE TESTS (CONTINUED)

NAME OF TEST	ADMINISTRATION	POSITIVE TEST MAY INDICATE
Pressure provocation test[42]	• The client begins seated with the examiner sitting in front. • Support the client's wrist with the left hand and palpate the cubital tunnel with the right hand. • Apply pressure over the ulnar nerve proximal to the cubital tunnel with your first and second fingers. The test is positive if pain or paresthesias is present along the ulnar nerve distribution.	Cubital tunnel syndrome
Tinel's sign (cubital)[42]	• The client begins seated. • Stabilize the client's wrist while applying 4 to 6 taps to the ulnar nerve at the cubital tunnel. • A reflex hammer or the first and second digits may be used to apply the stimulus. The test is positive if symptoms are reproduced along the ulnar nerve distribution.	Cubital tunnel syndrome

(continued)

UNIT 2-57 EVALUATION

UNIT 2-57 EVALUATION

PROVOCATIVE PERIPHERAL NERVE TESTS (CONTINUED)

NAME OF TEST	ADMINISTRATION	POSITIVE TEST MAY INDICATE
Wrist and Hand		
Median nerve compression test/ pressure provocation test[43,44]	• The client begins seated while the examiner is opposite of the client. • Support the client's hand while the forearm is in supination. • Apply pressure directly over the median nerve as it passes under the flexor retinaculum between the flexor carpi radialis and the palmaris longus (if present). • Sustain this gentle pressure with the thumbs for 15 seconds to 2 minutes. The test is positive if pain, paresthesia, or numbness is present along the median nerve distribution.	Carpal tunnel syndrome
Phalen's test[44]	• The client begins seated. • Instruct the client to bring both wrists into full flexion, and bring the wrists together so that the dorsal sides of the hand are touching, fingers pointing down toward the floor. • The client should maintain this position for 1 minute. The test is positive if numbness and tingling are present along the median nerve distribution (thumb, index finger, middle finger).	Carpal tunnel syndrome

(continued)

PROVOCATIVE PERIPHERAL NERVE TESTS (CONTINUED)

NAME OF TEST	ADMINISTRATION	POSITIVE TEST MAY INDICATE
Tinel's sign (carpal)[42,44]	• The client begins seated with his or her forearm supported on the table and his or her palm up. • The examiner then applies 4 to 6 taps to the median nerve at the area of the carpal tunnel in the wrist. The test is positive if numbness and tingling are present along the client's median nerve distribution (thumb, index finger, middle finger).	Carpal tunnel syndrome
Froment's sign[35]	• The client begins seated. • Instruct the client to hold a piece of paper between his or her thumb and index finger. • The examiner attempts to pull the paper out of the client's finger grasp. The test is positive if the client displays signs of adductor pollicis weakness by needing to flex the thumb interphalangeal joint to compensate, rather than the thumb interphalangeal joint remaining extended or flat.	Ulnar nerve palsy

(continued)

UNIT 2-57 EVALUATION

UNIT 2-57 EVALUATION

PROVOCATIVE PERIPHERAL NERVE TESTS (CONTINUED)

Name of Test	Administration	Positive Test May Indicate
Wartenberg's sign[45,46]	• The client begins seated with the testing hand pronated and resting on a surface. • The client may either actively abduct all fingers or the examiner may passively abduct the client's fingers. • The client is asked to adduct all fingers. The test is positive if the fifth digit remains abducted.	Ulnar nerve lesion

COMMON INTERVENTIONS ACROSS PRACTICE SETTINGS

INTERVENTION	ACUTE	INPATIENT	HOME HEALTH	SNF	OUTPATIENT
Common Interventions Across Practice Settings					
Sensory retraining/desensitization	✓	✓			✓
Mirror therapy	✓	✓			✓
Nerve glide exercises	✓	✓			✓
Low Vision Intervention Strategies	✓	✓			✓
Vestibular Rehabilitation		✓			✓
Pain Management	✓	✓	✓	✓	✓
Common Splints for the Peripheral Nervous System	✓	✓			✓
Peripheral Nervous System Precautions and Contraindications	✓	✓	✓	✓	✓

(continued)

UNIT 3-58 INTERVENTION

COMMON INTERVENTIONS
ACROSS PRACTICE SETTINGS (CONTINUED)

SENSORY RETRAINING/DESENSITIZATION[47]

- Description: *Sensory retraining* refers to exercises that reeducate the brain on how to interpret sensations. *Desensitization* refers to techniques that modify an area's oversensitivity to a particular stimulus.
- Approach: Manual techniques, electrical stimulation, and vibration are common applications.
- Precautions: Do not use this treatment on an open wound due to the risk of infection. Clean the equipment between uses.
- Significance: This intervention may be used following peripheral nerve damage or surgery to the body in order to help the client tolerate sensory experiences and improve participation in daily activities.

MIRROR THERAPY[48]

- Description: Mirror therapy is a motor imagery intervention that allows the client to observe the unaffected body part as it performs movements. The client observes the movement through the mirror, which conveys visual stimuli to the brain.
- Approach: The client begins seated at a table, and the mirror is positioned to block the client's view of the unaffected extremity. The client performs the same movements with both limbs, and observes the reflection of their unaffected limb in the mirror. The occupational therapy practitioner stands opposite of the client to supervise the movement on each side of the mirror and ensure that the client is watching the unaffected extremity in the mirror. The treatment duration is 30 minutes per day at minimum, and the protocol duration is 5 days a week for 1 month unless otherwise stated by a physician.
- Precautions: Some clients may become bored during mirror therapy.
- Significance: Mirror therapy positively affects motor function and participation in daily activities. Mirror therapy is also used to reduce phantom limb pain and unilateral spatial neglect.

(continued)

COMMON INTERVENTIONS
ACROSS PRACTICE SETTINGS (CONTINUED)

NERVE GLIDE EXERCISES[49]

- Description: Nerve glide exercises improve mobilization of peripheral nerves.

- Approach: Upper extremity nerve glide exercises may target the ulnar, median, or radial nerve. Exercises may include elbow flexion with forearm pronation, tilting the head to one side and stretching the opposite arm to the side with the elbow and wrist extended, and tilting the head to one side and stretching the opposite arm to the side with the wrist flexed. These exercises may be repeated for a few months.

- Precautions: Sharp pain may result from abnormal gliding through the surrounding sheath.

- Significance: Nerve glide exercises can help reduce discomfort.

UNIT 3-58 INTERVENTION

LOW VISION INTERVENTION STRATEGIES

The client's primary diagnosis may not be low vision, but many clients experience low vision and would benefit from a few of the strategies listed. A multicomponent intervention and multiple training sessions for the use of adaptive devices and techniques are recommended.

Refer the client to an optometrist, ophthalmologist, neuro-ophthalmologist, or an occupational therapist with a specialty in low vision whenever appropriate.[50]

STRATEGY	RECOMMENDATIONS[23,50,51]
General strategies	• Ask the client if he or she wears glasses, and make sure the client has access to them while in the hospital or facility. • Always announce yourself when walking into the client's room. • Do not move items in the client's room or home without permission, as they may be used as landmarks for the client's navigation or location of other objects. • Use a normal tone of voice when speaking to client. • Educate the client on safety.
Magnification	• Use enlarged print as needed for client education handouts and home exercise programs. • Connect the client with resources for purchasing enlarged print books and accessing built-in programs for enlargement on personal devices. • Ask the pharmacy for large-print labels for medications.

(continued)

LOW VISION INTERVENTION STRATEGIES (CONTINUED)

STRATEGY	RECOMMENDATIONS[23,50,51]
Lighting	• Ensure appropriate lighting during therapy treatment sessions. • Add floor lamps or task-specific lighting throughout the home. If possible, position lighting to come from the side to reduce glare. Otherwise, place the light source behind the client. • The therapist may want to recommend installing under-cabinet lighting in the kitchen and motion-sensitive lighting along pathways leading to the bathroom to help prevent falls. • Consider that halogen bulbs are hotter than other light sources and should be used with caution to prevent burns in clients with low vision.
Contrast	• Add colored tape to distinguish hospital call buttons, doorways, the edge of steps, light switches, or counters. • Use items such as colored dining place mats or colored bathroom towels to increase visibility during daily occupations. • Avoid patterned floors or tablecloths, as items on top may be difficult for the client to distinguish.
Adaptive devices	• Optical devices should always be prescribed by an optometrist. • Many adaptive devices are designed for clients with low vision. • Connect the client with local resources to view these devices or research specific needs: ◦ For example, low vision aids for clients with diabetes might include a talking blood glucose monitor.
Organization	• Reduce cluttered workspaces to help locate items, and identify and organize clothes with labels: ◦ For example, label dark blue vs black clothing. Remove cluttered pathways and floor rugs to prevent falls.

(continued)

UNIT 3-59 INTERVENTION

Low Vision Intervention Strategies (Continued)	
Strategy	**Recommendations**[23,50,51]
Sensory substitution	• Add tactile raised markers for the start buttons and preferred settings on microwaves, dishwashers, and laundry machines. • Tactile cues, such as rubber bands, can help the client identify pill bottles. • Voice-output adaptive devices or text-to-speech programs may be used as necessary.
Scanning	• Scanning may be used for peripheral visual field loss, hemianopsia, and hemi-inattention. • The lighthouse scanning strategy involves the client visualizing a lighthouse that sweeps from one side to the other. • The anchor scanning strategy may involve a colored line on the left side of the page or cues to scan toward an object. • The client should practice scanning for items while walking down the hallway.
Eccentric viewing (central scotoma)	• Eccentric viewing may be used for clients with central scotoma. Help the client become aware of the scotoma. Oftentimes, the body's visual system fills in space, and it is difficult to understand why things disappear and reappear. • A clock face or other method may be used to teach the client to voluntarily position his or her eye to look above, below, or to the side in order to visualize the target straight ahead.

UNIT 3-59 INTERVENTION

VESTIBULAR REHABILITATION

Treatment strategies for management of dizziness include fall prevention; education; passive movements and maneuvers; and balance, visual, and vestibular exercises. The chosen intervention is dependent on the underlying cause of dizziness. The goals of vestibular rehabilitation should minimize fall risk and maximize participation in functional daily activities.[1]

CENTRAL DIZZINESS INTERVENTIONS[1]	PERIPHERAL DIZZINESS INTERVENTIONS[1]
• Provide an ADL handout to minimize the potential for injury. • Refer the client to neurology. • Request vestibular rehabilitation, as exercise can make symptoms tolerable. • Provide an eye patch if the client has diplopia. • Make discharge recommendations. • Provide durable medical equipment or adaptive devices.	• Provide an ADL handout to minimize the potential for injury. • Refer the client to ear, nose, and throat doctor, or physical therapist. • Request vestibular rehabilitation such as BPPV, Brand-Daroff desensitization exercises, or an occupational therapist with vestibular training. • Make discharge recommendations. • Provide durable medical equipment or adaptive devices.

(continued)

VESTIBULAR REHABILITATION (CONTINUED)

VESTIBULAR INTERVENTION STRATEGIES

Strategy	Description
Fall prevention and dizziness education[1]	• It is recommended that the client sit whenever possible during toileting, bathing, grooming, cooking, and other ADLs. • The client should not drive while experiencing symptoms of dizziness. • The client should avoid rapid changes in head position, including leaning over to dress, bathe, or reach for items. • Adaptive equipment, such as a reacher, sock aid, transfer tub bench, long shoehorn, raised toilet seat, or handheld showerhead, may be beneficial for completing self-care activities. • The client's floor should be clear of obstacles or rugs that may result in falls.
Passive movements and maneuvers[1]	• For clients with BPPV, a trained therapist may use passive movements of the head to move loose stones out of the semicircular canals. • The therapist may educate clients on these positioning techniques. • Maneuvers for treating BPPV include the Canalith Repositioning Maneuver, Brandt-Daroff exercises, Liberatory/Semont's Maneuver, BBQ Roll, Casani Maneuver, and Modified Gufoni Maneuver. • In one study of elderly individuals, in which 36% of the sample reported dizziness, 11% were found to have BPPV.[52]

(continued)

VESTIBULAR REHABILITATION (CONTINUED)	
Strategy	Description
Balance exercises[1,53]	• Sitting balance exercises can range from static sitting on the mat to dynamic sitting that includes weight shifting and reaching. • Standing balance exercises can include weight shifting, standing on one leg, and marching in place. • Dynamic ambulation may include walking backward, walking heel to toe, and catching or kicking a ball while walking.
Visual and vestibular exercises[1]	• The client focuses on an object while performing vertical and/or horizontal head turns. • The client focuses on objects such as street signs while riding in a moving car. • The client passes a ball back and forth with another person while moving in a circle.
Grading activities[1]	• Consider altering the base of support: ◦ This includes altering the size of the base of support, static or dynamic balance requirements, stability of the surface, and client's position. For example, carpet, balance boards, and uneven terrain all provide different support surfaces. • Incorporate therapy balls or stairs. • Ask the client to perform the activity with eyes open or closed, with increased head motion, or while using a mirror.

UNIT 3-60 INTERVENTION

PAIN MANAGEMENT	
Occupational therapy can help clients manage their pain in various ways. Agent modalities are beneficial for treating nociceptor pain, while chronic pain can be managed by a number of strategies that involve physical and psychological interventions.[54]	
CRPS treatments[55]	• Stress loading • Contrast bath • Edema gloves, icing, elevation • Electrical stimulation, ultrasound • Fluidotherapy • Active and passive range of motion instruction • Pharmacologic intervention Refer to Section Four, Unit 3-74, for information about physical agent modalities.
Nonpharmacologic interventions[56]	• Comfort measures • Position change • Massage • Application of hot and cold • Adaptive devices • Transcutaneous electrical nerve stimulation • Surgical intervention
Cognitive behavioral interventions[56]	• Relaxation exercises • Guided imagery • Distraction • Complementary and alternative medicine
Occupational therapist's role in chronic pain management[57]	• Help clients recognize sources and triggers of increased pain. • Teach strategies to reduce duration and frequency of pain. • Reduce reliance on pain medications by implementing alternate pain management strategies. • Work with team members to select the best course of treatment. • Make adaptive equipment recommendations to reduce pain.

UNIT 3–61 INTERVENTION

COMMON SPLINTS FOR THE PERIPHERAL NERVOUS SYSTEM

Refer to Section Four, Unit 3-77, for information about orthotic guidelines.

CONDITION	TYPICAL SPLINTS USED	WEARING GUIDELINES
Carpal tunnel syndrome[55]	• A wrist immobilization splint should be used to hold the wrist in a neutral position and allow for full metacarpophalangeal and thumb movement. • Do not block the distal palmar crease or thenar eminence.	The splint can be used at night and with activities that irritate the median nerve in order to reduce the pressure on the nerve. During a flare-up stage, the client should wear the splint for 4 to 6 weeks. The splint may be removed temporarily for hygiene or exercise. Follow the surgeon's wearing schedule after surgery.
CRPS[55]	• Wrist immobilization splints should hold the wrist in a functional position or in a resting hand position	The splint should be worn during functional activities as needed to prevent pain.
Cubital tunnel syndrome[55]	• An elbow immobilization splint should hold the elbow in 30 to 45 degrees of extension as a volar splint.	The splint should be worn at night. Discuss positioning during daily activities with the client.
Radial nerve injury (wrist drop)[55]	• A wrist immobilization splint should position the wrist in 15 to 30 degrees of extension to improve function. • The metacarpophalangeal and thumb joints should maintain an extended position. • A dynamic splint may be used to increase finger extension.	A dynamic splint should be worn during the day, while a wrist immobilization static splint can be worn during the day or night.

UNIT 3-62 INTERVENTION

PERIPHERAL NERVOUS SYSTEM PRECAUTIONS AND CONTRAINDICATIONS	
PAIN CONDITIONS	
Cognitive status[58]	• Assess the client's cognitive status to ensure that any pain assessments and treatments are based on accurate client reports.
General precautions[58]	• Clients may avoid daily activities due to pain. • Addiction or abuse of pain medication may occur.
CRPS[58]	• Avoid using manual techniques, dynamic splinting, and casting during phase I as they may exacerbate pain symptoms • Check for pain and swelling if using splints • Introduce activities slowly. Be mindful about any increase in pain, swelling, or reduced circulation.
Back pain[58]	• Maintain BLT (bending, lifting, or twisting) precautions: no bending, lifting, or twisting the spine. • With acute back pain, the client should avoid prolonged bed rest and spinal tractions. • Clients with osteoporosis or disk disorders should be careful with spinal tractions.
Modalities[58]	• Follow precautions for modalities. Refer to Section Four, Unit 3-74, for information on physical agent modality precautions.

(continued)

PERIPHERAL NERVOUS SYSTEM PRECAUTIONS AND CONTRAINDICATIONS (CONTINUED)

LOSS OF SENSATION

Be aware of safety risks for injury or burns, and check the skin regularly in clients with loss of sensation.[58]

VISION

Fall risk[58]	• Clients with low vision are at an increased risk for falling. • Falling may result in an injury.

Retinal detachment[59,60]	• Be aware that retinal detachment is a medical emergency because cells can die quickly.
	• An emergency referral to the eye doctor is necessary if the client reports any of the following issues:
	  ◦ Distortion or wavy lines
	  ◦ Floaters
	  ◦ Bright light flashes
	  ◦ Sharp eye pain
	  ◦ Light sensitivity

VESTIBULAR AND DIZZINESS

Dizziness[58]	• Clients with dizziness are at an increased risk of falls.
BPPV[58]	• Clients should maintain a level position of the head for 48 hours following maneuvers. • Clients should sleep supine at a 45-degree angle for 2 nights.

UNIT 3-63 INTERVENTION

REFERENCES

1. Hamby JR. Appendix H: the dizzy patient. In: H. Smith-Gabai, ed. *Occupational Therapy in Acute Care*. Bethesda, MD: AOTA Pres; 2011:638-647.

2. Cohen HS. Specialized knowledge and skills in adult vestibular rehabilitation for occupational therapy practice. *Am J Occup Ther*. 2001;55(6):661-665. doi:10.5014/ajot.60.6.669

3. Lundy-Ekman L. *Neuroscience: Fundamentals for Rehabilitation*. 4th ed. St. Louis, Mo: Elsevier Saunders; 2013.

4. Bodranghien F, Bastian A, Casali C, et al. Consensus paper: revisiting the symptoms and signs of cerebellar syndrome. *Cerebellum*. 2016;15(3):369-391. doi:10.1007/s12311-015-0687-3

5. Jevon P. *Treating the Critical Care Patient*. Oxford, United Kingdom: Blackwell Publishing; 2007.

6. Bersten AD, Soni N. *Oh's Intensive Care Manual*. 5th ed. London, United Kingdom: Butterworth-Heinemann; 2003.

7. American Pain Society. Pain: current understanding of assessment, management, and treatments. American Pain Society. http://americanpainsociety.org/uploads/education/npc.pdf. Accessed April 26, 2019.

8. International Association for the Study of Pain. IASP terminology. https://www.iasp-pain.org/Education/Content.aspx?ItemNumber=1698. Updated December 14, 2017. Accessed April 26, 2019.

9. Acerra NE, Souvlis T, Moseley GL. Stroke, complex regional pain syndrome and phantom limb pain: can commonalities direct future management? *J Rehabil Med*. 2007;39(2):109-114. doi:10.2340/16501977-0027

10. Kirshblum SC. International standards for neurologic classification of spinal cord injury. *J Spin Cord Med*. 2011;34(6):535-546. doi:10.1179/204577211X13207446293695

11. Total Life Care Compounding by Lake Side Pharmacy. Printable dermatome chart. http://tlccrx.com/resources/printable-dermatome-chart/. Published 2016. Accessed April 26, 2019.

12. Gaubet CS, Mockett SP. Inter-rater reliability of the Nottingham method of stereognosis assessment. *Clin Rehabil*. 2000;14(2):153-159. doi:10.1191/026921500677422368

13. Ng CL, Ho DD, Chow SP. The Moberg pickup test: results of testing with a standard protocol. *J Hand Ther*. 1999;12:309-312. doi:10.1016/S0894-1130(99)80069-6

14. Damodaran O, Rizk E, Rodriguez J, Lee G. Cranial nerve assessment: a concise guide to clinical examination. *Clin Anat*. 2014;27(1):25-30. doi:10.1002/ca.22336

15. Gutman SA. The cranial nerves. In: *Quick Reference Neuroscience for Rehabilitation Professionals: The Essential Neurologic Principles Underlying Rehabilitation Practice*. 3rd ed. Thorofare, NJ: SLACK Incorporated; 2017:68-98.

16. Cohen HS. Specialized knowledge and skills in adult vestibular rehabilitation for occupational therapy practice. *Am J Occup Ther*. 2001;55(6):661-665. doi:10.5014/ajot.60.6.669

17. Ardiç FN, Tümkaya F, Akdag B, Senol H. The subscales and short forms of the dizziness handicap inventory: are they useful for comparison of the patient groups? *Disabil Rehabil*. 2017;39(20):2119-2122. doi:10.1080/09638288.2016.1219923

18. Agrawal Y, Carey JP, Hoffman HJ, Sklare DA, Schubert MC. The modified Romberg balance test: normative data in U.S. adults. *Otol Neurotol*. 2011;32(8):1309-1311. doi:10.1097/MAO.0b013e1822e5bee

19. Berg KO, Wood-Dauphinee SL, Williams JI, Maki B. Measuring balance in the elderly: validation of an instrument. *Can J Public Health*. 1992;82(suppl 2):S7-S11.

20. Powell LE, Myers AM. The activities-specific balance confidence (ABC) scale. *J Gerontol A Biol Sci Med Sci.* 1995;50A(1): M28-M34. doi:10.1093/gerona/50A.1.M28

21. Wrisley DM, Marchetti GF, Kuharsky DK, Whitney SL. Reliability, internal consistency, and validity of data obtained with the functional gait assessment. *Phys Ther.* 2004;84:906-918.

22. Shumway-Cook A, Baldwin M, Polissar NL, Gruber W. Predicting the probability for falls in community dwelling older adults. *Phys Ther.* 1997;77(8):812-819.

23. American Optometric Association. Low vision. American Optometric Association. https://www.aoa.org/patients-and-public/caring-for-your-vision/low-vision. Updated 2018. Accessed April 26, 2019.

24. Whittaker SG, Scheiman M, Sokol-McKay DA. *Low Vision Rehabilitation: A Practical Guide for Occupational Therapists.* 2nd ed. Thorofare, NJ: SLACK Incorporated; 2016.

25. Hyvärinen L. LEA vision test system for assessment and screening. LEA-Test Ltd. http://www.lea-test.fi/en/vistests/instruct/LEA_Vision_Test_System.pdf. Accessed April 26, 2019.

26. Mansfield JS, Ahn SJ, Legge GE, Leubeker A. A new reading acuity chart for normal and low vision. In: Ophthalmic Visual Optics/Non-Invasive Assessment of the Visual System. *OSA Technical Digest, 3.* Washington, DC: Optical Society of America; 1993:232-535.

27. MacKeben M, Nair UKW, Walker LL, Fletcher DC. Random word recognition chart helps scotoma assessment in low vision. *Optom Vis Sci.* 2015;92(4):421-428. doi:10.1097/OPX.0000000000000548

28. Trobe JD, Acosta PC, Krischer JP, Trick GL. Confrontation visual field techniques in the detection of anterior visual pathway lesions. *Ann Neurol.* 1981;10(1):28-34. doi:10.1002/ana.410100105

29. Warren M. *Brain Injury Visual Assessment Battery for Adults Test Manual.* Birmingham, AL: visAbilitiesRehabServices; 1998.

30. Hawker GA, Mian S, Kendzerska T, French M. Measures of adult pain: visual analog scale of pain (VAS pain), numeric rating scale for pain (NRS pain), McGill pain questionnaire (MPQ), short-form McGill pain questionnaire (SF-MPQ), chronic pain grade scale (CPGS), short form-36 bodily pain scale (SF-36 BPS), and measure of intermittent and constant osteoarthritis pain (ICOAP). *Arthritis Care Res (Honoken).* 2011;63(suppl 11):S240-S252. doi:10.1002/acr.20543

31. Melzack R. The McGill pain questionnaire: major properties and scoring methods. *Pain.* 1975;1(3):277-299.

32. Roach KE, Budiman-Mak E, Songsiridej N, Lertratanakul Y. Development of a shoulder pain and disability index. *Arthritis Care Res.* 1991;4(4)143-149.

33. Tracey EH, Greene AJ, Doty RL. Optimizing reliability and sensitivity of Semmes-Weinstein monofilaments for establishing point tactile thresholds. *Physiol Behav.* 2012;105(4):982-986. doi:10.1016/j.physbeh.2011.11.002

34. Dellon ES, Keller KM, Moratz V, Dellon AL. Validation of cutaneous pressure threshold measurements for the evaluation of hand function. *Ann Plast Surg.* 1997;38(5):485-492.

35. Rubinstein SM, Pool JJM, Tulder MW, Riphagen II, Vet HCW. A systematic review of the diagnostic accuracy of provocative tests of the neck for diagnosing cervical radiculopathy. *Eur Spine J.* 2007;16(3):307-319. doi:10.1007/s00586-006-022506

36. Konin JG, Wiksten DL, Isear JA, Brader H. *Special Tests for Orthopedic Examination.* Thorofare, NJ: SLACK Incorporated; 2006.

37. Davidson RI, Dunn EJ, Metzmaker JN. The shoulder abduction test in the diagnosis of radicular pain in cervical extradural compressive monoradiculopathies. *Spine.* 1981;6(5):441-446.

38. Wainner RS, Gill H. Diagnosis and nonoperative management of cervical radiculopathy. *J Ortho Sports Phys Ther.* 2000;30(12):728-744. doi:10.2519/jospt.2000.30.12.728

39. Malanga GA, Nadler S. *Musculoskeletal Physical Examination: An Evidence-Based Approach.* Philadelphia, PA: Mosby Elsevier; 2005:51.

40. Sanders RJ, Hammond SL, Rao NM. Diagnosis of thoracic outlet syndrome. *J Vasc Surg.* 2007;46(3):601-604. doi:10.1016/j.jvs.2007.04.050

41. Scaia V, Baxter D, Cook C. The pain provocation-based straight leg raise test for diagnosis of lumbar disc herniation, lumbar radiculopathy, and/or sciatica: a systematic review of clinical utility. *J Back Musculoskelet Rehabil.* 2002;25(4):215-223. doi:10.3233/BMR-2012-0339

42. Kuschner SH, Ebramzadeh E, Mitchell S. Evaluation of elbow flexion and Tinel tests for cubital tunnel syndrome in asymptomatic individuals. *Orthopedics.* 2006;29(4):305-308. doi:10.3928/01477447-20060401-06

43. Novak CM, Gilbert WL, Mackinnon SE, Lay L. Provocative testing for cubital tunnel syndrome. *J Hand Surg Am.* 1994;19(5):817-820. doi:10.1016/0363-5023(94)90193-7

44. Durkan JA. A new diagnostic test for carpal tunnel syndrome. *J Bone Joint Surg Am.* 1991;73(4):535-538.

45. MacDermid JC, Wessel J. Clinical diagnosis of carpal tunnel syndrome: a systematic review. *J Hand Ther.* 2004;17(2):309-319. doi:10.1197/j.jht.2004.02.015

46. Wartenberg R. A sign of ulnar nerve palsy. *JAMA.* 1939;112(17):1688. doi:10.1001/jama.1939.62800170002011a

47. Goldman SB, Brininger TL, Schrader JW, Curtis R, Koceja DM. Analysis of clinical motor testing for adult patients with diagnosed ulnar neuropathy at the elbow. *Arch Phys Med Rehabil.* 2009;90:1846-1852. doi:10.1016/j.apmr.2009.06.007

48. Goransson I, Cederlund R. A study of the effect of desensitization on hyperaesthesia in the hand and upper extremity after injury or surgery. *Hand Ther.* 2011;16(1):12-18. doi:10.1258/ht.2010.010023

49. Fitzgibbons P, Medvedev G. Functional and clinical outcomes of upper extremity amputation. *J Am Acad Orthop Surg.* 2015;12(23):751-760. doi:10.5435/JAAOS-D-14-00302

50. Kim SD. Efficacy of tendon and nerve gliding exercises for carpal tunnel syndrome: a systematic review of randomized controlled trials. *J Phys Ther Sci.* 2015;27(8):2645-2648. doi:10.1589/jpts.27.2645

51. Berger S. Effectiveness of occupational therapy interventions for older adults living with low vision. *Am J Occup Ther.* 2013;67:263-265. doi:10.5014/ajot.2013.007203

52. Liu CJ, Brost MA, Horton VE, Kenyon SB, Mears KE. Occupational therapy interventions to improve performance of daily activities at home for older adults with low vision: a systematic review. *Am J Occup Ther.* 2013;67:279-287. doi:10.5014/ajot.2013.005512

53. Kollén L, Frändin K, Möller M, Fagevik Olsén M, Möller C. Benign paroxysmal positional vertigo is a common cause of dizziness and unsteadiness in a large population of 75-year-olds. *Aging Clin Exp Res.* 2012;24(4):317-323.

54. Shahanawaz SD, Rathod PV. Adding visual and proprioceptive exercises to dizziness caused by BPPV: a randomized clinical trial. *Indian J Physiother Occup Ther.* 2015;9(4):235. doi:10.5958/0973-5674.2015.00178.1

55. McCormack GL. Pain management by occupational therapists. *Am J Occup Ther.* 1988;42:582-590. doi:10.5014/ajot.42.9.582

56. Smith-Gabai H, Holm SE. *Occupational Therapy in Acute Care.* 2nd ed. Bethesda, MD: AOTA Press; 2017:638-647.

57. American Occupational Therapy Association. Managing chronic pain: tips for living. American Occupational Therapy Association. https://static1.squarespace.com/static/5445aed2e4b010eb77c0fdfe/t/5660647de4b066b69a9364ce/1449157757146/Chronic+Pain.pdf. Revised December 2002. Accessed June 17, 2019.

58. Coppard BM, Lohman H. *Introduction to Orthotics: A Clinical Reasoning and Problem-Solving Approach.* 4th ed. St. Louis, MO: Elsevier Mosby; 2015.

59. Reed KL. *Quick Reference to Occupational Therapy.* 3rd ed. Austin, TX: Pro-Ed; 2014.

60. National Eye Institute. Facts about retinal detachment. National Institutes of Health. https://nei.nih.gov/health/retinaldetach/retinaldetach. Updated October 2009. Accessed April 26, 2019.

SECTION FOUR

Musculoskeletal System

Sit W, Neville M.
Handbook of Occupational Therapy for
Adults With Physical Disabilities (pp 283-369).
© 2020 SLACK Incorporated.

CASE

DIAGNOSIS: HETEROTOPIC OSSIFICATION DUE TO BURNS

At the start of each spring semester in the occupational therapy program where I teach, I like to ask my students the question, "Can a patient without hands feed themselves?" Most students respond "No," assuming that it is not possible. Unfailingly, I always then proceed to share a story that changes their minds.

This story is about a client I treated (we will call her Mary) at an inpatient rehabilitation hospital. Mary was a middle-aged woman and mom to a 3-year-old daughter. Unfortunately, Mary was the victim of a crime committed at her home: a man broke in, igniting a fire while Mary was inside a parked car in the garage. As a result, 90% of her body was covered in burns, and her face and body were now disfigured. Heterotopic ossification occurred in both her arms, leaving Mary unable to bend her elbows.

I decided to construct an adaptive splint to help Mary's occupational performance, so she could perhaps once again groom and feed herself. I created a soft brace positioned on Mary's bicep, and I constructed a detachable extension made of splinting material that could be attached to the brace with Velcro. The extension, when attached, reached from the anterior-medial side of the brace toward Mary's face. The free end of the extension could be exchanged to hold different objects: eating utensils, a toothbrush, or, as Mary would choose, something else entirely.

With the aid of the adaptive device and without the use of her hands, Mary could flex and horizontally adduct her shoulder to bring objects to her mouth. Once the brace was positioned on her bicep, I asked Mary if she would like to try brushing her teeth or eating. Her answer surprised me. "No," she said, "I want to put on lipstick." Having not seen her daughter in three months, Mary was concerned that her appearance might frighten her daughter. So, that is just what we did: Mary used the adaptive device to apply lipstick.

I will always remember Mary's story because it exemplifies the meaning behind occupations. Occupational therapy helped Mary apply lipstick on her own, so she could see her daughter again with greater confidence and peace of mind.

MYOTOMES

Myotomes refer to a group of muscles that are innervated by a shared spinal nerve.[1]

SPINAL NERVE	MOVEMENT[1]
C1/C2	Neck flexion and extension
C3	Neck lateral flexion
C4	Shoulder elevation
C5 C5/6	Shoulder abduction by the middle deltoid Elbow flexion by the biceps
C6	Wrist extension by extensor carpi radialis
C7	Elbow extension by the triceps Wrist flexion by the flexor carpi radialis (FCR) and flexor carpi ulnaris (FCU)
C8	Finger flexion by the flexor digitorum superficialis (FDS)
T1	Finger abduction by the dorsal interossei
L2	Hip flexion by the iliopsoas
L3	Knee extension by the quadriceps
L4	Ankle dorsiflexion by the anterior tibialis
L5	Great toe extension by the extensor hallucis longus
S1	Ankle plantarflexion by the gastrocnemius Ankle eversion Hip extension
S2	Knee flexion

MUSCLE FUNCTIONS

JOINT MOTION	KEY MUSCLES[2]	FUNCTIONAL MOVEMENT[3]
Shoulder		
Flexion	• Anterior deltoid • Pectoralis major • Biceps brachii • Coracobrachialis	• Reaching up to open a cabinet • Hanging clothes in the closet
Extension	• Posterior deltoid • Latissimus dorsi • Teres major • Pectoralis major • Triceps (long head)	• Reaching behind to pull luggage • Bringing a bowling ball back behind to bowl
Horizontal abduction	• Posterior deltoid	• Pulling open a door handle • Shooting a bow and arrow
Horizontal adduction	• Anterior deltoid • Pectoralis major	• Putting on earrings • Brushing teeth • Applying deodorant
Abduction	• Deltoid • Supraspinatus	• Shampooing hair • Putting on coat sleeves
Adduction	• Latissimus dorsi • Teres major • Infraspinatus • Teres minor • Pectoralis major • Triceps (long head) • Coracobrachialis	• Holding a purse at the side • Holding a book under the arm against the side
External rotation (lateral)	• Posterior deltoid • Infraspinatus • Teres minor	• Brushing the back of the hair
Internal rotation (medial)	• Anterior deltoid • Latissimus dorsi • Teres major • Subscapularis • Pectoralis major	• Tucking in a shirt • Clasping a bra *(continued)*

UNIT 1–66 NEED TO KNOW

MUSCLE FUNCTIONS (CONTINUED)		
JOINT MOTION	KEY MUSCLES[2]	FUNCTIONAL MOVEMENT[3]
Scapula		
Elevation	• Upper trapezius • Rhomboid major • Rhomboid minor • Levator scapula	• Shrugging the shoulders
Depression	• Lower trapezius • Serratus anterior • Pectoralis minor	• Pushing up from a surface (eg, using a sliding board) • Reaching into pockets
Protraction/ abduction	• Serratus anterior • Pectoralis minor	• Lifting weights in supine • Throwing a snowball across a field
Retraction/ adduction	• Middle trapezius • Rhomboid major • Rhomboid minor	• Climbing a rock wall • Scratching mid-back
Upward rotation	• Upper and lower trapezius • Serratus anterior	• Hiking one shoulder with a backpack strap on
Downward rotation	• Rhomboid major • Rhomboid minor • Levator scapula • Pectoralis minor	• Putting down a backpack from shoulders
Elbow		

Flexion	• Biceps brachii
	• Brachialis
	• Brachioradialis
	• Assistance from:
	  ○ FCR
	  ○ FCU
	  ○ Palmaris longus
	  ○ Pronator teres
	  ○ ECRL
	  ○ ECRB
		• Bicep curls
		• Bringing eating utensils to the mouth

(continued)

Muscle Functions (continued)

Joint Motion	Key Muscles[2]	Functional Movement[3]
Extension	• Triceps (all heads) • Anconeus	• Reaching for an item on a shelf • Pulling off pants
Supination of forearm	• Biceps brachii • Supinator • Assistance from: ○ Brachioradialis	• Turning a doorknob or key • Applying shampoo to a hand or obtaining hand soap
Pronation of forearm	• Pronator teres • Pronator quadratus • Assistance from: ○ Brachioradialis	• Turning a doorknob or key • Stabilizing a piece of paper • Typing on a keyboard • Playing the piano
Wrist		

Flexion	• FCR
	• FCU
	• Palmaris longus
	• FDS
	• Assistance from:
	   ○ FDP
	   ○ FPL
		• Pouring a drink
		• Holding an object, such as a book, toward you

Extension	• ECRL
	• ECRB
	• ECU
	• Assistance from:
	   ○ Extensor digitorum
	   ○ Extensor indicis
		• Using a tenodesis grip
		• Scratching back of neck
		• Scooping ice cream

(continued)

MUSCLE FUNCTIONS (CONTINUED)		
JOINT MOTION	KEY MUSCLES[2]	FUNCTIONAL MOVEMENT[3]
Radial deviation/ abduction	• ECRL • ECRB • EPL • EPB • FCR • APL	• Waving • Opening a jar
Ulnar deviation/ adduction	• ECU • FCU	• Waving • Opening a jar
Digits 2 to 5		

Flexion (MCP, PIP, and DIP)	• FDS
	• FDP
	• Flexor digiti minimi brevis (fifth)
	• Lumbricals
	• Assistance from:
	  ○ Dorsal interossei (second to fourth)
	  ○ Palmar interossei (second, fourth, and fifth)
		• Making a fist
		• Carrying a mug
		• Holding a fork

Extension (MCP, PIP, and DIP)	• Extensor digitorum
	• Lumbricals
	• Extensor indicis (second)
	• Assistance from:
	  ○ Dorsal interossei (second to fourth)
	  ○ Palmar interossei (second, fourth, and fifth)
		• Typing, such as reaching the keys on a keyboard
		• Releasing objects held in a hand

Abduction (MCP)	• Dorsal interossei (second to fourth) • Abductor digiti minimi (fifth)	• Positioning the hand to paint the nails • Reaching across a keyboard

(continued)

Muscle Functions (continued)		
Joint Motion	Key Muscles[2]	Functional Movement[3]
Adduction (MCP)	• Palmar interossei (second, fourth, and fifth) • Extensor indicis (second)	• Holding out the hand to receive an item • Scooping water into the hands
Thumb		

Flexion (CMC and MCP)	• FPL
	• FPB
	• Assistance from:
	  ◦ Adductor pollicis
	  ◦ Palmar interossei (first)
		• Texting
		• Holding ski poles

Extension (CMC and MCP)	• EPL • EPB • APL • Assistance from: ◦ Palmar interossei (first)	• Giving a thumbs-up

Opposition (CMC and MCP)	• Opponens pollicis
	• Assistance from:
	  ◦ FPB
	  ◦ APB
		• Holding items in your hand

Abduction (CMC and MCP)	• APL • APB	• Making an OK sign
Adduction (CMC and MCP)	• Adductor pollicis • Palmar interossei (first)	• Giving a salute

(continued)

Muscle Functions (continued)

Joint Motion	Key Muscles[2]	Functional Movement[3]
Vertebral Column		
Flexion	• Rectus abdominis • External oblique • Internal oblique • Psoas major • Iliacus	• Doing sit-ups • Bending to put on one's shoes

Extension	• Longissimus
	• Iliocostalis
	• Multifidi
	• Rotatores
	• Semispinalis capitis
	• Spinalis
	• Interspinales
	• Intertransversarii
	• Assistance from:
	   ◦ Quadratus lumborum
	   ◦ Latissimus dorsi (when arm is fixed)
		• Bridging in bed
		• Sitting up straight
		• Standing up

Rotation	• External oblique (opposite side) • Internal oblique (same side) • Multifidi (opposite side) • Rotatores (opposite side)	• Turning to look behind you while sitting • Kayaking

(continued)

MUSCLE FUNCTIONS (CONTINUED)

JOINT MOTION	KEY MUSCLES[2]	FUNCTIONAL MOVEMENT[3]

Lateral flexion	• Iliocostalis
	• External oblique
	• Internal oblique
	• Longissimus
	• Quadratus lumborum
	• Intertransversarii
	• Spinalis
	• Assistance from:
	   ◦ Psoas major
	   ◦ Latissimus dorsi
		• Transferring to or from a car
		• Stretching to one side

Neck (Cervical Spine)

JOINT MOTION	KEY MUSCLES[2]	FUNCTIONAL MOVEMENT[3]
Flexion	• Sternocleidomastoid • Anterior scalene • Longus capitis • Longus colli	• Looking down at the feet when walking up stairs • Looking down to button a shirt

Extension	• Upper trapezius
	• Levator scapula
	• Splenius capitis
	• Splenius cervicis
	• Rectus capitis posterior major
	• Rectus capitis posterior minor
	• Oblique capitis superior
	• Semispinalis capitis
	• Multifidi
	• Rotatores
	• Intertransversarii
	• Interspinales
	• Assistance from:
	   ◦ Longissimus capitis
	   ◦ Longissimus cervicis
	   ◦ Iliocostalis cervicis
		• Leaning the head back to look up
		• Nodding the head to indicate "yes"

(continued)

MUSCLE FUNCTIONS (CONTINUED)		
JOINT MOTION	KEY MUSCLES[2]	FUNCTIONAL MOVEMENT[3]
Rotation	• Levator scapula • Splenius capitis • Splenius cervicis • Rectus capitis posterior major • Oblique capitis inferior • Longus colli • Longus capitis • Longissimus cervicis • Iliocostalis cervicis • Upper trapezius (opposite side) • Sternocleidomastoid (opposite side) • Scalenes (opposite side) • Multifidi (opposite side) • Rotatores (opposite side) • Assistance from: ○ Longissimus capitis	• Turning the head to look over the shoulder when driving or while backing out • Shaking the head to indicate "no"
		(continued)

MUSCLE FUNCTIONS (CONTINUED)

JOINT MOTION	KEY MUSCLES[2]	FUNCTIONAL MOVEMENT[3]

Lateral Flexion	• Upper trapezius
	• Levator scapula
	• Sternocleidomastoid
	• Scalenes
	• Splenius capitis
	• Splenius cervicis
	• Longus capitis
	• Longus colli
	• Oblique capitis superior
	• Intertransversarii
	• Assistance from:
	   ○ Longissimus capitis
	   ○ Longissimus cervicis
	   ○ Iliocostalis cervicis
		• Putting in ear drops

APB: abductor pollicis brevis; APL: abductor pollicis longus; CMC: carpometacarpal; DIP: distal interphalangeal; ECRB: extensor carpi radialis brevis; ECRL: extensor carpi radialis longus; ECU: extensor carpi ulnaris; EPB: extensor pollicis brevis; EPL: extensor pollicis longus; FDP: flexor digitorum profundus; FPB: flexor pollicis brevis; FPL: flexor pollicis longus; MCP: metacarpophalangeal; PIP: proximal interphalangeal.

UNIT 2-67 EVALUATION

COMMON ASSESSMENTS ACROSS PRACTICE SETTINGS

ASSESSMENT	ACUTE	INPATIENT	HOME HEALTH	SNF	OUTPATIENT
Common Assessments Across Practice Settings					
Timed Up and Go	✓	✓			✓
Berg Balance Scale		✓			✓
Arm Motor Ability Test		✓			✓
Quick Disabilities of the Arm, Shoulder and Hand		✓			✓
Oswestry Low Back Pain Disability Questionnaire					✓
Grip and pinch strength	✓	✓			✓
Range of Motion	✓	✓	✓	✓	✓
Manual Muscle Testing Guidelines	✓	✓	✓	✓	✓
Dexterity and Coordination Assessments					
Box and Blocks Test		✓			✓
Jebsen-Taylor Hand Function Test					
Minnesota Manual Dexterity Test					
Nine-Hole Peg Test					
Purdue Pegboard Test					
Provocative Tests					
External rotation lag sign		✓			✓
Empty Can Test					
Neer Impingement Test					
Hawkins–Kennedy Test					

(continued)

COMMON ASSESSMENTS ACROSS PRACTICE SETTINGS (CONTINUED)

ASSESSMENT	ACUTE	INPATIENT	HOME HEALTH	SNF	OUTPATIENT
Speed test		✓			✓
Drop arm test					
Cozen's test					
Finklestein's test					
Murphy's sign					
Flexion, abduction, and external rotation test (Patrick's test)					
Grind (scouring) test					
Piriformis test					
Click test					
Anterior labral tear test					
Resisted straight leg raise test					
McMurray's test					
Apley's test					
Patellar apprehension test					
Clarke's sign					
Noble Compression Test					
Anterior drawer test					
Talar tilt test					

SNF: skilled nursing facility.

(continued)

Common Assessments Across Practice Settings (continued)

Timed Up and Go[4]

- Purpose: Assesses mobility, balance, and walking ability
- Context: Clients across diagnoses and who are elderly in inpatient and outpatient settings
- Format: Timed, performance-based test
- Time to administer: 3 minutes
- Materials: Armchair and stopwatch
- Cost: Free
- Website: https://www.cdc.gov/steadi/pdf/TUG_Test-print.pdf

Berg Balance Scale[5]

Refer to Section Two, Unit 2-26, for information about the Berg Balance Scale.

Arm Motor Ability Test[6]

Refer Section Two, Unit 2-26, for information about the Arm Motor Ability Test.

Quick Disabilities of the Arm, Shoulder and Hand[7]

- Purpose: Assesses physical function of the upper extremity
- Context: Clients with musculoskeletal disorders of the upper extremity
- Format: Self-report questionnaire
- Time to administer: 10 minutes
- Materials: Questionnaire form and writing utensil
- Cost: Free
- Website: https://www.hss.edu/physician-files/fufa/Fufa-quickdash-questionnaire.pdf

(continued)

COMMON ASSESSMENTS
ACROSS PRACTICE SETTINGS (CONTINUED)

OSWESTRY LOW BACK PAIN DISABILITY QUESTIONNAIRE[8]

- Purpose: Assesses impact of low back pain on functional activities and disability
- Context: Clients with back pain
- Format: Self-report questionnaire
- Time to administer: 3 to 6 minutes
- Materials: Questionnaire form and writing utensil
- Cost: Free
- Website: http://www.rehab.msu.edu/_files/_docs/ oswestry_low_back_disability.pdf

GRIP AND PINCH STRENGTH[9]

- Purpose: Assesses muscular strength of hand
- Context: Clients across diagnoses in acute, inpatient, and outpatient settings
- Format: Physical gauge of strength
- Time to administer: Less than 5 minutes
- Materials: Dynamometer and pinch gauge
- Cost: $360 and up for both
- Website: https://www.protherapysupplies.com/Shop-by-Brand/ Patterson-Medical/Jamar-Hydraulic-Hand-Dynamometer

UNIT 2-67 EVALUATION

UNIT 2-68 EVALUATION

RANGE OF MOTION

Range of motion (ROM) is a measurement of joint function.[10]

Use of a goniometer-based smartphone application has not yet been found to provide accurate measurement of ROM. Thus, use of a physical goniometer device is recommended.[11]

The following chart outlines the normal ROM for movements performed at each joint, the position that the client should be in while measuring ROM, the placement of the fulcrum for measurement, and the normal end feel of the motion.[10]

JOINT	NORMAL ROM	CLIENT POSITION	FULCRUM LOCATION	END FEEL
Shoulder				
Flexion	0 to 180 degrees	Supine or sitting	Lateral acromion process	Firm
Extension/hyperextension	0 to 60 degrees	Prone or sitting	Lateral acromion process	Firm
Abduction	0 to 180 degrees	Sitting	Anterior acromion process	Firm
Adduction	180 to 0 degrees	Sitting	Anterior acromion process	Soft
External rotation	0 to 90 degrees	Prone or sitting	Olecranon process	Firm
Internal rotation	0 to 70 degrees	Prone or sitting	Olecranon process	Firm
Horizontal abduction	0 to 45 degrees	Sitting	Superior acromion process	Firm
Horizontal adduction	0 to 135 degrees	Sitting	Superior acromion process	Firm

(continued)

RANGE OF MOTION (CONTINUED)

JOINT	NORMAL ROM	CLIENT POSITION	FULCRUM LOCATION	END FEEL
Elbow				
Flexion	0 to 135 degrees	Supine or sitting	Lateral epicondyle of humerus	Soft
Extension	135 to 0 degrees	Supine or sitting	Lateral epicondyle of humerus	Firm
Supination	0 to 90 degrees	Sitting	Pisiform	Firm
Pronation	0 to 90 degrees	Sitting	Ulnar styloid process	Hard
Wrist				
Flexion	0 to 80 degrees	Tabletop (supinated)	Ulnar styloid process	Firm
Extension	0 to 70 degrees	Tabletop (pronated)	Ulnar styloid process	Firm
Radial deviation	0 to 20 degrees	Tabletop (pronated)	Base of third metacarpal (MC) over capitate	Hard
Ulnar deviation	0 to 30 degrees	Tabletop (pronated)	Base of third MC over capitate	Firm
Digits and Thumb				
MCP flexion of the finger	0 to 90 degrees	Tabletop (neutral)	Dorsal MCP of the tested joint	Hard
MCP extension	90 to 0 degrees	Tabletop (neutral)	Dorsal MCP of the tested joint	Firm
MCP hyperextension	0 to 30 degrees	Tabletop (neutral)	Dorsal MCP of the tested joint	Firm
MCP adduction	Compare	Tabletop (pronated)	Dorsal MCP of the tested joint	Firm
MCP abduction	Compare	Tabletop (pronated)	Dorsal MCP of the tested joint	Soft

(continued)

UNIT 2-68 EVALUATION

UNIT 2-68 EVALUATION

RANGE OF MOTION (CONTINUED)

JOINT AND MOTION	NORMAL ROM	CLIENT POSITION	FULCRUM LOCATION	END FEEL
PIP flexion	0 to 100 degrees	Tabletop (neutral)	Dorsal PIP of the tested joint	Hard
PIP extension	90 to 0 degrees	Tabletop (neutral)	Dorsal PIP of the tested joint	Firm
DIP flexion and extension	0 to 90 to 0 degrees	Tabletop (neutral)	Dorsal DIP of the tested joint	Firm
CMC flexion	0 to 20 degrees	Tabletop (neutral)	Base of the CMC joint	Soft
CMC extension	0 to 45 degrees	Tabletop (supinated)	Base of the CMC joint	Firm
CMC abduction	0 to 70 degrees	Tabletop (neutral)	Lateral/dorsal CMC joint	Firm
CMC adduction	Compared/70 to 0 degrees	Tabletop (neutral)	Lateral/dorsal CMC joint	Soft
Interphalangeal (IP) flexion and extension of the thumb	0 to 90 to 0 degrees	Tabletop (neutral)	Dorsal thumb at the IP joint	Firm
MCP flexion of the thumb	0 to 50 degrees	Tabletop (neutral or supinated)	Dorsal thumb at the MCP joint	Hard
MCP extension of the thumb	50 to 0 degrees	Tabletop (neutral or supinated)	Dorsal thumb at the MCP joint	Firm
Digit opposition	0 cm	Tabletop (supinated)	Measure from the tip of the digit	Soft

MANUAL MUSCLE TESTING GUIDELINES

The manual muscle test is performed as a test of the forces generated by individual muscles and muscle groups.

GRADING SCALE

The following scale is used to record the client's strength for each muscle. When testing the client's muscle strength against gravity, apply minimum resistance by applying a steady force in the direction opposite of the motion once. Apply moderate resistance by applying a steady force opposing the motion once, then pause, then apply force a second time. Apply maximum resistance by applying an opposing force 3 times.[12]

Note: Manual muscle test grading scales may vary slightly between sites.

Score	Description
5	The client demonstrates full ROM against gravity and withstands maximum resistance.
4	The client demonstrates full ROM against gravity and withstands moderate resistance.
4-	The client demonstrates full ROM against gravity and withstands minimum resistance.
3+	The client demonstrates full ROM against gravity and can hold at the end range without resistance.
3	The client demonstrates full ROM against gravity but is unable to hold at end range.
3-	The client demonstrates partial ROM against gravity.
2+	The client initiates movement against gravity.
2	The client demonstrates full ROM with gravity eliminated.
2-	The client demonstrates partial ROM with gravity eliminated.
1	Muscle contraction can be felt through palpation of the muscle with gravity eliminated, but the client demonstrates no motion at the joint.
0	The client demonstrates no joint motion and no muscle contraction.

(continued)

MANUAL MUSCLE TESTING GUIDELINES (CONTINUED)

In the following chart, the left column lists the muscles responsible for movements at each joint and the position the client should assume for testing the muscle against gravity or with gravity eliminated. The right column specifies where the therapist should palpate the muscle if no movement is observed at the joint.

JOINT MOVEMENT MUSCLE AND RELATED POSITIONS	PALPATION
Shoulder	
Flexion Against gravity: Sitting Gravity eliminated: Side-lying	
Coracobrachialis	Not palpated
Anterior deltoid	Front of the humerus
Pectoralis major	Clavicular fibers located below midclavicle
Extension Against gravity: Prone or sitting Gravity eliminated: Side-lying	
Teres major	Lower border of the scapula
Latissimus dorsi	Lower border of the scapula
Posterior deltoid	Dorsal, proximal one-third of the humerus
Internal rotation Against gravity: Prone Gravity eliminated: Prone with elbow extended or sitting	
Subscapularis	Deep axilla insertion
	(continued)

MANUAL MUSCLE TESTING GUIDELINES (CONTINUED)

JOINT MOVEMENT MUSCLE AND RELATED POSITIONS	PALPATION
External rotation Against gravity: Prone Gravity eliminated: Prone with elbow extended or sitting	
Teres minor	Not palpated (located below infraspinatus)
Infraspinatus	Inferior to the spine of the scapula
Abduction Against gravity: Sitting Gravity eliminated: Supine	
Middle deltoid	Below acromioclavicular joint, lateral proximal one-third of humerus belly
Supraspinatus	Not palpated
Adduction Against gravity: Sitting Gravity eliminated: Supine	
Pectoralis major	Below midclavicle
Latissimus dorsi	Lower border of the scapula
Horizontal abduction Against gravity: Prone Gravity eliminated: Sitting	
Posterior deltoid	Below acromioclavicular joint, dorsal and proximal one-third of humerus
	(continued)

UNIT 2-69 EVALUATION

MANUAL MUSCLE TESTING GUIDELINES (CONTINUED)

JOINT MOVEMENT MUSCLE AND RELATED POSITIONS	PALPATION
Horizontal adduction Against gravity: Supine Gravity eliminated: Sitting. Shoulder abducted and elbow flexed to 90 degrees	
Pectoralis major	Palpate clavicular fibers below middle of clavicle. Palpate sternal anterior surface.
Scapula	
Elevation Against gravity: Sitting Gravity eliminated: Supine or prone	
Upper trapezius	Belly on top shoulder or C7 or lateral one-third of clavicle
Levator scapulae	Superior border of scapula or C1 to C3
Depression Against gravity: Sitting Gravity eliminated: Prone	
Lower trapezius	Inferior medial border of scapula or T6 to T12 vertebrae
Adduction/retraction (downward rotation) Against gravity: Prone Gravity eliminated: Sitting	
Middle trapezius	Above spine of scapula or medial to vertebral border of scapula
Rhomboids	Medial to vertebral border of scapula
	(continued)

MANUAL MUSCLE TESTING GUIDELINES (CONTINUED)

JOINT MOVEMENT MUSCLE AND RELATED POSITIONS	PALPATION
Abduction/protraction (upward rotation) Against gravity: Supine Gravity eliminated: Sitting	
Serratus anterior Shoulder flexed 90 degrees	From lateral scapular border, anterior to rib
Elbow	
Flexion Against gravity: Supine or sitting Gravity eliminated: Resting on table	
Biceps brachii (in supinated position)	Volar distal surface of medial humerus
Brachialis (in pronated position)	Medial to bicep
Brachioradialis (in neutral position)	Distal/lateral humerus
Extension Against gravity: Supine Gravity eliminated: Resting on table	
Triceps	Posterior midhumerus
Anconeus	Not palpated
Forearm	
Supination Against gravity: Sitting Gravity eliminated: Tabletop; performing the queen wave	
Supinator	Posterior proximal surface of forearm over radius
	(continued)

UNIT 2–69 EVALUATION

UNIT 2-69 EVALUATION

MANUAL MUSCLE TESTING GUIDELINES (CONTINUED)

JOINT MOVEMENT MUSCLE AND RELATED POSITIONS	PALPATION
Pronation Against gravity: Sitting Gravity eliminated: Tabletop; performing the queen wave	
Pronator teres	Anterior proximal forearm between radius and ulna
Pronator quadratus	Not palpated
Wrist	
Flexion Against gravity: Tabletop; forearm supinated Gravity eliminated: Tabletop; forearm neutral	
FCR	Anterior surface of forearm, in line with second MC
FCU	Proximal to fifth MC or pisiform on anterior/distal forearm
Palmaris longus	Tested with flexor carpi ulnaris and flexor carpi radialis. Absent in about 20% of population.
Extension Against gravity: Tabletop; forearm pronated Gravity eliminated: Tabletop; forearm neutral	
ECRL	Distal/dorsal forearm, base of second MC

(continued)

MANUAL MUSCLE TESTING GUIDELINES (CONTINUED)

JOINT MOVEMENT MUSCLE AND RELATED POSITIONS	PALPATION
ECRB	Distal/dorsal forearm, base of third MC
ECU	Dorsal wrist between fifth MC and ulnar styloid

Finger (Digits 2 to 5)

Flexion

Against gravity: Forearm supinated

Gravity eliminated: Forearm neutral

Lumbricals: MCP	Not palpated
FDS: PIP	Proximal phalanx, volar wrist
FDP: DIP	Middle phalanx

Extension

Against gravity: Forearm pronated

Gravity eliminated: Forearm neutral

Extensor digitorum: MCP	Dorsal surface of MCP heads
Lumbricals: IP	Not palpated

Adduction

Forearm pronated. The test was not performed against gravity or with gravity eliminated.

Palmar interossei	Not palpated

Abduction

Forearm pronated. The test was not performed against gravity or with gravity eliminated.

Dorsal interossei	Not palpated

(continued)

UNIT 2-69 EVALUATION

MANUAL MUSCLE TESTING GUIDELINES (CONTINUED)

JOINT MOVEMENT MUSCLE AND RELATED POSITIONS	PALPATION
Opposition Against gravity: Forearm supinated Gravity eliminated: Forearm neutral	
Opponens digiti minimi	Volar shaft of fifth MC
Thumb	
Flexion Against gravity: Forearm supinated Gravity eliminated: Forearm neutral	
FPB: MCP	First MCP phalanx
FPL: IP	First proximal phalanx; palmar
Extension Against gravity: Forearm neutral Gravity eliminated: Forearm supinated	
EPB: MCP	Radial border of anatomical snuffbox; medial to APL
EPL: MCP and IP	Ulnar border of anatomical snuffbox; dorsal surface of proximal phalanx of thumb
Abduction Against gravity: Forearm supinated Gravity eliminated: Forearm neutral	
APB	Center of thenar eminence
APL	Distal to radial styloid; lateral to EPB
Adduction Against gravity: Forearm pronated Gravity eliminated: Forearm neutral	
Adductor pollicis	Palmar surface of thumb web space
Opposition Against gravity: Forearm supinated Gravity eliminated: Forearm neutral	
Opponens pollicis	Lateral side of first MC

DEXTERITY AND COORDINATION ASSESSMENTS

The following table summarizes assessment tools that can be used to evaluate the client's dexterity and coordination.

TOOL	DESCRIPTION
Box and Blocks Test[13]	• Purpose: Measures gross manual dexterity • Context: Individuals with coordination impairments, including stoke, hemiplegia, traumatic brain injury, spinal cord injury (SCI), and geriatric populations • Format: Performance based • Time to administer: Less than 5 minutes • Materials: Wooden text box, 150 wooden cubes, stopwatch, test booklet with instructions, and table • Cost: More than $200 • Website: https://www.sralab.org/sites/default/files/2017-06/Box%20and%20Blocks%20Test%20Instructions.pdf
Jebsen-Taylor Hand Function Test[14]	• Purpose: Assesses hand functions necessary for activities of daily living using common task items • Context: Clients with stroke, arthritic conditions, joint conditions, and SCIs • Format: Performance based • Time to administer: 15 to 45 minutes • Materials: Test kit containing wooden board and items, stopwatch, chair, table, and record sheet • Cost: More than $300 • Website: https://www.performancehealth.com/jamar-hand-function-test

(continued)

DEXTERITY AND COORDINATION ASSESSMENTS (CONTINUED)

TOOL	DESCRIPTION
Minnesota Manual Dexterity Test[15]	• Purpose: Assesses rapid hand-finger-eye movements and dexterity • Context: Clients in rehabilitation settings • Format: Performance based • Time to administer: Up to 1 hour • Materials: Test kit (includes folding board and discs) and score sheets • Cost: More than $200 • Website: http://www.prohealthcareproducts.com/complete-minnesota-manual-dexterity-test-rate-of-manipulation
Nine-Hole Peg Test[16]	• Purpose: Assesses finger dexterity for assembly tasks and gross movement of upper extremity • Context: Clients with rheumatoid arthritis, stroke, Parkinson's disease, multiple sclerosis, and traumatic brain injury • Format: Performance based • Time to administer: 5 to 10 minutes • Materials: Square peg board, nine pegs, table, stopwatch, record sheets, and instructions • Cost: $50 • Website: https://www.sralab.org/sites/default/files/2017-07/Nine%20Hole%20Peg%20Test%20Instructions.pdf
Purdue Pegboard Test[17]	• Purpose: Assesses heart rate, blood pressure, respiratory rate, and oxygen saturation during strenuous activity • Context: Clients with stroke, Parkinson's disease, and other neurological or musculoskeletal conditions • Format: Ordinal scale • Time to administer: 5 to 10 minutes • Materials: Pegboard, pins, collars, washers, manual, score sheets, stopwatch, and table • Cost: $150 • Website: http://lafayetteevaluation.com/products/purdue-pegboard

PROVOCATIVE TESTS

Provocative tests are administered with the intent to provoke symptoms. These tests help practitioners understand and diagnose conditions of the musculoskeletal system.

NAME OF TEST	ADMINISTRATION	POSITIVE TEST MAY INDICATE
Shoulder		
External rotation lag sign[18]	• Stand behind the client, who begins seated. • Abduct the client's arm about 30 degrees, then hold the elbow (in about 90 degrees of flexion) with one hand and the wrist in the other hand. • Passively externally rotate the shoulder to end range, and ask the client to hold the position. • Release the client's wrist while still providing gentle support at the elbow. The test is positive if there is a lag that occurs due to the client's inability to maintain near full external rotation.	Supraspinatus or infraspinatus tear

(continued)

UNIT 2-71 EVALUATION

UNIT 2-71 EVALUATION

PROVOCATIVE TESTS (CONTINUED)

NAME OF TEST	ADMINISTRATION	POSITIVE TEST MAY INDICATE
Empty Can Test[19]	• Stand behind the client, who begins seated. • Abduct the client's arms to 90 degrees with the thumbs facing up and elbows extended. • Instruct the client to resist while providing a downward pressure on the client's arms, noting his or her strength. • Instruct the client to rotate the arms so that the thumbs are facing downward (as if emptying a can). • Instruct the client to resist as the examiner provides a downward pressure on the arms. The test is positive if there is more weakness in the empty can position as opposed to the full can position. The test is also positive if pain is present while performing the test.	Torn rotator cuff or all stages of impingement from bursitis
Neer Impingement Test[20,21]	• Stand on the client's involved side while the client is seated. • Passively flex the client's shoulder to end range while keeping the arm internally rotated (the palm of the client's hand should face outward). The test is positive if pain is present.	Subacromial impingement or subacromial bursitis

(continued)

PROVOCATIVE TESTS (CONTINUED)

NAME OF TEST	ADMINISTRATION	POSITIVE TEST MAY INDICATE
Hawkins–Kennedy Test[20,21]	• Stand in front of the client, who begins seated. • Passively raise the client's arm to approximately 90 degrees of shoulder flexion. • Use one hand to support the scapula. Apply an internal rotation force at the humerus to reproduce pain symptoms. The test is positive if pain is present.	Subacromial impingement, subacromial bursitis, rotator cuff tear, or superior labral tear
Speed test[21]	• Stand in front of the client, who begins standing. • Extend the client's arm and supinate the forearm. Instruct the client to perform active shoulder flexion. • Apply resistance from 0 to 60 degrees. The test is positive if pain is present over the bicipital groove.	Subacromial impingement, any labral lesion, or biceps pathology
Drop arm test[20]	• While the client is standing or seated, abduct the client's arm to 90 degrees. The client attempts to slowly lower the arm back to the side. The test is positive if the client reports pain when lowering the arm, is unable to lower the arm slowly, or is unable to control movement of the adductors.	Rotator cuff tear

(continued)

UNIT 2-71 EVALUATION

PROVOCATIVE TESTS (CONTINUED)

NAME OF TEST	ADMINISTRATION	POSITIVE TEST MAY INDICATE
Elbow and Forearm		
Cozen's test[22]	• While the client is seated, palpate the lateral epicondyle. • Instruct the client to make a fist with the forearm in pronation and radial deviation of the wrist. • Provide resistance while the client extends the wrist. The test is positive if pain is present along the lateral epicondyle.	Lateral epicondylitis (Note: No diagnostic accuracy studies are available at this time.)
Wrist and Hand		
Finkelstein's test[23]	• While the client is seated or standing, instruct the client to position his or her hand into a fist with the thumb on the inside. • Move the client's wrist into ulnar deviation (downward). The test is positive if pain is present over the area of the abductor pollicis longus and EPB.	de Quervain's tenosynovitis
Murphy's sign[24]	• While the client is seated, ask the client to make a fist. The test is positive if the third MC is at the same level as the second and fourth MC, rather than being raised.	Dislocation of lunate

(continued)

PROVOCATIVE TESTS (CONTINUED)

NAME OF TEST	ADMINISTRATION	POSITIVE TEST MAY INDICATE
Hip		
Flexion, abduction, and external rotation test (Patrick's test)[25]	• While the client is lying supine, passively flex, abduct, and externally rotate the testing hip so that the foot is resting just above the opposite knee. • Slowly lower the testing knee down toward the table surface. The test is positive when the involved knee is unable to assume the position and/or the painful symptoms are reproduced.	Hip dysfunction and intra-articular pathology
Grind (scouring) test[23]	• While the client is lying supine, position the involved hip in 90 degrees of flexion with the knee maximally flexed. • Apply a compressive load onto the femur via the knee joint. The test is positive when pain within the hip joint is reproduced. Pain may refer to the knee and elsewhere.	Degenerative joint disease
Piriformis test[25]	• While the client is lying supine, passively place the foot of the testing leg lateral to the opposite knee. • Adduct the testing hip till the testing knee passes over the opposite knee. The test is positive if the testing knee is unable to pass over the resting knee, and/or pain in the buttock (or along sciatic nerve) is reproduced.	Piriformis syndrome

(continued)

UNIT 2-71 EVALUATION

UNIT 2-71 EVALUATION

PROVOCATIVE TESTS (CONTINUED)

NAME OF TEST	ADMINISTRATION	POSITIVE TEST MAY INDICATE
Flexion, adduction, and internal rotation • Click test • Anterior labral tear test also known as the *apprehension test*[26]	• While the client is lying supine, position the testing hip into full flexion, lateral rotation, and full abduction as the starting position. • Extend the hip, combined with internal rotation and adduction. The test is positive if pain is reproduced.	Anterior labral tear
Resisted straight leg raise test[23]	• While the client is lying supine, position the testing leg with the knee extended and the hip externally rotated and adducted. • Raise the testing leg by the ankle, and maintain knee extension by holding the anterior leg above the knee. The test is positive if pain is reproduced in the back of the leg or the back.	Intra-articular pathology

(continued)

PROVOCATIVE TESTS (CONTINUED)

NAME OF TEST	ADMINISTRATION	POSITIVE TEST MAY INDICATE
Knee		
McMurray's test[27]	• While the client is lying supine, position the testing knee in maximal flexion. • Position the tibia in either internal rotation (to test medical meniscus) or external rotation (to test lateral meniscus). • To test the medial meniscus, externally rotate the tibia while extending the knee. • To test the lateral meniscus, internally rotate the tibia while extending the knee. The test is positive if pain is reported or a "click" is felt.	Meniscal tear
Apley's test[27]	• While the client is lying prone, flex the testing knee to 90 degrees, and stabilize the testing thigh to the table (with the examiner's knee). • Distract the testing knee joint passively, then slowly rotate the tibia internally and externally. • Compress the knee joint and slowly rotate the tibia internally and externally. The presence of pain or increased motion during distraction indicates a ligamentous lesion. The presence of pain or decreased motion during compression indicates a meniscal tear.	Meniscal tears or ligamentous lesions

(continued)

UNIT 2-71 EVALUATION

PROVOCATIVE TESTS (CONTINUED)

NAME OF TEST	ADMINISTRATION	POSITIVE TEST MAY INDICATE
Patellar apprehension test[28]	• While the client is lying supine with the testing knee flexed to 30 degrees, passively glide the testing patella laterally. The test is positive if the client does not allow or like the patella to move in a lateral direction.	History of patella dislocation
Clarke's sign[29]	• While the client is lying supine, extend the testing knee as it is resting on the table. • Push posteriorly on the superior border of the patella, and instruct the client to actively contract the quadriceps. The test is positive if pain is produced.	Patellofemoral dysfunction
Noble Compression Test[30]	• While the client is lying supine, position the testing leg in 45 degrees of hip flexion and 90 degrees of knee flexion. • Apply pressure to lateral femoral epicondyle, then extend the knee. The test is positive when pain is reproduced at the lateral femoral condyle during extension motion.	Iliotibial band friction syndrome

(continued)

PROVOCATIVE TESTS (CONTINUED)

NAME OF TEST	ADMINISTRATION	POSITIVE TEST MAY INDICATE
Ankle		
Anterior drawer test[31]	• While the client is lying supine with the testing heel on the edge of the table, position the testing ankle in 20-degree plantar flexion. • Grasp the foot and pull the talus anteriorly while stabilizing the lower leg with the other hand. The test is positive if excessive anterior motion or pain is noted.	Anterior talofibular ligament instability
Talar tilt test[32]	• While the client is lying on his or her side with the testing leg on the top, slightly flex the testing knee with the ankle in neutral. • Move the foot into adduction (calcaneofibular ligament) and abduction (deltoid ligament). The test is positive if excessive motion or pain is noted.	Ligament instability

UNIT 2-71 EVALUATION

UNIT 3-72 INTERVENTION

COMMON INTERVENTIONS ACROSS PRACTICE SETTINGS

Intervention	Acute	Inpatient	Home Health	SNF	Outpatient
Common Interventions Across Practice Settings					
Muscle strengthening	✓	✓	✓	✓	✓
Stretching	✓	✓			✓
Joint mobilization	✓	✓			✓
Joint protection	✓	✓			✓
Pain management	✓	✓	✓	✓	✓
Inhibition and Facilitation Techniques	✓	✓	✓	✓	✓
Physical Agent Modalities					
Thermal physical agent modalities (PAMs)	✓	✓			✓
Electrical PAMs					
Ultrasound PAMs					
Kinesio Taping		✓		✓	✓
Orthopedic Serial Casting					
Orthotic Guidelines	✓	✓			✓
Prostheses	✓	✓			✓
Wheelchair Prescription	✓	✓			
Musculoskeletal System Precautions and Contraindications	✓	✓			

(continued)

COMMON INTERVENTIONS
ACROSS PRACTICE SETTINGS (CONTINUED)

MUSCLE STRENGTHENING[33]

- Description: *Muscle strengthening* refers to exercises that move muscles against resistance.
- Approach: Walking on a treadmill or riding on a stationary bike are 2 aerobic activities used by therapy programs. The cardiovascular demand increases with the addition of resistance exercises using handheld weights or TheraBands (Performance Health) resistance training products. Increase handheld weight or TheraBand resistance gradually over treatment sessions.
- Precautions: Limit the weight to 10 pounds (lbs) to maintain sternal precautions. For patients with smaller upper extremity musculature, lifting an object that is too heavy results in unsafe working demands on the heart.
- Significance: Benefits of strengthening include improved posture and balance, increased muscle strength, improved metabolism, injury prevention, improved mental integrity, and weight management.

STRETCHING[33]

- Description: *Stretching* refers to flexing or stretching of a specific muscle or tendon in order to increase elasticity and improve muscle tone. Stretching is considered a form of exercise.
- Approach: Static stretching is beneficial for mild muscle soreness. The client may hold the stretch longer by counting "One thousand and one, one thousand and two, one thousand and three..." in place of "One, two, three..." Warm up the muscles prior to stretching by walking in place for a few minutes.
- Precautions: Rest for 1 day, modify the intervention, and decrease the load by half if the client reports a 6-out-of-10 pain level that persists overnight with pain medication following stretching.
- Significance: Stretching improves ROM, flexibility, and muscle control.

(continued)

COMMON INTERVENTIONS # ACROSS PRACTICE SETTINGS (CONTINUED)
JOINT MOBILIZATION[33]
• Description: *Joint mobilization* refers to manual therapy that carries the joints to their end range. • Approach: The therapist passively and slowly moves the joint to the end range. The therapist holds the joint at end range for a few seconds as long as the client is within his or her pain limit. The client may require pain medication in order to tolerate joint mobilization. Consult with the nurse and physician if it seems the client will benefit from pain medication. • Precautions: The client should not perform active or passive ROM within 2 weeks of soft tissue repair or exposed tendon operation unless otherwise stated by the physician. • Significance: Joint mobilization focuses on synovial joints to reduce pain due to nonuse and tightness.
JOINT PROTECTION[33]
• Description: *Joint protection* refers to strategies that help manage pain due to rheumatoid arthritis in order to perform functional activities. • Approach: Joint protection is performed by the client as a form of self-management. Strategies may include energy conservation, altering movement patterns, losing weight, improving posture to reduce stress placed on joints, splinting, using safety gear, and activity pacing. • Precautions: Avoid repetitive movement during joint flare-ups. • Significance: Joint protection can reduce pain and increase the client's independence in performing daily activities.
PAIN MANAGEMENT[33]
Refer to Section Three, Unit 3-61, for information on pain management.

UNIT 3–72 INTERVENTION

INHIBITION AND FACILITATION TECHNIQUES

INHIBITION TECHNIQUES

Inhibition techniques are used to relax a muscle in order to reduce spasticity or release unwanted contractions.[34]

Technique	Description
Joint compression	Use one hand to stabilize, and apply force with the other hand.
Reciprocal inhibition	Contract an agonist muscle to inhibit the motor neurons of the antagonist.
	For example, the bicep (ie, the agonist) contracts while the tricep (ie, the antagonist) relaxes to produce elbow flexion.
Pressure at muscle insertion	Apply pressure at the muscle insertion to relax the muscle.
Weightbearing and Cocontraction	Weightbearing through the lower extremity and pelvis helps to reduce spasticity.
	Cocontraction in the upper extremity assists in restoring normal muscle tone.
Reflex-inhibiting postures	For example, to inhibit abnormal upper extremity flexion pattern, extend the neck and spine, externally rotate the shoulder, extend the elbow, supinate the forearm, and abduct the thumb.
Inversion	When the head is positioned lower than the rest of the body, the carotid sinus inhibits all stretch reflexes except the labyrinthine reflex.
Mobilization of proximal joints	Mobilizing the shoulder girdle or pelvis assists in reducing abnormal muscle tone.
Sensory stimuli	Present auditory stimuli with a regular rhythm lower than the heart rate. Other inhibitory stimuli include dimmed lighting, pleasant odors, and warm fluids to inhibit hyperactive swallowing.

(continued)

UNIT 3-73 INTERVENTION

INHIBITION AND FACILITATION TECHNIQUES (CONTINUED)

Technique	Description
Slow rocking	Rhythmically and slowly rock in a rocking chair or on a large ball.
Slow rolling	Place one hand on the client's shoulder and one hand on the client's pelvis, and slowly roll the client from supine to side-lying then back to supine for several minutes.
Slow stroking	While the client is prone, place your index and middle finger on either side of the posterior rami of the spinal cord. Apply a light but firm touch slowly from the client's neck to the coccyx, directly to skin.
Neutral warmth	Wrap the client's body in a cotton blanket for 10 to 20 minutes.

(continued)

UNIT 3-73 INTERVENTION

INHIBITION AND FACILITATION TECHNIQUES (CONTINUED)

FACILITATION TECHNIQUES

Facilitation techniques are used to assist a muscle to contract.[34]

Technique	Description
Brushing	Apply a stimulus for 10 to 15 seconds to the skin over the muscle belly of the muscle that is to be facilitated.
Tapping, rubbing, or quick stretching	Do not apply pressure or quick stretch to a spastic muscle.
Resistance	Apply resistance in a pattern as follows: apply resistance, hold, release, apply resistance, hold, and release.
Joint traction (pulling apart at the joint)	Joint traction facilitates flexor patterns. Do not use joint traction if there is a fracture in any bone involved with the joint.
Joint approximation (pressing together at the joint)	When joint approximation is applied with more than body weight, it facilitates extensor patterns and cocontracting patterns. Do not use joint approximation if there is a fracture in any bone involved with the joint.
Icing	Wrap an ice cube in a towel and rub with pressure over the muscle belly in 3 quick swipes from a distal to proximal direction. Do not ice the forehead, anterior midline of trunk, or posterior trunk because blood pressure may increase.
Sensory stimuli	Present bright colors, salty and oily fluids, and noxious odors.

(continued)

UNIT 3-73 INTERVENTION

INHIBITION AND FACILITATION TECHNIQUES (CONTINUED)

Technique	Description
Change in postures	Positions that allow the client to work against gravity may increase muscle tone.
Successive induction	Alternate contractions of agonist and antagonist muscles. For example, if wrist flexors are weak, then give maximum resistance to the wrist extensors and then resistance to wrist flexors.
Vestibular stimulation (fast rolling, spinning, tilting, and swinging)	Vestibular stimulation increases muscle tone. Do not use spinning with clients who are prone to seizures.
Vibration	Use a battery-operated device. The effect of vibration wears off in about 3 minutes. Do not use vibration with clients who are prone to seizures.

PHYSICAL AGENT MODALITIES

PAMs are interventions or technologies that produce a response in soft tissue using temperature, light, sound, water, and electricity. Use of PAMs in occupational therapy is somewhat controversial. PAMs are used to facilitate outcomes and healing in a quick and cost-effective manner, but consider them carefully and only when appropriate in conjunction with functional activity.[35]

Best practice for using PAMs includes these steps:

- Question the client to determine prior negative reactions to PAMs in past treatments.
- Inform the client of the procedure, expected outcomes, and sensations that he or she may experience during the treatment.
- Inform the client that the expected outcome is to alleviate pain and stiffness.
- Inspect the client's skin integrity.
- Know and observe the contraindications.

Be sure to document the following issues:

- Inspection of the client's skin integrity
- Physical agents applied and treatment parameters
- Treatment duration and site of application
- Client's knowledge of the expected outcome
- Subjective responses from the client including tolerance, reaction, and clinical effectiveness

Prior to using PAMs, the occupational therapist should know local, state, and institutional rules and guidelines, as well as reimbursement issues and certified occupational therapy assistant and occupational therapist registered roles. Continued training and education are necessary for using PAMs safely.[35]

(continued)

UNIT 3-74 INTERVENTION

PHYSICAL AGENT MODALITIES (CONTINUED)

THERMAL PHYSICAL AGENT MODALITIES[36]

PAMs	Application	
Superficial heat agent • Any modality that raises the skin and superficial subcutaneous tissue temperature • Therapeutic effects at depths of 1 cm or less	**Purpose and effects** • Decreases pain and stiffness • Improves ROM/tendon excursion • Improves viscosity of synovia • Promotes healing and reduces spasms	**Conditions** • Muscle spasms and pain • Subcutaneous adhesion • Contractures • Chronic arthritis • Trauma • Wounds • Subacute and chronic inflammation **Administration** • Therapeutic temperature range is 105°F to 110°F. • Temperatures of more than 120°F will cause destruction of collagen.

Precautions	Contraindications
• Diminished sensation • Compromised circulation • Anticoagulant medication use • Bleeding tendency • Acute inflammation or swelling	• Impaired sensation due to skin graft or scarring • Tumors or cancer diagnosis • Advanced cardiac disease • Acute inflammation or swelling • Deep vein thrombophlebitis • Pregnancy • Bleeding tendency • Infection • Primary repair of tendon or ligament • Semi-coma or impaired cognitive status • Rheumatoid arthritis

(continued)

UNIT 3-74 INTERVENTION

PHYSICAL AGENT MODALITIES (CONTINUED)

PAMs	Application

Hot packs	Purpose and effects	Conditions
• Mild heat • Passive treatment	• Relieves pain • Reduces muscle spasms • Improves connective tissue extensibility when combined with ROM • Assists with wound healing	• Muscle spasms • Subcutaneous adhesions • Contractures • Subacute inflammation **Administration** • Therapeutic temperature range is 102°F to 113°F. • Requires dry padding between the hot pack and skin to avoid burns. • Fold paper towels so that there are 6 to 8 layers. • Treatment duration is 15 to 20 minutes. • May be given daily or more often.

Precautions	Contraindications
• Use tongs, and do not lie on the hot pack • Already existing edema • Sensory loss • Clients who are confused • Compromised circulation	• Acute inflammation or edema conditions • Fever • Malignancies • Anticoagulant medication use • Active bleeding • Bleeding tendency • Absent sensation • Severely impaired circulation • Cardiac insufficiency • Extreme elder adults and children under 4 years of age, due to unreliable thermoregulatory systems • Peripheral vascular disease • Tissues that have just had x-ray therapy • Deep vein thrombophlebitis

(continued)

PHYSICAL AGENT MODALITIES (CONTINUED)

PAMs	Application	

Fluidotherapy and whirlpool bath
• Superficial thermal modality
• Form of heat transfer that utilizes convection
	Purpose and effects
	• Mobilizes or desensitizes
	Conditions
	• Whirlpool bath:
	  ○ Inflammatory conditions
	  ○ Peripheral vascular disease
	  ○ Status post fractures (stiffness and excessive skin dryness)
		Administration
		• Fluidotherapy:
		  ○ Therapeutic temperature range is 105°F to 118°F.
		  ○ Treatment duration is 15 to 20 minutes.
		• Whirlpool bath:
		  ○ Therapeutic temperature range for a whirlpool bath is 79°F to 104°F.
		  ○ Can be used on hands or feet.

Precautions	Contraindications
• Decreased sensation • Decreased circulation • Respiratory problems • Swelling	• Open, draining wounds • Allergy to corn

PAMs	Application	
Paraffin bath • Delivers heat • Effective for areas difficult to heat • Passive treatment	**Purpose and effects** • Helps soften skin • Decreases joint stiffness • Improves ROM • Relieves pain • Useful for distal extremities **Conditions** • Arthritis • Healed amputation • Strains and sprains	**Administration** • Therapeutic temperature range is 113°F to 129°F. • Dip and wrap (dip 8 times, plastic wrap, towel). • Dip and reimmerse (dip and hold for 5 minutes).

Precautions	Contraindications
• Check thermostat • Decreased sensation • Decreased circulation • Existing edema • Sensory loss • Clients who are confused • Compromised circulation	• Infections • Absent sensation • Skin lesions • Open wounds

(continued)

UNIT 3-74 INTERVENTION

Physical Agent Modalities (continued)

PAMs	Application	

Cryotherapy
 	
• Application of a superficial cold agent that lowers the temperature of the tissue
• Includes ice massage, cold packs, and ice towels
	Purpose and effects
	
	• Slows healing process
	• Reduces swelling
	• Reduces pain
	• Ice massage:
	  ○ Effectively treats small areas
	• Ice towels:
	  ○ Provides circumferential cooling
	• Cold packs:
	  ○ Apply single layer of moist towel to area.
	  ○ Apply the pack and mold it to fit the body part.
	  ○ Cover the pack with several layers of dry toweling.
	  ○ Treatment duration is 10 to 20 minutes.
		○ Treatments up to several hours are acceptable in emergency situations, such as following a burn.
		○ Remove pack and check for skin condition and physiological response.
		• Ice towels:
		  ○ Treatment duration is 5 to 6 minutes.
		Conditions
		• Painful conditions
		• Arthritis exacerbation
		• Acute injury
		• Swelling and internal bleeding
		Administration
		• Ice massage:
		  ○ Treatment duration is 5 to 10 minutes.

Precautions	Contraindications
• Superficial main nerve branch • Open wound • Hypertension • Poor sensation • Very young or very old • Impaired circulation and acute edema	• Cold hypersensitivity or intolerance • Cold sensitivity • Raynaud's disease • Regenerating nerve • Swelling of unknown cause • Systemic lupus • Peripheral vascular disease • Unable to respond or feel cold • Decreased circulation • Decreased sensation • Healing wounds • Leukemia • Cold intolerance associated with rheumatic diseases, crush injuries, and amputations

(continued)

UNIT 3-74 INTERVENTION

PHYSICAL AGENT MODALITIES (CONTINUED)

PAMs	Application	
Contrast baths • A type of vascular exercise alternating between heat and cold	**Purpose and effects** • Promotes healing • Increases blood flow • Has benefits of heat and cold therapies with a reduction of adverse effects **Conditions** • Subacute or chronic traumatic and inflammatory conditions • Sinus or congestive headaches • Reflex sympathetic dystrophy • Complex regional pain syndrome	**Administration** • Prepare 2 pails of water to a depth that will cover the treatment area. • Warm bath temperature is 100°F to 110°F. • Cold bath temperature is 55°F to 65°F. • Immerse the part in the warm bath for 3 to 5 minutes. • Immerse the part in the cold bath for up to 1 minute. • Repeat alternating heat and cold immersion for 20 to 30 minutes.

Precautions	Contraindications
• Anesthetic skin • May cause client with no apparent contraindications to develop chest pains or become chilled. If this occurs, have the client lie down and gently warm with heat application to the chest, head, and neck area.	• Malignancies • Tendency to hemorrhage • Active bleeding • Cold hypersensitivity • Raynaud's disease • Peripheral arterial disease • Cardiac and respiratory instability • Fever • Very young or very old clients • Tissues that have recently had an x-ray

(continued)

UNIT 3-74 INTERVENTION

Physical Agent Modalities (continued)

Electrical Physical Agent Modalities[36]

PAMs	Application	
NMES • Uses current to stimulate innervated muscle to restore muscle function	**Purpose and effects** • Reduces muscle spasms • Strengthens muscle • Pumps edema • Prevents atrophy • Reeducates muscle • Restores muscle function • Facilitates voluntary movement • Corrects contracture • Preserves or increase ROM • Reduces spasticity	**Conditions** • Neuromuscular and musculoskeletal conditions • Cortical neuron lesion • SCI • Orthopedic surgery • Lower motor neuron disorders • Guillain-Barré syndrome • Brachial plexus injury
Functional electrical stimulation (Bioness) • Uses current to stimulate muscle groups for orthotic substitution	**Purpose and effects** • Strengthens muscle • Increases ROM • Enhances effects of botulinum toxin • Reduces spasticity • Reeducates movement • Improves sensory awareness • Reduces pain with spasticity	**Conditions** • Shoulder subluxation • Foot drop • Hemiplegia • Tetraplegia
Transcutaneous electrical nerve stimulation	**Purpose and effects** • Controls pain • Strengthens muscle • Cares for a wound • Heals a fracture • Manages edema • Increases ROM • Delivers medication through skin • Replaces orthotics • Reduces spasticity • Reduces scoliosis	**Conditions** • Neuromuscular and musculoskeletal conditions • Cortical neuron lesion • SCI • Orthopedic surgery

(continued)

UNIT 3-74 INTERVENTION

Physical Agent Modalities (continued)

PAMs	Application	
Electrical muscle stimulation • Uses current to stimulate denervated muscle	**Purpose and effects** • Prevents atrophy and degeneration • Potentially facilitates nerve regeneration and muscle reinnervation	
Iontophoresis • Ionizes topical medication into tissue	**Purpose and effects** • Manages scars	**Conditions** • Inflammatory conditions • Wrist tendonitis • Epicondylitis • Carpal tunnel syndrome • Glenohumeral bursitis
High-voltage pulse galvanic stimulation	**Purpose and effects** • Heals wounds • Reduces edema	

Precautions	Contraindications
• Obesity (fat is an electrical insulator and stimulation is not well-tolerated) • Areas of absent or diminished sensation • Peripheral neuropathies may prevent generation of muscle contractions • In presence of metal, electrodes should be positioned with metal outside path of current • Client not yet cleared for active exercise • Client unable to follow instructions or provide feedback • Spinal cord injury (may induce an episode of dysreflexia)	• Cardiac pacemakers • Over carotid sinus • Pregnancy • Undiagnosed pain • Cancerous lesions • Sensitive skin • Adjacent to or distal to an area of thrombophlebitis or phlebothrombosis • Presence of active tuberculosis • Area of active hemorrhage • Pain of unknown origin • Use near abdominal area in a client who is pregnant

(continue)

Physical Agent Modalities (continued)

Ultrasound Physical Agent Modalities[36]

PAMs	Application	

Continuous ultrasound (thermal)
• Heat effects
	Purpose and effects
	• Increases blood flow
	• Increases cellular activity
	• Reduces pain
	• Decreases muscle spasms
	• Reduces joint stiffness
	• Increases local metabolism
	• Stretch
		Conditions
		• Chronic inflammatory conditions
		• Chronic pain
		• Carpal tunnel syndrome
		• Tight tendons, capsules, ligaments, fascia, or scarring
		Administration
		• Typical protocol:
		  ○ Frequency: 1 MHz
		  ○ Intensity: 1.0 W/cm^2
		  ○ Duty cycle: 100% duty cycle
		  ○ Duration: 5 to 10 minutes

Pulsed ultrasound (nonthermal)
• Healing effects
	Purpose and effects
	• Facilitates tissue healing and repair
	• Decreases inflammation
	• Very local treatment
	Conditions
	• Acute and subacute inflammation
	• Tendonitis
	• Bursitis
	• Lateral epicondylitis
	• Overuse injuries
	• Acute soft tissue injuries
	• Acute pain
		Administration
		• Typical protocol:
		  ○ Frequency: 3 MHz
		  ○ Intensity: 0.5 W/cm^2
		  ○ Duty cycle: 20% duty cycle
		  ○ Duration: 1 to 2 minutes
		  ○ Effective radiating area

(continued)

UNIT 3-74 INTERVENTION

PHYSICAL AGENT MODALITIES (CONTINUED)

Precautions	Contraindications
• Never stay stationary; keep the sound head moving with slow, gentle, and constant pressure • Pregnancy • Unhealed fracture sites • Circulatory problems • Osteoporosis • Infections • Primary repair of a tendon or ligament • Pacemakers • People with diminished sensitivity to pain • Plastic and metal implants	• Malignancy or cancer diagnosis or cancer and cancerous lesions • Reduced sensation • Acute infections • Risk of hemorrhage, bleeding, or swelling • Severely ischemic tissue • Recent history of venous thrombosis or suspected deep vein thrombophlebitis • Exposed neural tissue • Do not use over a cardiac pacemaker or adjacent tissue • Pregnancy (do not use over a pregnant belly) • Do not use in the region of the active bone growth plates of children • Very old or very young clients due to compromised body temperature regulation • Metal implants • Do not use over brain, eyes, heart, spinal column, or reproductive organs • Deep vein thrombosis • Fractures • Tissue under therapy with radiation • Spinal cord after a laminectomy • Infection (heat can accelerate) and edema • Acute joint pathologies • Implanted joint • Plastics (they selectively absorb ultrasound waves and may cause an implanted joint component to become unseated)

KINESIO TAPING

Kinesio taping is a method that uses Kinesio Tex Tape with a particular application technique to target muscles that control movement and tissue pathology. With Kinesio tape, treatment is targeted to the cause of the pathology.[37-39]

Kinesio Tex Tape differs from athletic tape as indicated in the following chart.[37-39]

KINESIO TAPE	ATHLETIC TAPE
• Allows ROM	• Immobilizes
• Supports or corrects joints	• Inhibits joint or muscle movement
• Educates and supports a weakened muscle	• Provides pressure support and confinement to reduce pain
• Relieves pain	• Rests the muscle
• Reduces inflammation, edema, and fluid congestion	
• Decreases over-extension or over-contraction of a muscle	
• Mobilizes scar tissue and fascia	

The clinical goals of Kinesio tape are to assist with movement, enhance movement, enhance performance, and improve quality of life. Kinesio tape should be used as part of a complete therapeutic approach, and a thorough evaluation is necessary in order to obtain the best results. Remember to treat both the pain as well as the cause of the pain. It is recommended to keep the taping applications to a minimum and to educate the family on application techniques if the client requires long-term taping.[37-39]

(continued)

KINESIO TAPING (CONTINUED)

APPLICATION	DESCRIPTION
Taping patterns	 I Y X Buttonhole Fan
Tape application	• Clean the client's skin. Alcohol preparation is acceptable. Dry the skin before application. • Once tape is applied, lightly rub the tape to stimulate the adhesive. • Wait 10 minutes to check for any reactions or effects. • Use tape adherent (tincture of benzoin) prior to any sport activities. • Use extra water-resistant tape on hands and feet. • Remove tape if any blistering or increased pain occurs. Blistering is indicative of a true allergic reaction.
Taping to reduce tightness, restrictions, and spasms	• To inhibit or relax a muscle, position the client so that the muscle is fully elongated. The targeted tissue must be stretched. • Tape with light (15% to 20%) stretch. • When the muscle is relaxed, the tape will form convolutions. This increases circulation and helps allow the muscle to return to a normal length.

(continued)

Kinesio Taping (continued)

Application	Description
Taping to support a weakened or injured muscle or ligament	**Weakened Muscle** • To facilitate contractile tissue in a weakened muscle, position the client so that the muscle is fully elongated. • Tape with light to moderate (25% to 50%) stretch. • The tape provides support, facilitates movement, and compensates for muscle weakness. **Injured Muscle or Ligament** • To support non-contractile tissue, such as an injured joint or ligament, position the client so that the muscle is fully elongated and the joint is in full ROM. • Tape with moderate to maximum (50% to 75%) stretch. • The tape provides stability and facilitates joint function.
Taping for lymph drainage, bruising, and postural corrections	**Lymph Drainage and Bruising** • To tape for bruising or edema, position the client in full comfortable ROM. • Place the tape from proximal to distal over the injured area in order to pull fluid proximally. • Tape with very light (0% to 15%) stretch. **Postural Corrections** • To tape for postural corrections, position the client in the correct functional position. • Place anchors where the practitioner would use his or her hands to cue the client for correct positioning. • Tape with light to moderate (20% to 30%) stretch. • The tape cues the client to reposition when he or she is not in the correct position.
Wear and care	• Wash the tape often during the day with soap and water. • Pat the tape dry; do not rub. Do not use a blow dryer unless on the air setting without heat. • To remove Kinesio tape, use soap and water, baby oil, vegetable oil, or lotion. Roll the tape or pull skin away from the tape. Do not pull the tape off vigorously.

(continued)

UNIT 3-75 INTERVENTION

Kinesio Taping (continued)

Limitations

- Areas with excessive hair may need to be shaved.
- Apply at least 20 to 30 minutes before activity or exposure to heat and perspiration.
- Client may be unwilling to wear in public or for the recommended wearing schedule.

Precautions

- Clients with carotid artery disease
- Pregnant clients (avoid taping the acupuncture points of the upper trapezius and the medial lower leg as this may induce labor)

Contraindications

- Similar to those for PAMs
- Fragile or healing tissue
- Areas of infection

ORTHOPEDIC SERIAL CASTING

Orthopedic serial casting is used to facilitate or inhibit joint ROM, inhibit abnormal spasticity, promote neutral warmth, and increase ROM while decreasing spasticity.[40] The difference between a cast and a dynamic splint is that the cast offers circumferential neutral warmth and slow, long progressive stretch that allows changes to occur at the sarcomere level. Orthopedic serial casting is highly recommended after the client receives Botox (onabotulinumtoxinA) or phenol injections performed by a physician.[40]

The following supplies are needed:
- 3-inch plaster or fiberglass
- 2- or 3-inch stockinette
- 3-inch cotton cast padding (2 inches for pediatric)
- Cast saw
- Cast spreaders
- Bandage scissors

The client should be casted one joint at a time in one extremity at a time. Be sure to coordinate with the physical therapist.

(continued)

UNIT 3-76 INTERVENTION

ORTHOPEDIC SERIAL CASTING (CONTINUED)

SERIAL CASTING PROCEDURE[40]

1. Measure and cut the stockinette above the joint that is to be casted to cover the length of the area (eg, for the elbow, measure above the acromion process and past the radial and ulnar styloids).

2. Stretch the joint that is to be casted at maximum range, then back off 5 degrees.

3. Apply the stockinette.

4. Add extra padding to the bony prominences and skin against areas of increased resistance to force or shearing.

5. Continue to wrap the area with padding, layering each layer with half of the width of previous layer. You may roll up or down, but remove areas that can be pressure points. Do not dog ear or fold areas to create loops in the padding, and do not roll tightly.

6. Dip the plaster or fiberglass roll into a bucket of very warm water by holding onto the end of the roll until it bubbles. Stop, squeeze, and roll the plaster or fiberglass after laying it onto the extremity. Do not layer tightly as material will shrink with drying. Create negative space on each end of the cast to allow for circulation.

7. Fold back the edges of the stockinette to create a cuff, and secure the edges in casting material.

8. Smooth out the plaster or fiberglass to remove any rough textures.

9. Remove the cast by cutting up and down. Do not cut side to side.

10. Bivalve (ie, cut in half) to maintain stretch.

(continued)

ORTHOPEDIC SERIAL CASTING (CONTINUED)

AFTER SERIAL CASTING

Elevate the upper extremity after casting, in wheelchair and in bed, and avoid dependent positions. Ensure that the client, caregivers, and nursing staff are aware of precautions for the new cast. One way to ensure this is to post the precautions at the head of the bed. Once casting is completed, the practitioner should engage the client in active upper extremity exercises and meaningful, functional occupations and activities of daily living.[40]

Schedule[40]	• The first cast should be on for 24 hours to assess skin and overall tolerance to procedure, then remove the cast.
	• The second cast should be left on for 3 to 5 days and then re-casted until there are no gains in ROM.
	• Even if the skin integrity is really good, a serial cast should never be left on more than 7 days.
	• Cease casting after 3 consecutive casts if there has been no increase in ROM.
Signs of distress[40]	• Severely decreased circulation in the extremity, indicated by cold and cyanotic extremities
	• Profuse sweating
	• Increased agitation
	• Severe increase in edema
	• Unexplained spike in blood pressure
	• Unexplained spike in temperature/fever
	• May warrant immediate removal of the cast without exception

UNIT 3-76 INTERVENTION

ORTHOTIC GUIDELINES	
GENERAL SPLINTING TIPS[41]	
Practicing splinting	• Students and practitioners should practice splinting to become more comfortable and competent. • A good place to build skills is to practice molding the C-bar in a thumb spica splint with the thumb in palmar abduction instead of midway in opposition. • Practice being more flexible in splint construction using partial sheets or scrap pieces. • Try wearing the splint design yourself for at least 20 minutes to find typical pressure areas so that you will know where to pay careful attention and where to look with a client.
Preparing for splinting	• Prepare ahead for the worst situation. • Keep the heat pan clean and at a temperature between 160°F and 180°F, and maintain the water level to at least 3 inches. • Place a trash can next to the working area to collect scrap pieces of material. • Consider preparing the client's joint for the splinting position by using PAMs, such as paraffin, hot pack, or whirlpool, to increase the joint's range. • After creating a paper pattern of the splint, test the pattern on the client to adjust the tracing before cutting the material. • Use gravity when possible to assist in your splint construction. • Use padding to prevent pressure areas, especially with rough edges and limited time. • Use high-density padding as moleskin can trap dirt over time, and low-density padding typically flattens out very rapidly. Account for padding space in the splint design. *(continued)*

ORTHOTIC GUIDELINES (CONTINUED)

GENERAL SPLINTING TIPS[41]

Making adjustments and adding straps	• Reimmerse the splint for making major changes. Use a cup to pour hot water onto the splint to smooth out areas. • Use a heat gun for small adjustments by applying heat on both sides of the orthosis, and turn the heat gun to cool before turning it off. Use a spoon for smoothing out areas. • Chlorine can sometimes remove ink marks on the orthosis. • Use a heat gun on the area where the strapping adhesive will be placed, as well as on the back of the adhesive, to increase adhesion.
Cleaning scissors	• Clean your scissors with an alcohol swab. This will help keep the tool clean between clients, and will also remove residual glue from self-adhesive Velcro to keep scissors sharp.
Educating the patient	• Give the client or caregiver clear written instructions and, if available, a photo for donning and doffing. • As appropriate, provide instructions to nursing staff for splint donning and doffing. • Include the purpose of the splint, when to wear it, how to clean it, and how to cover it if it must be worn while bathing.
Edema	• Use soft, wide straps rather than rigid straps to help distribute the pressure and to accommodate for edema. • A wide elastic strap may be used to help maintain orthosis position. • Remold the splint as edema volume changes.
Considering a wound	• First place a stockinette over client's bandages to avoid having splinting material stick to the bandage. • Fabricate the orthosis over the client's dressings, and use gauze bandages to hold it in place.

(continued)

UNIT 3-77 INTERVENTION

ORTHOTIC GUIDELINES (CONTINUED)

GENERAL SPLINTING TIPS[41]

Considering the skin	• If the client has fragile skin or is at risk of burning, use a stockinette to protect his or her skin.
	• Pre-pad bony prominences; use flaring, wide straps; and smooth edges to reduce pressure.
	• If the client has scars, then a gel lining on the inside of the orthosis may be beneficial.
	• Check the client's skin frequently to assess for areas of excess pressure.

STATIC ORTHOSES[41]

After the person wears the static orthosis for 20 minutes, check for the following specifications:

Design	• The joint is positioned at the correct angle.
	• The joint involved in the orthosis has adequate medial and lateral support (ie, one-half of the circumference of the joint).
	• The trough is of adequate length distally and proximally (ie, two-thirds of the length of the forearm)
Function	• The orthosis accomplishes its goal (eg, immobilization or functional positioning).
	• The orthosis allows full motion at joints proximal and distal to the orthosis.
	• The orthosis provides adequate length and support to properly secure the joint in the orthosis without migrating or slipping off.
Straps	• The straps are securely held in place, and corners are rounded.
	• The strap length and width are adequate for the joint.
	• The Velcro is covered by the straps so that it does not catch on clothing.

(continued)

ORTHOTIC GUIDELINES (CONTINUED)

Comfort	• Edges of the orthotic device are smooth, and the corners are rounded. • Proximal and distal edges of the orthosis are flared and do not dig in to skin. • There are no areas of impingement or pressure sores. • Special care is taken to not irritate bony prominences. Padding may be used if needed.
Cosmetic appearance	• There are no visible fingerprints, dirt, or pencil and pen marks on the orthosis. • The splinting material is not buckled, warped, or wavy.
Therapeutic regimen	• The client understands the wearing schedule, including whether the orthosis is worn all the time or just at night, and for how many hours per day. • The client understands orthotic precautions. • The client understands how to clean the orthosis. • The client can don and doff the orthosis or can instruct others to do so.

UNIT 3-77 INTERVENTION

ORTHOTIC GUIDELINES (CONTINUED)

DYNAMIC ORTHOSES[41]

After the person wears the dynamic orthosis for 20 minutes, check for the following specifications:

Design	• The trough is an appropriate length and width. • The arches are supported but not compressed. • The trough permits full motion of the appropriate joints.
Function	• The finger cuffs are pulled in the correct direction, and perpendicular forces are used. • The orthosis accomplishes its goal, and the monofilament permits full motion when pulled. • The orthosis allows full motion as indicated at the joints proximal and distal to the orthosis. • The orthosis, finger cuff, and outrigger provide adequate length and support to properly secure the joint in the orthosis without migrating or slipping off. • The hook used for the monofilament and the outrigger are secured to the orthotic trough in the proper position and angle, so the hook will not be inadvertently pulled off.
Straps	• The straps are securely held in place, and the corners are rounded. • The strap length and width are adequate for the joint. • The Velcro is covered by straps so that it does not catch on clothing.
Comfort	• The edges of the orthotic device are smooth, and the corners are rounded. • Proximal, distal, and thenar edges of the orthosis are flared and do not dig in to skin. • There are no areas of impingement or pressure sores. • Special care is taken to not irritate bony prominences. Padding may be used if needed. • The finger cuff is smooth and wide to prevent irritation and to disperse forces. • Tension in the finger cuffs is appropriately adjusted for force.

(continued)

UNIT 3-77 INTERVENTION

ORTHOTIC GUIDELINES (CONTINUED)

Cosmetic appearance	• There are no visible fingerprints, dirt, or pencil and pen marks on the orthosis. • The material is not buckled, warped, or wavy.
Therapeutic regimen	• The client understands the wearing schedule, including whether the orthosis is worn all the time or just at night and for how many hours per day. • The client understands the orthotic precautions. • The client understands how to clean the orthosis. • The client can don and doff the orthosis or can instruct others to do so, including adjusting finger cuffs.

(continued)

ORTHOTIC GUIDELINES (CONTINUED)

COMMON SPLINTS[41]

Typical Splints Used	Wearing Guidelines
Boutonniere Deformity	
• The finger splint should hold the PIP joint in extension and maintain MCP and DIP joint movement. • Serial casting may also be used.	The splint should be worn continuously.
Burns on Hand	

• During the emergent phase, splint the hand in the antideformity position.
• Elevate and position in order to reduce edema.
• During the acute phase, splint the hand in the intrinsic plus position:
    ○ Wrist in 20 to 40 degrees of extension
    ○ MCP in 60 to 90 degrees of flexion
    ○ PIP and DIP joints in full extension
    ○ Thumb is positioned midway between radial and palmar abduction
• During the rehabilitation phase, use a static splint at night and dynamic splints in the daytime.
• Compression garments may also be used.
	The splint should be worn continuously.

de Quervain's Tenosynovitis	

• A thumb immobilization splint should be used to position the hand as follows:
    ○ 15 degrees of wrist extension
    ○ 40 to 45 degrees of CMC palmar abduction
    ○ Neutral thumb at the MCP joint
	The splint should be worn at night and during painful activities.

(continued)

UNIT 3-77 INTERVENTION

Orthotic Guidelines (continued)

Typical Splints Used	Wearing Guidelines
Dupuytren's Disease	
• A hand immobilization splint or resting hand splint should hold the wrist in neutral or slight extension. • Maintain full extension of the MCP, PIP, and DIP joints.	The splint should be worn following surgery during the day and at night. The splint may be removed temporarily for ROM exercises or hygiene.
Mallet Finger	
• A finger splint should hold the DIP joint in extension with the PIP joint able to flex. • The DIP joint should not be in flexion or able to flex.	The splint should be worn continuously for approximately 6 weeks while the tendon is healing, and then it should be worn only at night. The splint should be covered during showers. When the splint is removed in order to be cleaned, support the finger fully extended on a tabletop.
Osteoarthritis of the Thumb	
• A thumb immobilization splint should position the CMC in palmar abduction. • The thumb MCP joint may or may not be immobilized.	A forearm-based orthosis may be worn at night. The thumb orthosis should be worn during activities that require additional support for thumb stabilization or pain prevention. The splint should be worn continuously during an acute flare-up. It may be temporarily removed for ROM exercises or hygiene. *(continued)*

UNIT 3-77 INTERVENTION

ORTHOTIC GUIDELINES (CONTINUED)

Typical Splints Used	Wearing Guidelines
Rheumatoid Arthritis	

• A wrist immobilization splint should hold the wrist in 0 to 30 degrees of extension
 	
• A thumb immobilization splint, including a short opponens or thumb spica splint, can compensate for weak thenar muscles to increase thumb opposition for functional grasp.
 	
• A hand immobilization splint, also known as a *resting hand splint*, should position the hand to the following specifications:
   ◦ 0 to 15 degrees of wrist extension
   ◦ 15 to 45 degrees of MCP flexion
   ◦ Finger IPs in slight flexion
• The lateral borders of the thumb immobilization splint should be flared to block ulnar or radial deviation.
• Finger separators can also be used as needed.
• Ring splints are used for finger deformities (see swan neck and Boutonniere deformity in this table).
	The wrist immobilization splint or resting hand splint should be worn at night.
	
	Splints should be worn during painful daytime activities or to allow functional use of the hand.
	
	(continued)

ORTHOTIC GUIDELINES (CONTINUED)

Typical Splints Used	Wearing Guidelines
Scaphoid Fracture	

• A thumb immobilization splint should position the hand to these specifications:
   ◦ Wrist in a neutral position
   ◦ 0 to 10 degrees of thumb MCP flexion
   ◦ CMC palmar abduction
• The thumb can be positioned in a pincer grasp for functional use.
	Follow physician protocols.

Spasticity	

• A hand immobilization splint/resting hand splint should maintain a functional position as described here:
   ◦ The wrist in 20 to 30 degrees of extension
   ◦ MCP joints in 15 to 45 degrees of flexion
   ◦ 45 degrees of thumb palmer abduction
   ◦ IP joints in slight flexion
• A cone orthosis or ball orthosis with a finger spreader may be used.
• A hand paddle to encourage finger extension while weightbearing during therapy may also be encouraged.
• Create a palmer splint with a washcloth or a pool noodle and Velcro:
   ◦ First, place the middle of the Velcro into the washcloth, and roll the washcloth like a hotdog.
	The client can wear the resting hand splint at night and wear functional splints during therapy activities.

(continued)

UNIT 3-77 INTERVENTION

ORTHOTIC GUIDELINES (CONTINUED)

Typical Splints Used	Wearing Guidelines
• The other option is to cut a pool noodle to the width of the client's palm, and insert Velcro through the noodle: ◦ Crisscross Velcro around the dorsal wrist, and connect it at the volar wrist, overlapping the ends to hold the palmar piece in place. • Serial casting may also be used.	

Spinal Cord Injury

Refer to Section Two, Unit 3-44, for information about splinting for an SCI.

Swan Neck Deformity

| • A finger splint may include a ring splint to prevent PIP hyperextension and promote DIP extension.
• PIP flexion should not be restricted. | The splint should be worn continuously. |

Ulnar Collateral Ligament Injury (Skier's Thumb or Gamekeeper's Thumb)

| • A thumb orthosis should keep the MCP joint immobilized in neutral or slight ulnar deviation.
• CMC joint should be in 40 degrees of palmar abduction. | For microscopic tears, the splint should be worn continuously for 2 to 3 weeks.

For partial tears, the splint should be worn for more than 3 weeks.

For complete tears, follow the surgeon's postoperative protocols. |

UNIT 3-77 INTERVENTION

PROSTHESES

Prosthetics are designed to replace an extremity and may also be referred to as an *artificial limb.*[42,43]

PRESCRIPTION[42,43]	GOALS[42,43]

A prescription for an upper extremity prosthesis includes the following considerations:
 • Design
 • Strategy for control:
  ◦ Passive prosthesis
  ◦ Task-specific prosthesis
  ◦ Hybrid prosthesis
  ◦ Body-powered prosthesis
  ◦ Electrically powered prosthesis
 • Side and level of amputation
 • Socket interface
 • Socket frame
 • Mechanism for suspension:
  ◦ Suction
  ◦ Harness
  ◦ Anatomical
 • Terminal device
 • Wrist, elbow, or shoulder unit if applicable
	Occupational therapy related to a prosthesis in amputation rehabilitation may include the following goals:
	 • Minimize risks associated with use of prosthesis.
	 • Prevent overuse injuries in extremities.
	 • Promote care of residual limb.
	 • Maintain ROM in residual limb above amputation.
	 • Strengthen core, trunk, and extremities for use of prosthesis.
	 • Increase client satisfaction regarding prosthesis comfort and functionality.
	 • Increase independence in occupations with and without prosthesis.
	 • Improve quality of life.
	 • Maximize participation.

A prosthesis is custom made for the client and requires care. A prosthetist should be contacted if there are any questions or problems.

(continued)

UNIT 3-78 INTERVENTION

Prostheses (continued)

Types of Upper Extremity Prostheses

Control Strategy	Description[42,43]
Passive prosthesis	• If silicone, may resemble normal extremity • Cosmetically appealing for some clients • May be used to passively assist with functional tasks • Lightweight • Low maintenance • Easy to don • Difficult to perform activities requiring grasp
Task-specific prosthesis	• Enables function for specific activities • Low maintenance • Easy to don • Durable • Not functional for activities outside of intended use
Hybrid prosthesis	• Combines electric and body-powered control • Body-powered elbow and electrically powered wrist • Allows control of elbow and wrist or terminal device • Not as heavy as fully electric prosthesis • Allows increased grip strength • Requires a harness for the elbow prosthesis, which may be restrictive
Body-powered prosthesis	• Includes a harness, cable, socket, and hook or other terminal device • Durable and may be used in harsh environmental conditions • Provides the client with proprioceptive input • Cost effective • Clients may find the harness restrictive • Grip strength is decreased • Function may be limited, or may be difficult to control • Cosmetic appearance of hook and cables may bother some clients

(continued)

PROSTHESES (CONTINUED)

Control Strategy	Description[42,43]
Electrically-powered prosthesis	• Cosmetically has a natural appearance • Easy to don • May be fit during early rehabilitation • Allows more function than body-powered prosthesis • Requires less force to operate • Requires battery • Heavy • Requires complex maintenance and repairs • May be damaged by harsh environmental conditions

CARE OF YOUR PROSTHESIS[43]

Skin care	• Wash the limb at night with a mild soap. Rinse and dry the limb completely. • Do not use creams or powders unless instructed to by the physician or prosthetist. • Make sure the limb is clean and dry. • Inspect the skin for rashes, sores, or cracks. • The client should not wear the prosthesis if sores are present. The physician and/or prosthetist must be contacted first.
Socks and liners (Skip this section if the client does not use socks or liners.)	• Wash socks and liners daily. • Use mild soap and warm or cool water. Let socks and liners air dry, unless other specific instructions have been given. • Inspect the socks and liners before using. • Contact the prosthetist if socks or liners are damaged.

(continued)

UNIT 3-78 INTERVENTION

UNIT 3-78 INTERVENTION

PROSTHESES (CONTINUED)	

Before putting on the prosthesis	• Inspect the prosthesis for wear:
	   ○ Are there any loose parts?
	   ○ Is there an unusual noise?
	   ○ Is anything cracked or broken?
	• Call the prosthetist if any problems are found.
	• Do not wear a damaged prosthesis, as this may lead to a fall.

Shoes	• Make sure that the prosthesis has a shoe on it. • The heel height needs to be the same as the shoe that the prosthesis was made for. • The shoe must be laced tightly to the foot. • Do not wear a shoe that has a worn heel or a slippery sole.
Care of your prosthesis	• Keep the prosthesis dry. Do not wear the prosthesis in the water or shower, unless it was specifically made for that purpose. • If the prosthesis gets wet, immediately remove the shoe and towel dry the prosthesis. • Clean the inside of the socket daily. Use soap and water on a washcloth, or rubbing alcohol. • Keep the prosthesis away from high heat, which may damage the plastics. • Do not try to adjust or repair the prosthesis at home. Doing so may cause more expensive damage.
Putting on the prosthesis	• Sit in a chair with arms or on a bed with rails. • Put on the socks or liner, if any. • Ensure that the foot is pointing in the correct direction. • Place the limb in the socket as taught by the prosthetist. • Roll the suspension sleeve up onto the thigh, if there is one. • Push weight onto the prosthesis while still sitting to make sure that the limb is all of the way in the socket.

(continued)

PROSTHESES (CONTINUED)	
Getting up with the prosthesis	• Make sure that there is something sturdy to hold onto, such as the arms of a chair.
	• Push up through the arms and the unaffected leg(s).
	• The prosthesis should be positioned under the body and bear weight on it.
	• Before walking, the client should stand while holding onto something for a few seconds to be sure that he or she is balanced.

For more information, the Amputee Coalition provides online, phone, and person-to-person support for people with limb loss. The organization also advocates and lobbies on behalf of amputees. You may reach the Coalition at http://www.amputee-coalition.org

WHEELCHAIR PRESCRIPTION

MANUAL VERSUS POWER WHEELCHAIRS[44]

Manual Wheelchairs	Power Wheelchairs
• Manual wheelchairs require ROM, strength, and endurance in upper extremities. • The frames may be folding, rigid, standard, or lightweight. • Manual wheelchairs may have long-term effects on upper extremities. • Consider the client's need for camber or sport options. • Power assistance on a manual frame may be available.	• Power wheelchairs can be controlled through a hand joystick, head and neck controls, pneumatic controls, or other areas where a switch is placed. • Standing wheelchair options are available. • Power wheelchairs are heavier and more difficult to transport. • They must be charged and are generally more expensive than manual wheelchairs. • Consider the client's cognitive ability to operate a power wheelchair and the client's ability to maneuver in his or her environmental context, including car transportation options.

SEATING AND PREVENTION OF SKIN BREAKDOWN

Recline or tilt frames may be necessary for pressure redistribution breaks.

Pressure on the client's ischial tuberosity can lead to pressure ulcers. Cushions can help distribute the pressure. Types of cushions include air, foam, gel/liquid, honeycomb, hybrid, and custom molded cushions that can accommodate fixed contractures.[44]

(continued)

WHEELCHAIR PRESCRIPTION (CONTINUED)

WHEELCHAIR FITTING MEASUREMENTS

Note the client's body position and posture throughout measurements. Take fitting measurements while the client is sitting up straight with both feet flat on the floor, such as on a mat.[44]

Seat width	The seat width measures from the widest part of the thighs and hips with 0.5 inch to 1 inch added on each side.
	Consider accessibility through narrow spaces, and potential weight gain.
Seat depth	The seat depth measures from the base of the back to the inside of the bent knee with 1 to 2 inches subtracted.
	If the client has kyphosis or will slide forward throughout the day, then the client may need a longer measurement.
Seat height from floor	The seat height from the floor measures from the popliteal fossa to the bottom of the heel. The thighs should remain parallel to the floor.
Footplates	Footplates must clear the floor by at least 2 inches at their lowest point.
Backrest height	For full trunk support, the backrest height measures from the bottom of the seat to the top of the client's shoulders.
	For minimum trunk support, the backrest height measures from the bottom of the seat to below the inferior angle of the scapula.
Armrest height	The armrest height measures from the bottom of the seat to the bottom of the client's bent elbow.

UNIT 3-79 INTERVENTION

MUSCULOSKELETAL SYSTEM
PRECAUTIONS AND CONTRAINDICATIONS

WEIGHTBEARING

Always refer to the physician's orders for weightbearing precautions. Examples of weightbearing allowances and restrictions include the following[44]:

Weightbearing Status	Description
Nonweightbearing	The client may not put any weight on the extremity. He or she may need a sliding board for transfers.
Toe-touch weightbearing	The client can place his or her toe onto the ground for balance purposes, but cannot support more than 10% to 15% of his or her weight on the extremity. A tip for toe-touch weightbearing is to imagine that there is an egg underneath the foot.
Partial weightbearing	The client can support 30% to 50% of his or her weight on the extremity.
Weightbearing as tolerated	The client may place as much weight as tolerated with pain on the extremity.
Full weightbearing	There are no weightbearing restrictions.

(continued)

MUSCULOSKELETAL SYSTEM
PRECAUTIONS AND CONTRAINDICATIONS (CONTINUED)

TOTAL HIP REPLACEMENT[44,45]

Total hip replacement precautions are usually taken for 6 to 12 weeks after surgery. Always refer to the physician's orders. Hip dislocation can result from failure to follow precautions. The precautions vary according to the surgery approach.

Surgical Approach	Precautions
Anterior approach	• No hip extension is permitted. If the client has a long stride length, use a "wedding march" step technique. The client may not bridge in bed. • No hip adduction is permitted, including crossing of the legs. The client may use a hip abductor wedge when lying in the bed. • No external rotation is permitted. The toes must not be turned outward. The client should be cautious when getting out of bed or turning with a walker.

Posterior approach	• No hip flexion past 90 degrees is permitted:
	  ○ The client should use a hip kit reacher, sock aid, and elastic shoelaces for lower body dressing.
	  ○ A long-handled sponge should be used for bathing the lower body.
	  ○ When transferring, keep the client's legs extended and have the client lean backward.
	  ○ When getting into bed, the client should approach the bed backward and toward the midline.
	  ○ A tub bench, leg lifter, and raised toilet seat may also be used.
	
	• No hip adduction is permitted, including crossing of the legs. The client may use a hip abductor wedge when lying in the bed.
	
	• No external rotation is permitted. The toes must not be turned outward. The client should be cautious when getting out of bed or turning with a walker.

(continued)

UNIT 3-80 INTERVENTION

MUSCULOSKELETAL SYSTEM
PRECAUTIONS AND CONTRAINDICATIONS (CONTINUED)

INTERNAL FIXATION[44,45]

- Do not perform electrical stimulation over an area with metal, such as internal fixation screws.

EXTERNAL FIXATION[44,45]

- If the client has externally fixated extremities, move the extremities using the hardware.
- If there is a fracture in the middle of the limb, hold the limb proximally, distally, or both when moving the limb.
- Avoid holding the limb at the fracture site, but the limb may be picked up by the external fixator.

CERVICAL[44,45]

- The client should always wear a cervical collar unless he or she has been cleared by a doctor.
- Cervical precautions include no neck rotation, no bending at hips, no lifting objects weighing more than 8 lbs, and no driving.

LUMBAR[44,45]

- A client with lumbar precautions may need to wear a brace or corset when he or she is out of bed. The client may need to use a hip kit to perform functional activities.
- A client with lumbar precautions may not lift objects weighing more than 8 lbs, should not bend or twist at the hip, and should not pull on hospital bed side rails (to avoid straining the back).
- The client should avoid straining the abdomen when coughing, sneezing, or using the toilet.
- The client should not perform excessive physical activities until his or her surgeon clears the activity.

ORTHOTICS[44,45]

- A thoracic lumbosacral orthosis is typically donned and doffed while the client is supine. This brace can be worn while showering.
- A Philadelphia collar can be worn while showering.
- A Miami J collar must be removed and replaced with clean padding regularly.

UNIT 3–80 INTERVENTION

REFERENCES

1. OMICS International. Myotome. OMICS International. http://research.omicsgroup. org/index.php/Myotome. Published 2014. Accessed May 2, 2019.
2. Javed O, Ashmyan R. *Anatomy, Upper Limb, Muscles.* Treasure Island, FL; StatPearls Publishing; 2018.
3. Escamilla RF, Yamashiro K, Paulos L, Andrews JR. Shoulder muscle activity and function in common shoulder rehabilitation exercises. *Sports Med.* 2009;39(8):663-685. doi:10.2165/00007256-200939080-00004
4. Podsiadlo D, Richardson S. The timed up & go: a test of basic functional mobility for frail elderly persons. *J Am Geriatr Soc.* 1991;39(2):142-148.
5. Berg KO, Wood-Dauphinee SL, Williams JI, Maki B. Measuring balance in the elderly: validation of an instrument. *Can J Public Health.* 1992;82(suppl 2):S7-S11.
6. Kopp B, Kunkel A, Flor H, et al. The arm motor ability test: reliability, validity, and sensitivity to change of an instrument for assessing disabilities in activities of daily living. *Arch Phys Med Rehabil.* 1997;78(6):615-620.
7. Beaton DE, Wright JG, Katz JN. Development of the quickDASH: comparison of three item-reduction approaches. *J Bone Joint Surg Am.* 2005;87(5):1038-1046. doi:10.2106/JBJS.D.02060
8. Fairbank JC, Pynsent PB. The Oswestry disability index. *Spine.* 2000;25(22):2940-2952.
9. Mathiowetz V, Kashman N, Volland G, Weber K, Dowe M, Rogers S. Grip and pinch strength: normative data for adults. *Arch Phys Med Rehabil.* 1985;66(2):69-74.
10. Whelan LR. Assessing abilities and capacities: range of motion, strength, and endurance. In: Radomski MV, Trombly-Latham CA, eds. *Occupational Therapy for Physical Dysfunction.* 7th ed. Baltimore, MD: Lippincott Williams & Wilkins/Wolters Kluwer; 2014:145-241.
11. Calk P, Stewart L, Thomas S, Reichardt E. Accuracy and clinical usability of goniometer applications. *Am J Occup Ther.* 2016;70(7011500079p1). doi:10.5014/ ajot.2016.70S1-PO7074
12. Conable KA, Rosner AL. A narrative review of manual muscle testing and implications for muscle testing research. *J Chiropr Med.* 2011;10(3):157-165. doi:10.1016/j/ jcm.2011.04.001
13. Mathiowetz V, Volland G, Kashman N, Weber K. Adult norms for the box and blocks test of manual dexterity. *Am J Occup Ther.* 1985;39(6):386-391. doi:10.5014/ ajot.39.6.386
14. Jebsen RH, Taylor N, Trieschmann RB, Trotter MJ, Howard LA. An objective and standardized test of hand function. *Arch Phys Med Rehabil.* 1969;50(6):311-319.
15. Surrey L, Nelson K, Delelio C, et al. A comparison of performance outcomes between the Minnesota rate of manipulation test and the Minnesota manual dexterity test. *Work.* 2003;20(2):97-102.
16. Mathiowetz V, Weber K, Kashman N, et al. Adult norms for the nine hole peg test of finger dexterity. *OTJR.* 1985;5(1): 24-38. doi:10.1177/153944928500500102
17. Tiffin J, Asher EJ. The Purdue pegboard: norms and studies of reliability and validity. *J Appl Psychol.* 1948;32(3):234-247. doi:10.1037/h0061266
18. Hertel R, Ballmer FT, Lombert SM, Gerber C. Lag signs in the diagnosis of rotator cuff rupture. *J Shoulder Elbow Surg.* 1996;5(4):307-313.
19. Michener LA, Walsworth MK, Doukas WC, Murphy KP. Reliability and diagnostic accuracy of 5 physical examination tests and combination of tests for subacromial impingement. *Arch Phys Med Rehabil.* 2009;90(11):1898-1903. doi:10.1016/j. apmr.2009.05.015

20. Caliş M, Akgün K, Birtane M, Karacan I, Caliş H, Tüzün F. Diagnostic values of clinical diagnostic tests in subacromial impingement syndrome. *Ann Rheum Dis.* 2000;59:44-47.

21. Hegedus EJ, Goode A, Campbell S, et al. Physical examination tests of the shoulder: a systematic review with meta-analysis of individual tests. *Br J Sports Med.* 2008;42:80-92. doi:10.1136/bjsm.2007.038406

22. Marx RG, Bombardier C, Wright JG. What do we know about the reliability and validity of physical examination tests used to examine the upper extremity? *J Hand Surg.* 1999;24A:185-193. doi:10.1052/jhsu.1999.jhsu24a0185

23. Magee DJ. *Orthopedic Physical Assessment.* 5th ed. St. Louis, MO: Saunders Elsevier; 2008.

24. Konin JG, Wiksten DL, Isear JA, Brader H. *Special Tests for Orthopedic Examination.* Thorofare, NJ: SLACK Incorporated; 2006.

25. Flynn T, Cleland J, Whitman J. *User's Guide to the Musculoskeletal Examination: Fundamentals for the Evidence-based Clinician.* Buckner, KY: Evidence in Motion; 2008.

26. Fitzgerald RH. Acetabular labrum tears. Diagnosis and treatment. *Clin Orthop Relat Res.* 1995;(311):60-68.

27. Hegedus EJ, Cook C, Hasselblad V, Goode A, McCrory DC. Physical examination tests for assessing a torn meniscus in the knee: a systematic review with meta-analysis. *J Orthop Sports Phys Ther.* 2007;37(9):541-550. doi:10.2519/jospt.2007.2560

28. Ahmad CS, McCarthy M, Gomez JA, Shubin Stein BE. The moving patellar apprehension test for lateral patellar instability. *Am J Sports Med.* 2009;37(4):791-796. doi:10.1177/0363546508328113

29. Baxter R. *Pocket Guide to Musculoskeletal Assessment.* 2nd ed. Philadelphia, PA: Elsevier; 2003.

30. Noble CA. The treatment of iliotibial band friction syndrome. *Br J Sports Med.* 1979;13(2):51-54.

31. Lee KT, Park YU, Jegal H, Park JW, Choi JP, Kim JS. New method of diagnosis for chronic ankle instability: comparison of manual anterior drawer test, stress radiography and stress ultrasound. *Knee Surg Sports Traumatol Arthrosc.* 2014;22:1701-1707. doi:10.1007/s00167-013-2690-x

32. Cook CE, Hegedus EJ. *Orthopedic Physical Examination Tests: An Evidence-Based Approach.* New Jersey, NJ: Prentice Hall/Pearson; 2007.

33. Marik TL, Roll SC. Effectiveness of occupational therapy interventions for musculoskeletal shoulder conditions: a systematic review. *Am J Occup Ther.* 2016;71(1):7101180020p1-7101180020p11. doi:10.5014/ajot.2017.023127

34. Reed KL. Inhibition and facilitation techniques. In: Reed K, Zukas R, eds. *Quick Reference to Occupational Therapy.* 2nd ed. Pro-Ed, Inc; 2001:844-846

35. American Occupational Therapy Association. Physical agent modalities: a position paper. *Am J Occup Ther.* 2008;62(6):691-693. doi:10.5014/ajot.62.6.691

36. Bracciano AG. *Physical Agent Modalities: Theory and Application for the Occupational Therapist.* Thorofare, NJ: SLACK Incorporated; 2008.

37. Coopee RA. Elastic Taping (Kinesio Taping Method). In: Skirven TM, Osterman AL, eds. *Rehabilitation of the Hand and Upper Extremity.* 5th ed. Philadelphia, PA: Mosby; 2002.

38. Kase K, Hashimoto T, Okane T. *Kinesio Taping Perfect Manual.* Tokyo, Japan: Ken Ikai; 1996.

39. Kase K. *Illustrated Kinesio Taping.* 3rd ed. Tokyo, Japan: Ken Ikai; 1996.

40. Coppard BM, Lohman H. *Introduction to Orthotics: A Clinical Reasoning & Problem-Solving Approach.* 3rd ed. St. Louis, MO: Elsevier Mosby; 2008.

41. Coppard BM, Lohman H. *Introduction to Orthotics: A Clinical Reasoning & Problem-Solving Approach.* 4th ed. St. Louis, MO: Elsevier Mosby; 2015.

42. Fitzgibbons P, Medvedev G. Functional and clinical outcomes of upper extremity amputation. *J Am Acad Orthop Surg.* 2015;12(23):751-760. doi:10.5435/JAAOS-D-14-00302

43. Baird J. Overview of limb prosthetics. Merck Manual Professional Version. https://www.merckmanuals.com/professional/special-subjects/limb-prosthetics/overview-of-limb-prosthetics. Updated July 2015. Accessed May 2, 2019.

44. Pendleton HM, Schultz-Krohn W. *Pedretti's Occupational Therapy: Practice Skills for Physical Dysfunction.* 7th ed. St. Louis, MO: Elsevier Mosby; 2013.

45. Reed KL. *Quick Reference to Occupational Therapy.* 3rd ed. Austin, TX: Pro-Ed; 2014.

SECTION FIVE

Cardiovascular, Lymphatic, Respiratory, and Integumentary Systems

Sit W, Neville M.
*Handbook of Occupational Therapy for
Adults With Physical Disabilities* (pp 371-428).
© 2020 SLACK Incorporated.

CASE

DIAGNOSIS: SKIN CANCER

This story comes from a memorable experience I had while working in the intensive care unit (ICU) at a local hospital. My client had a diagnosis of skin cancer and was undergoing leech therapy treatment in the ICU. The leeches were being used to remove the drainage from the man's face, which was misshapen with swelling due to the removal of half his tongue. The ICU room was equipped with a bear shield positioned over the man, to keep the leeches warm. On the wall was a container where all the leeches swam in blood that had been drained from the client.

As I spoke to the client, he confided in me that he did not like the leech shield; specifically, he did not want to be covered. This gave me an idea, so I asked the client, "Why don't we draw on the bear shield to make it a bear?" He consented, and it worked: this made the bear shield more comfortable for him. While we could not change the client's circumstance, we were able to change an aspect of the environment to improve his level of comfort.

VITAL SIGNS

Pay close attention to the client's vital signs before, during, and after therapy. Stop therapy immediately if there is any sudden change in vital signs. Defer therapy if the value is outside the client's normal range. Always pay attention to the client's chart and doctor's orders.

NORMAL ADULT VALUES[1]

Heart rate	60 to 100 beats per minute (beats/min)
Blood pressure	120/80 mm Hg (systolic 100 to 140, and diastolic 60 to 90)
Mean arterial pressure	70 to 110 mm Hg
Respiration rate	12 to 20 breaths per minute
Pulse oximetry	95% to 100% saturation
Oral temperature	98.6°F
Rectal temperature	99.6°F
Intracranial pressure (ICP)	Less than 20 mm Hg

PULSE SCALE[1]

0	Absent pulse
1+	Weak and thready pulse
2+	Normal pulse
3+	Strong pulse
4+	Bounding pulse

VITAL SIGNS (CONTINUED)

FACTORS IMPACTING VITAL SIGN READINGS AND THERAPY IMPLICATIONS

Vital Sign	Factors	Therapy Implications
Heart rate[1]	• Resting heart rate may be increased to 90 to 110 beats/min in clients who have undergone a heart transplant. • Beta blockers may cause lower heart rate responses.	Monitor heart rate and blood pressure for signs of exercise intolerance.
Pulse oximetry[1]	• Carboxyhemoglobin, methemoglobin, low hemoglobin levels, or fever may result in a false high reading. • Peripheral vascular disease, poor circulation, cold tested extremity, bruising under the nail bed or dark nail polish, and environmental light interference may result in a false low reading. • Consider using earlobe or forehead probes for pulse oximetry to avoid false low readings.	Stop therapy if oxygen saturation drops below 90%, unless the physician has set individual parameters for the patient. *(continued)*

VITAL SIGNS (CONTINUED)

FACTORS IMPACTING VITAL SIGN READINGS AND THERAPY IMPLICATIONS

Vital Sign	Factors	Therapy Implications

Blood pressure[1]	• For the most accurate measure, blood pressure should always be taken on the same arm in the same position.
	• Bed rest may cause blood pressure to drop when the client changes position. Within 3 minutes of orthostatic stress, the following may occur:
	  ○ Systolic blood pressure may drop 20 mm Hg.
	  ○ Diastolic blood pressure may drop 10 mm Hg.
	• The client may benefit from gradually increasing the bed angle by 20 to 30 degrees until he or she is upright.
		Monitor heart rate and blood pressure for signs of exercise intolerance.

ICP[1]	• ICP may increase in the following situations:
	  ○ Increased blood pressure
	  ○ Agitation
	  ○ Nausea or vomiting
	  ○ Increased physical exertion
	  ○ Lying in a supine position with the head of the bed flat
	  ○ Attempting the Valsalva maneuver
	  ○ Compression of the abdomen
		In patients whose ICP is being closely monitored, do not change the angle of the head of bed without clearance from medical staff.

HEMATOLOGY VALUES

The following chart includes normal ranges for common lab values in a complete blood count.

Therapy is normally deferred in patients with critical values.

WHITE BLOOD CELLS AND LEUKOCYTES[1]

Measure of blood components responsible for fighting infections	Normal range: 4500 to 11,000/mm³ • Below normal values: Client is highly susceptible to infection. Observe neutropenic precautions, including washing hands and wearing a mask and gown. • Above normal values: Client may have decreased exercise tolerance. Critical values: • Less than 2000/mm³ • More than 30,000/mm³

HEMOGLOBIN[1]

Measure of the blood's capacity to carry oxygen	Normal range: Males: 13 to 18 g/dl Females: 12 to 16 g/dl • Less than 8.0: No exercise is permitted. • 8 to 10: Light exercise/activities of daily living (ADLs)/gait will be permitted. Allow frequent rest breaks Critical values: • Less than 5 • More than 20

HEMATOCRIT[1]

Measure of red blood cell percentage in total blood volume	Normal range: Males: 37% to 49% Females: 36% to 46% • Less than 25%: Do not mobilize the client. Critical values: • Less than 20% • More than 60%

(continued)

HEMATOLOGY VALUES (CONTINUED)

PLATELET[1] Measure of blood component involved in coagulation	Normal range: 140,000 to 440,000/mm^3 <ul><li>Less than 20,000: No therapy</li><li>20,000 to 50,000: Do not use resistive exercises, but may use active range of motion (AROM), ADLs, and ambulation</li><li>More than 50,000: May do resistive exercise</li><li>Below normal range: Increased risk of bleeding</li><li>Above normal range: Increased risk of blood clots</li></ul> Critical values: <ul><li>Less than 20,000</li></ul>

ELECTROCARDIOGRAM INTERPRETATION

An electrocardiogram (ECG) records the electrical activity of the heart by placing electrodes in specific locations.[1,2]

The electrode cables, or leads, measure the voltage difference between the electrodes. The 12 leads typically used include 6 limb leads and 6 chest leads.[1,2]

- Limb leads may be placed on wrists and ankles, or on the chest corners:
    - Limb leads include leads I, II, III, aVR, aVL, and aVF.
- Chest leads include leads V_1, V_2, V_3, V_4, V_5, and V_6.

If the ECG paper is calibrated at 25 mm/s, each large square is equivalent to 5 mm (0.2 seconds), and each small square is equivalent to 1 mm (0.04 seconds).[1,2]

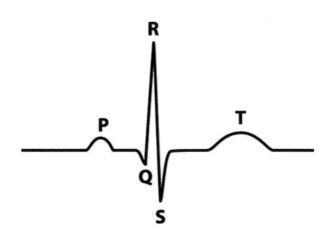

P Wave: Atrial contraction

QRS: Ventricular depolarization and contraction

PR interval: Time for electrical signal to travel from sinus node to ventricles

T wave: Ventricles repolarizing

(continued)

UNIT 1–84 NEED TO KNOW

ELECTROCARDIOGRAM INTERPRETATION (CONTINUED)

STEPS FOR ANALYZING AN ELECTROCARDIOGRAM READING[1,2]

1. Rhythm	• The ventricular rhythm is the distance between each R: 　o Is the ventricular rhythm regular? • The atrial rhythm is the distance between each P: 　o Is the atrial rhythm regular? • The sinus rhythm is the heart rhythm that originates in the sinus node: 　o Is the sinus rhythm regular? Is there a P wave before each QRS?
2. Heart rate	• The heart rate is the number of QRS segments in 1 minute or multiplied over a shorter time.
3. Axis	• Left axis deviation is evident when QRS is positive in lead I but negative in lead III. • Right axis deviation is evident when QRS is negative in lead I but positive in lead III.
4. P wave	• Normal amplitude: 0.05 to 0.25 mV • Normal duration: 0.06 to 0.11 seconds • Normal shape: Smooth and rounded • Normal frequency: One per QRS segment • Tall P wave may indicate right atrial enlargement. • Bifid "M" P wave may indicate left atrial enlargement.
5. PR interval	• Normal interval: 0.12 to 0.20 seconds: 　o The interval may be longer in elderly adults. 　o The interval will appear shorter if the heart rate is faster. • Long PR interval: Indicative of slowed conduction from atria to ventricles • Short PR interval: Indicative of another pathway of conduction

(continued)

Electrocardiogram Interpretation (continued)

Steps for Analyzing an Electrocardiogram Reading[1,2]

6. QRS interval	• Normal interval: 0.08 to 0.10 seconds
	• Large Q wave: Indicative of previous myocardial infarction (MI) or even an MI within the last 6 hours
	• R wave: The height from baseline to R in V1 should be less than baseline to S. If not, it may indicate right ventricular hypertrophy or posterior infarction
7. T wave	• Note if the T wave is deflected downward or has a tall, sharp peak. It may be followed immediately by a small rounded U wave.
	• T wave inversion: Indicative of possible ischemia or previous infarction
	• Tall T waves: Indicative of hyperkalemia or hyperacute MI
8. QT interval	• Normal interval: 0.36 to 0.44 seconds from the beginning of the Q to the end of the T wave, or less than half of the R-R interval
9. ST segment	• The ST segment is the end of QRS to the beginning of the T wave
	• Normal shape: Typically flat
	• ST elevation: Indicative of possible acute MI (ST elevated myocardial infarction), acute pericarditis, or aneurysm
	• ST depression: Indicative of acute ischemia
	(continued)

ELECTROCARDIOGRAM INTERPRETATION (CONTINUED)

THERAPY IMPLICATIONS

Look at the client's telemetry monitor prior to and during therapy to determine if you need to stop or if you can proceed with therapy.

Premature ventricular contraction	Premature ventricular contraction is a premature heartbeat that occurs in the ventricles.
Ventricular tachycardia	Ventricular tachycardia presents as a heart rate of more than 100 beats/min. Defer therapy because the client is medically unstable; sudden death can occur. Ventricular tachycardia on an ECG
Ventricular fibrillation	Defer therapy.
Other conditions: • Premature ventricular contractions • Atrial arrhythmias • Atrioventricular block • Junctional arrhythmia	Talk with medical staff about holding therapy and monitor closely.

ECHOCARDIOGRAM

Echocardiography, or *diagnostic cardiac ultrasound*, is a cardiac imaging test that uses sound waves to create an echocardiogram (ie, an image of the heart). The test informs cardiologists about the structure and function of the heart.[3] Results from the echo may be included on the client's chart.

One function that the echo measures is the ejection fraction (EF), which indicates how the heart is pumping out blood.[1,3]

- Normal EF levels are between 50% and 70%.

- EF levels between 41% and 49% are considered borderline and may be due to heart damage.

- EF levels below 40% may indicate heart failure.

METABOLIC EQUIVALENTS AND ACTIVITIES

Metabolic equivalent (MET) levels measure the amount of oxygen required for an activity. More oxygen is required to meet increased activity demands, indicating that the heart and lungs are working harder. MET levels describe the amount of energy expended by the client.[1,4] Understanding MET levels can help the practitioner identify the client's activity tolerance and are useful during cardiac rehabilitation.

The following chart describes the intensity level of the activity and sample activities.

(continued)

METABOLIC EQUIVALENTS AND ACTIVITIES (CONTINUED)

ACTIVITY INTENSITY (METABOLIC EQUIVALENT LEVEL)	ACTIVITY EXAMPLES
Minimal (1 to 1.5 METs)[1,4]	• Sleeping • Sitting at the edge of the bed • Typing at a computer • Watching TV • Riding in a car
Light (1.5 to 3.0 METs)[1,4]	• Grooming • Dressing • Eating • Getting in or out of bed • Cooking • Washing dishes • Driving • Sewing • Playing cards • Writing
Moderate (3.0 to 6.0 METs)[1,4]	• Sweeping floors • Vacuuming • Carrying light laundry • Raking a lawn or digging in a garden • Moving furniture • Having a bowel movement • Taking care of children • Walking upstairs • Playing golf • Practicing yoga • Walking 3 mph
Vigorous (More than 6.0 METs)[1,4]	• Jogging or running • Carrying groceries upstairs • Playing sports such as soccer, basketball, or football • Quickly climbing stairs

UNIT 2-87 EVALUATION

COMMON ASSESSMENTS ACROSS PRACTICE SETTINGS

ASSESSMENT	ACUTE	INPATIENT	HOME HEALTH	SNF	OUTPATIENT
Common Assessments Across Practice Settings					
Vital signs	✓	✓	✓	✓	
Borg Rating of Perceived Exertion Scale	✓	✓			✓
Stages of a Pressure Ulcer Wound	✓	✓		✓	
Edema Scale	✓	✓		✓	

SNF: skilled nursing facility.

(continued)

COMMON ASSESSMENTS
ACROSS PRACTICE SETTINGS (CONTINUED)

VITAL SIGNS

Refer to Unit 1-82 in this section for information about vital signs.

BORG RATING OF PERCEIVED EXERTION SCALE[5]

- Purpose: Assesses physical activity intensity
- Context: Clients across diagnoses in an acute, inpatient, or outpatient setting
- Format: Verbal rating scale
- Time to administer: Varies by the duration of the physical activity
- Materials: None
- Cost: Free
- Website: https://www.cdc.gov/physicalactivity/basics/measuring/exertion.htm

UNIT 2-87 EVALUATION

STAGES OF A PRESSURE ULCER WOUND

The following scale can be used to describe skin integrity and rate the severity of a pressure ulcer wound.[6]

STAGE 1

- The skin is intact with redness that does not blanch. The area may be warmer, cooler, painful, firm, or soft to the touch.
- Note: Stage 1 may be difficult to detect in individuals who have darkly pigmented skin.

STAGE 2

- There is partial-thickness skin loss. A shallow open ulcer may appear red or pink, and a blister may be present.
- No slough or bruising is present.

STAGE 3

- There is full-thickness skin loss. Subcutaneous fat may be visible, but bone and muscle are not visible.
- Slough may be present.

STAGE 4

- There is full-thickness skin and tissue loss with exposed bone, tendon, or muscle.
- Epibole (rolled edges), undermining, and tunneling are often present.
- Slough or eschar may be present.

UNSTAGEABLE

- There is full-thickness skin and tissue loss, but the base of the ulcer is covered by slough or eschar, so the true depth and stage (3 or 4) cannot be determined until its removal.
- Stable eschar on heels, that which is dry, adherent, and intact without erythema, should not be removed.

(continued)

STAGES OF A PRESSURE ULCER WOUND (CONTINUED)

DEEP-TISSUE PRESSURE INJURY

- There is purple or maroon discoloration over intact or non-intact skin that is non-blanchable or has a blood-filled blister. This indicates damage to underlying soft tissue from pressure or shear forces.
- Deep-tissue pressure injury is often preceded by pain and temperature change.
- Does not describe vascular, traumatic, neuropathic, or dermatologic conditions.
- Note: Deep-tissue pressure injuries may be difficult to detect in individuals who have darkly pigmented skin.

UNIT 2-88 EVALUATION

EDEMA SCALE

Pitting edema refers to swelling that leaves an indentation or pit when pressed. The following scale is used to rate the severity of edema, and requires the practitioner to press on the swollen area and observe the indentation depth, quality, and rebound time.[7]

0	• None
+1	• Trace • Barely noticeable pit indentation • Disappears immediately • Normal contours of foot and leg
+2	• Mild • Pit indentation of less than 5 mm • Rebounds within a few seconds • Fairly normal contours of foot and leg
+3	• Moderate • Deep pit indentation of 5 to 10 mm • Rebounds within several seconds • Noticeable foot and leg swelling
+4	• Severe • Pit indentation of more than 1 cm • Rebounds in 20 seconds or longer • Severe foot and leg swelling

COMMON INTERVENTIONS ACROSS PRACTICE SETTINGS

Intervention	Acute	Inpatient	Home Health	SNF	Outpatient
Common Interventions Across Practice Settings					
Ventilatory techniques (positioning, pursed lip breathing, and diaphragmatic breathing)	✓	✓			✓
Pressure ulcer prevention	✓	✓		✓	
Lymphedema management	✓	✓	✓	✓	✓
Phase 1 Cardiac Rehabilitation Guidelines and Precautions	✓	✓			✓
Energy Conservation Tips	✓	✓	✓	✓	✓
Burn Care	✓	✓			✓
Passy-Muir Valve (PMV)	✓	✓			
Common ICU Equipment	✓	✓			
Cardiovascular, Lymphatic, Respiratory, and Integumentary Systems Precautions and Contraindications	✓	✓	✓	✓	

(continued)

UNIT 3-90 INTERVENTION

COMMON INTERVENTIONS
ACROSS PRACTICE SETTINGS (CONTINUED)

VENTILATORY TECHNIQUES[8]

- Description: Ventilatory techniques help the client to breathe better. Noninvasive ventilation supports breathing through the upper airway by using a mask or other device. Invasive ventilation supports breathing by bypassing the upper airway and includes laryngeal mask, tracheostomy, or tracheal tube.

- Approach: Ventilatory techniques include pursed-lip breathing, deep breathing, and diaphragmatic breathing. Count inspirations and expirations slowly with, "One thousand and one, one thousand and two, one thousand and three ..." as opposed to "One, two, three ..." Education may include energy conservation, smoking cessation, and dressing lightly. The therapist may record the client's cardiac rhythm and heart rate at each session.

- Precautions: Clients with cardiac conditions need to monitor their heart rate and blood pressure closely. Early in rehabilitation, the client may work at 50% of maximum capacity in order to protect healing cardiac tissue. Stop therapy immediately and report to the physician if the client experiences chest pain, dizziness, shortness of breath, nausea, or extreme fatigue. Other symptoms that may warrant stopping therapy include angina, confusion, light-headedness, and nausea. Sternal precautions must be maintained for 6 to 8 weeks after open-chest surgery. Consider preexisting medical conditions while planning treatments.

- Significance: Higher activity levels result in the heart pumping harder and faster in order to meet the body's demand for more oxygen. Strain on the heart muscle may result in damage or a heart attack. Ventilatory techniques aid the body in taking in more oxygen to meet demands and prevent damage.

(continued)

UNIT 3-90 INTERVENTION

COMMON INTERVENTIONS
ACROSS PRACTICE SETTINGS (CONTINUED)

PRESSURE ULCER PREVENTION[9]

- Description: *Pressure ulcer prevention* refers to reduction of pressure on the skin, proper caring for wounds, pain management, infection prevention, and nutrition education.

- Approach: For clients on bed rest, pressure ulcers can be prevented through AROM or passive range of motion (PROM) exercises, skin integrity maintenance, pressure mapping, and caregiver training. Pillows and cushions may be used for elevation, positioning, and postural support.

- Precautions: Pressure ulcers tend to form over bony prominences, including elbows, lower back, hips, and ankles. Facilities may be penalized if clients acquire pressure ulcers.

- Significance: Blood flow containing oxygen and nutrients to the skin is reduced as a result of pressure secondary to lack of movement.

LYMPHEDEMA MANAGEMENT[10]

- Description: *Lymphedema management* refers to interventions that manage swelling associated with fluid of the lymphatic system.

- Approach: Exercise, retrograde massage, and manual lymphatic drainage are techniques that manage lymphedema. Leg elevation is important to assist with lymph flow, and compression stockings, isotonic gloves, pneumatic pumps, and multilayer bandages may also be used.

- Precautions: For clients with deep vein thrombosis, avoid intervention for 48 hours following the start of Coumadin (warfarin) in order to reduce risk of stroke.

- Significance: Lymphedema can result in disability, amputation, infection, pain, or death over time. Although lymphedema cannot be cured in every case, it can be managed to reduce the risk of complications.

UNIT 3-90 INTERVENTION

PHASE 1 CARDIAC REHABILITATION GUIDELINES AND PRECAUTIONS

Phase 1 of cardiac rehabilitation occurs in the hospital. Phase 2 of cardiac rehabilitation occurs in outpatient therapy. Phase 3 of cardiac rehabilitation is the maintenance phase.[1,11]

Phase 1 Intervention Guidelines[1,11]	• Rehabilitation may begin when physician orders are received after surgery.
	• Assess the client's vital signs in a resting position before any activity.
	• Perform 5 minutes of warm-up exercises prior to ambulation or activity sessions.
	• Monitor vital signs throughout the activity.
	• Perform 5 minutes of cool-down exercises.
	• Assess the client's vital signs in a resting position after activity.
	• Higher level activities and distances may be incorporated once the client is able to maintain a stable hemodynamic status.
	• Provide the client and any family members with education on precautions, activity levels, and exercise monitoring.

(continued)

PHASE 1 CARDIAC REHABILITATION GUIDELINES AND PRECAUTIONS (CONTINUED)	
Phase 1 Precautions[1,11]	• Stop Phase 1 activities, and notify the physician if any of the following occur:
	◦ The client experiences angina (chest pain).
	◦ The client has an increase in heart rate by more than 25 beats/min during exercise.
	◦ The client has a drop in blood pressure by more than 20 mm Hg.
	◦ Systolic blood pressure is less than 90 mm Hg or more than 180 mm Hg.
	◦ The client experiences excess fatigue, dyspnea, or dizziness.
	• Observe these sternal precautions:
	◦ Sternotomy, about 8 to 10 weeks
	◦ Mini-sternotomy, about 4 weeks
	◦ Minimally invasive direct coronary artery bypass, refer to pain level
	• Observe these radial graft precautions:
	◦ Pain levels guide activity level.
	◦ The client's arm should be kept supported, but constant elevation is not necessary.
	• Oxygen is needed during ambulation if the client's oxygen saturation rate is less than 90% or if the client is on 2 liters of oxygen.
	• Mediastinal and pleural chest tubes may need to be put to water seal when ambulating.
	• Observe this pacemaker removal precaution:
	◦ The client should not perform more than minimal activity for 4 hours after the pacemaker wires are removed.
	• Observe these precautions for the client's showering:
	◦ Permitted 48 hours after chest tube removal, but no sooner than the fourth day after surgery
	◦ Remove temporary pacemaker wires
	◦ No sooner than 10 days after an internal cardiac defibrillator is placed

UNIT 3-91 INTERVENTION

ENERGY CONSERVATION TIPS

Educating clients on energy conservation strategies can help reduce fatigue for clients with diagnoses including cardiovascular disease, multiple sclerosis, spinal cord injury, and rheumatoid arthritis.[12]

When suggesting specific energy conservation tips, it is important to collaborate with clients on areas in which they may wish to conserve energy and areas that are highly meaningful in which energy conservation tips may impede their occupational identity.[12]

Prioritizing[12]	• Eliminate unnecessary tasks (as determined by the client):
	    ○ Air dry dishes rather than hand drying.
	    ○ Use precut vegetables when cooking.
	 • Delegate tasks to family members or hired staff, if able.
	 • Consider using resources such as Meals on Wheels or grocery store deliveries.

Planning[12]	• Consider the best time of day for each activity with typical energy levels. • Spread out activities evenly throughout the week. • To minimize trips, gather all supplies and equipment needed before starting an activity.

Positioning[12]	• Sit during activities when possible:
	    ○ Use a shower chair.
	    ○ Use a chair while folding laundry, cooking, dressing, and grooming.
	 • Rather than lifting, slide objects across a counter or use wheeled carts.
	 • Arrange commonly used items in areas of easy reach.
	 • Use long-handled tools to minimize bending and reaching.
	 • Use a long-handled sponge in the shower.

Pacing[12]	• Take frequent breaks. • Avoid rushing.

BURN CARE

GENERAL OCCUPATIONAL THERAPY GUIDELINES

- Burns should be evaluated by an occupational therapist within the first 24 hours after injury for early positioning and splinting treatments.[1,13]
- It may be beneficial to complete the evaluation during a dressing change to more accurately observe the wound.[1]
- Coordinate range of motion (ROM) evaluations and occupational therapy treatments with administration of pain medication.[1]
- Be aware of physiological responses to occupational therapy treatment, and look for signs of pain if the patient cannot verbally communicate. Watch for facial expressions and vital sign changes.[1]
- A variety of dressing types may be used depending on the physician's specifications.[1]
- Dressings may include topical antimicrobial ointments, and dressings that include silver, biologic dressings, or biosynthetic products.[1]
- Hydrotherapy is a method of whirlpool used to remove necrotic tissue and improve circulation. Hydrotherapy may provide an opportunity for ROM exercises and simple ADL participation unencumbered by dressings.[1]

PHASE 1: EMERGENT PHASE

- The emergent phase is the first 72 hours after a burn.[14]
- Total body surface area affected and depth of burn are determined.[14]
- Intubation may be required.[14]

Interventions[1,13]

- Splinting
- Positioning
- ROM (specifically PROM)

(continued)

UNIT 3-93 INTERVENTION

BURN CARE (CONTINUED)

BED POSITIONING AND SPLINTING

- Position the area affected by the burn in an anti-contracture position, using splints as needed.[13,14]
- Anti-contracture positions of joints are described as follows:

Affected Body/ Joint Area	Anti-Contracture Splinting Positions
Neck[1,13,14]	• In midline, extended • No pillows if burn includes neck area or ears
Shoulders, axilla[1,13,14]	• Abducted 90 degrees with 10 degrees of flexion • Airplane splint • If the axilla region is involved in the burn, the arm may be further placed in scaption • External rotation
Elbows[1,13,14]	• Extended • Forearm supinated
Wrists[1,13,14]	• Extended up to 45 degrees • In instances of circumferential burns, alternate splints may be needed in positions of flexion and extension

Hands[1,13,14]	• Splinted, palms up
	• Hand splint:
	  ∘ Intrinsic plus hand orthosis, antideformity, position of safe immobilization
	  ∘ Wrist slightly extended 0 to 30 degrees
	  ∘ Metacarpophalangeal flexed 70 to 90 degrees
	  ∘ Proximal interphalangeal and distal interphalangeal joints fully extended

Hips[1,13,14]	• Extended, avoid rotation • Abducted approximately 20 degrees
Knees[1,13,14]	• Extended
Feet[1,13,14]	• Flexed 90 degrees to neutral position

(continued)

UNIT 3-93 INTERVENTION

BURN CARE (CONTINUED)

RANGE OF MOTION EXERCISES AND STRETCHING

- Perform AROM exercises (active assistive ROM or PROM as necessary) multiple times a day.[13]
- Stretches should be held long enough to provide a sustained stretch, but should be low repetitions.[14]

  Follow precautions when performing ROM of hand with extensor tendon injury. Avoid placing the extensor tendon on maximal stretch by first placing the wrist in 45 to 90 degrees of extension and completing only isolated joint PROM exercises. Do not perform composite ROM exercises.[1]

PHASE 2: ACUTE PHASE

- The acute phase begins after the emergent phase and may include a surgical or postoperative phase.[14]
- Wound healing and closure occurs.[14]

Interventions

- Continued splinting, anti-contracture positioning, and ROM:
  - Splinting may be used to immobilize a skin graft during the first 3 to 7 days after the graft until it is stable.[14]
  - After skin grafting procedures, do not perform ROM for 3+ days until it has been cleared by the physician, including holding ambulation in cases of lower extremity grafting.[14]
  - Hydrotherapy may be an appropriate time to perform ROM exercises.[14]
- Client and caregiver education[1,13]
- Psychological support[1,13]
- Exercise to prevent muscular atrophy of nonimmobilized areas:
  - Contraindications to aerobic exercise may include exposed tendons, flaps, reconstruction, regrafting, k-wires, or other conditions.[14]
- Promote independence in self-care using adaptive equipment if needed[1,13]
- Hydrotherapy may be an appropriate time to perform some ADLs[14]

(continued)

UNIT 3-93 INTERVENTION

BURN CARE (CONTINUED)

PHASE 3: REHABILITATION PHASE

- The rehabilitation phase begins after wounds are healed.[14]

Interventions

- Restore muscle strength and activity tolerance.
- Consider effects of long-term restrictive lung injury from inhalation injuries.[15]
- Begin compression therapy and scar management program to prevent contractures.[13,14]
- Educate the client and caregiver about scar care.[13,14]
- Promote independence in self-care. Aim to reduce the amount of adaptive equipment used.[1,14]

Skin Care Education

- Moisturize skin daily.[14]
- Protect skin from the sun through sunscreen and clothing until scars have matured.[15]
- Teach clients or caregivers to massage the area with firm pressure in slow, circular motions to desensitize, prevent scar adhesions, decrease itching, and stretch the tissue.[14]

Hypertrophic Scarring

- Initially appears 6 to 8 weeks after wound closure and can take 12 to 24 months to fully mature.[14]

Compression Garments

- Compression garments or bandaging help prevent raised scarring.[13]
- Measuring and prescribing a compression garment is a specialized skill, and remeasuring occurs every 3 to 6 months.[14]
- Recommended pressure of garments is between 24 and 40 mm Hg. The garment is to be worn at all times except during bathing, massaging, or moisturizing the skin.[14]
- Compression garments should be worn until scars have fully matured (approximately 12 to 18 months).[14]
- Compression garments should be washed daily. Two garments should available for this purpose.[14]

PASSY-MUIR VALVE

A PMV is placed on the end of a tracheostomy tube to allow clients to speak. In addition, clinical benefits of PMVs include improved swallowing, increased oxygen intake, stronger cough, and improved secretion control.[16]

Candidates for PMV[16]	• A client may be a candidate for PMV if:
	  ○ Tracheostomy placement was at least 48-hours prior.
	  ○ Vital signs are stable.
	  ○ Cuff deflation is tolerated.
	  ○ The client is alert and attempting to communicate.

PMV in a nonventilated client[16]	• To use a PMV in a nonventilated client, fully deflate the cuff prior to placing the PMV, and monitor to ensure that the client's oxygen saturation stays above 92%.
Maintenance and safety[16]	• The PMV should be cleaned daily with warm soapy water and allowed to air dry. • If a PMV comes off due to the client's coughing, then clear secretions with suctioning and place the valve back on the tracheostomy tube using a quarter turn.

COMMON INTENSIVE CARE UNIT EQUIPMENT

Clients in the ICU may have cords, tubes, drains, and/or lines connected to them. Certain lines have critical consequences if distributed; therefore, it is important for the occupational therapy practitioner to understand how to manipulate cords, tubes, and lines while performing occupational therapy with the client. Client safety is everyone's responsibility, and ICU clients are considered highly vulnerable due to sedation, unconsciousness, or disorientation. Communication with nursing staff, health care providers, and the family is crucial.[17]

(continued)

COMMON INTENSIVE CARE UNIT EQUIPMENT (CONTINUED)

RESPIRATORY EQUIPMENT

Endotracheal Tube

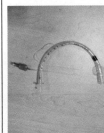

Description[17]

An endotracheal tube (ETT) is a commonly used device that is critical for client safety, so it is important that you understand its design and use.

ETTs come in various sizes and shapes, but the basic concepts underlying them is the same for all.

Purpose[17]

• Provides a passage for gases to flow between a client's lungs and an anaesthesia breathing system

• Allows one to provide positive pressure ventilation

• Protects the lung from contamination from gastric contents and nasopharyngeal matter, such as blood

Precautions[17]

• Never remove the tube or connected hose.

• Kinks in the tube will result in a loss of airflow.

(continued)

UNIT 3-95 INTERVENTION

UNIT 3-95 INTERVENTION

COMMON INTENSIVE CARE UNIT EQUIPMENT (CONTINUED)

Tracheostomy Tube

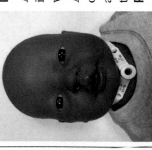

Description[17]

A tracheostomy (trach) tube is a curved tube that is inserted into a tracheostomy stoma (ie, the hole made in the neck and windpipe, or trachea).

A commonly used tracheostomy tube consists of three parts: outer cannula with flange (neck plate), inner cannula, and an obturator. The outer cannula is the outer tube that holds the tracheostomy open.

Purpose[17]

• Provides a passage for gases to flow between a client's lungs and an anaesthesia breathing system

• Allows one to provide positive pressure ventilation

• Protects the lung from contamination from gastric contents and nasopharyngeal matter, such as blood

• Suitable for long-term ventilatory management

Precautions[17]

• Oxygen is connected; do not remove.

• Be aware of leaks and blockages.

• Do not cover the tracheostomy.

• Beware of the coughing client.

(continued)

COMMON INTENSIVE CARE UNIT EQUIPMENT (CONTINUED)

Nasal Canula

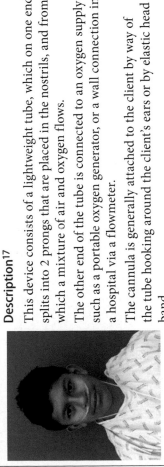

Description[17]

This device consists of a lightweight tube, which on one end splits into 2 prongs that are placed in the nostrils, and from which a mixture of air and oxygen flows.

The other end of the tube is connected to an oxygen supply such as a portable oxygen generator, or a wall connection in a hospital via a flowmeter.

The cannula is generally attached to the client by way of the tube hooking around the client's ears or by elastic head band.

Purpose[17]

• Delivers low levels of supplemental oxygen or airflow to a client in need of respiratory help

• Sometimes used to deliver high levels of oxygen

Precautions[17]

• Watch for kinks or leaks in airflow.

• Only interrupt the flow of oxygen for a couple of seconds while changing sources.

(continued)

UNIT 3–95 INTERVENTION

COMMON INTENSIVE CARE UNIT EQUIPMENT (CONTINUED)

Face Mask

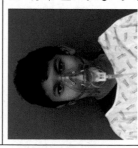

Description[17]

Simple face mask covering the nose and mouth with a long thin tube that connects to an oxygen source.

Purpose[17]

• Used to deliver oxygen to people who do not otherwise get enough oxygen

• Commonly used to provide relief to people with respiratory disorders

Precautions[17]

• Do not remove for more than 1 minute.

• Keep the mask connected to the oxygen source.

• Avoid kinks and obstruction in the air flow.

Venti-Mask

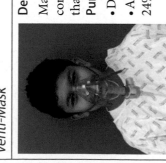

Description[17]

Mask that covers nose and mouth with a long thin tube that connects to an oxygen source. Various adapters are attached that determine the percentage of oxygen delivered.

Purpose[17]

• Delivers higher levels of oxygen than simple face mask

• Allows for varying percentage of oxygen delivered from 24% to 50% FiO_2

Precautions[17]

• Venti-masks have variable levels of oxygen flow.

• Do not touch the knobs.

(continued)

COMMON INTENSIVE CARE UNIT EQUIPMENT (CONTINUED)

Non-Rebreather Mask

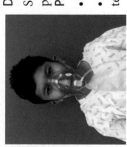

Description[17]

SpO_2 is an estimation of oxygen in the blood. It is the percentage of oxygenated hemoglobin vs total hemoglobin

Purpose[17]

- Oxygen saturation is the single most important vital sign.
- Refer to Unit 3-90 of this section under ventilatory techniques, for information on oxygen saturation.

Precautions[17]

- The bag must be inflated.
- Do not remove the mask for more than 1 minute.

Tracheostomy Mask

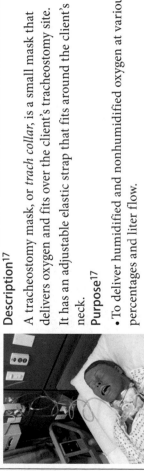

Description[17]

A tracheostomy mask, or *trach collar*, is a small mask that delivers oxygen and fits over the client's tracheostomy site. It has an adjustable elastic strap that fits around the client's neck.

Purpose[17]

- To deliver humidified and nonhumidified oxygen at various percentages and liter flow.

Precautions[17]

- Do not remove the tracheostomy mask.
- Kinks will obstruct airflow.

(continued)

UNIT 3-95 INTERVENTION

UNIT 3–95 INTERVENTION

COMMON INTENSIVE CARE UNIT EQUIPMENT (CONTINUED)

Chest Tube

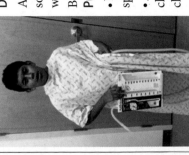

Description[17]

A chest tube (or chest drain) is a clear, plastic-like PVC and soft silicone. It is flexible and is inserted through the chest wall and into the pleural space or mediastinum.

Bubbling in the canister is normal.

Purpose[17]

• Used to remove air, fluid, or pus from the intrathoracic space

• A chest drainage canister device is typically used to collect chest drainage. Most commonly, drainage canisters use 3 chambers, which are based on the 3-bottle system.

Precautions[17]

• Do not remove the tubing.

• Disconnect the wall suctioning prior to moving the client.

• Keep the collection unit positioned upright at all times.

• The canister sits on the floor next to the bed. Be careful not to accidently kick the canister over.

• Use Vaseline-soaked gauze to cover the area if the tube is accidently dislodged.

(continued)

COMMON INTENSIVE CARE UNIT EQUIPMENT (CONTINUED)

Continuous Positive Airway Pressure

Description[17]

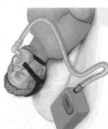

A continuous positive airway pressure (CPAP) machine increases air pressure in the throat so the airway does not collapse when the person breathes in.

A person can use CPAP at home every night while sleeping. The CPAP machine has a mask that covers the nose and mouth.

CPAP also may be used to treat preterm infants whose lungs have not fully developed. For example, doctors may use CPAP to treat infants who have respiratory distress syndrome or bronchopulmonary dysplasia.

Purpose[17]

- CPAP therapy uses a machine to help a person who has obstructive sleep apnea breathe more easily during sleep.

- Sleep apnea is a common disorder that causes pauses in breathing or shallow breaths while sleeping. As a result, not enough air reaches the lungs.

- In obstructive sleep apnea, the airway collapses or is blocked during sleep. When the person tries to breathe, any air that squeezes past the blockage can cause loud snoring.

Precautions[17]

- Do not remove the CPAP machine from the client.
- Kinks will obstruct airflow.
- Power failure is a concern for individuals with home units.

(continued)

UNIT 3-95 INTERVENTION

UNIT 3–95 INTERVENTION

COMMON INTENSIVE CARE UNIT EQUIPMENT (CONTINUED)

Oxygen Saturation

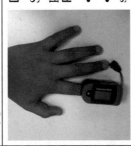

Description[17]

SpO$_2$ is an estimation of oxygen in the blood. It is the percentage of oxygenated hemoglobin vs total hemoglobin.

Purpose[17]

• Oxygen saturation is the single most important vital sign.
• Refer to Unit 3-90 of this section for information on oxygen saturation.

Precautions[17]

• There is no harm to the client if the oxygen saturation monitor is removed.
• Inform the nurse if you remove the oxygen saturation monitor.

Peripheral Intravenous

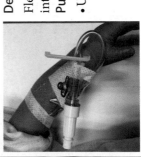

Description[17]

Flexible catheters of various lengths and diameters inserted into veins

Purpose[17]

• Used for medications and fluid replacement therapy

Precautions[17]

• Keep the line taped in place.
• Keep the line dry.
• Do not tug at it.
• Do not allow kinks in it.

(continued)

COMMON INTENSIVE CARE UNIT EQUIPMENT (CONTINUED)

CIRCULATORY EQUIPMENT

Peripherally Inserted Intravenous Central Catheter Lines

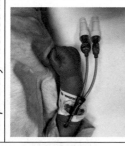

Description[17]

Flexible catheters of longer length inserted into veins that can terminate in the central venous system

Purpose[17]

• Used for a prolonged period of time

• Chemotherapy regimens, extended antibiotic therapy, or total parenteral nutrition

Precautions[17]

• Do not pull.

• Do not disconnect.

• Watch the bed rails for pinching.

• If the line is accidently dislodged and bleeding, apply firm pressure.

Central Venous Lines

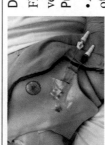

Description[17]

Flexible catheters inserted into the subclavian or jugular vein that terminate in the central venous system

Purpose[17]

• Allows concentrated solutions to be infused with less risk of complications

• Remains in place for a longer period of time than other venous access devices

• A number of uses; long-standing use includes total parenteral nutrition in a chronically ill patient

Precautions[17]

• Do not pull or tug; line is sutured in place.

• Do not disconnect any fluids.

• Keep dressing clean and dry.

(continued)

UNIT 3-95 INTERVENTION

UNIT 3–95   INTERVENTION

COMMON INTENSIVE CARE UNIT EQUIPMENT (CONTINUED)

Arterial Lines

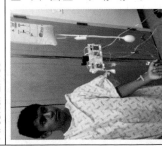

Description[17]

Flexible catheter inserted into an artery and attached to a pressure line/transducer then connected to a monitor

Purpose[17]

- Used for continuous monitoring of arterial blood pressure and for withdrawal of arterial blood for diagnostic sampling

- Arterial line placement can be in the arm, wrist, or groin

Precautions[17]

- Accidental removal is a medical emergency.
- Do not pull or kink.
- Do not disconnect for exercise.

(continued)

COMMON INTENSIVE CARE UNIT EQUIPMENT (CONTINUED)

Mediport (Also Known as Port-a-Cath or Perm-a-Cath)

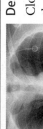

Description[17]

Closed system consisting of a flat septum inserted under the skin in the upper chest connected to a line inserted in the central venous system

Purpose[17]

- Carries nutrients and medicine through the body
- Used to take blood for blood tests
- Used for chemotherapy, antibiotics, total parenteral nutrition
- Used for clients with difficult vein access, including sickle

Precaution[17]

- Do not pull or kink.

Intravenous Pumps

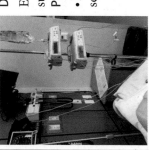

Description[17]

Electronic pump with a tubing set and key pad for settings such as rate and volume to be infused

Purpose[17]

- Deliver intravenous fluids and medications at a constant set rate

Precautions[17]

- Do not pull or kink.
- Plug back in after exercise; must be plugged in to charge due to battery life.
- Notify the nurse if the intravenous pump beeps, as beeping indicates kinks, empty intravenous fluid bag, or air in the line.

(continued)

UNIT 3-95   INTERVENTION

UNIT 3–95 INTERVENTION

COMMON INTENSIVE CARE UNIT EQUIPMENT (CONTINUED)

Syringe Pump

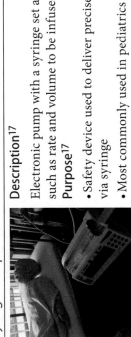

Description[17]

Electronic pump with a syringe set and key pad for settings, such as rate and volume to be infused

Purpose[17]

• Safety device used to deliver precise metered doses of therapy via syringe

• Most commonly used in pediatrics

Precautions[17]

• Do not pull or kink.

• Plug pump back in after exercise.

Patient-Controlled Analgesia Pump

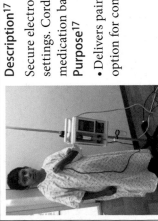

Description[17]

Secure electronic pump with a syringe set locking key pad for settings. Cord with button held by patient for demand dosing of medication based on settings and limits for safety.

Purpose[17]

• Delivers pain medication when client pushes a button, with option for continuous rate

Precautions[17]

• Client is at higher risk of falls.

• Plug pump back in after exercise.

• Ensure the client can reach the button.

(continued)

COMMON INTENSIVE CARE UNIT EQUIPMENT (CONTINUED)

Electrocardiogram

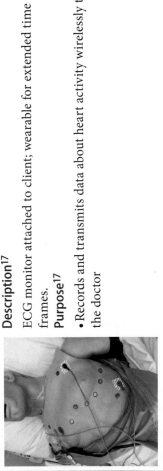

Description[17]

ECG monitor with gel pads, placed on client's chest, attached to a monitor.

Purpose[17]

- Measures the electrical activity of the heart
- Indicator of the client's cardiopulmonary status

Precautions[17]

- Keep the leads attached to the client.
- Keep electrodes dry.
- Alert nurse if the monitor is off for any reason.

Holter Monitor

Description[17]

ECG monitor attached to client; wearable for extended time frames.

Purpose[17]

- Records and transmits data about heart activity wirelessly to the doctor

Precaution[17]

- Keep the monitor dry.

(continued)

UNIT 3-95 INTERVENTION

UNIT 3-95 INTERVENTION

COMMON INTENSIVE CARE UNIT EQUIPMENT (CONTINUED)

Telemetry Monitors

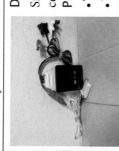

Description[17]

Small wearable ECG monitors that transmit data to a central monitoring station staffed by trained personnel.

Purpose[17]

• Type of cardiac monitor

• Used in therapy to indicate how the client is tolerating activity by changes in heart rate and rhythm

Precautions[17]

• Keep telemetry box in the pocket of the client's gown.

• Turn the monitor off if going on a walk without the telemetry box.

Sequential Compression Device

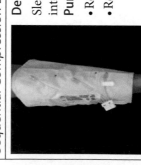

Description[17]

Sleeves or foot pads attached to a pump that inflates intermittently.

Purpose[17]

• Returns blood from the legs back to the heart

• Reduces edema

Precaution[17]

• Remove sequential compression devices from the client before exercise.

(continued)

COMMON INTENSIVE CARE UNIT EQUIPMENT (CONTINUED)

Left Ventricle Assist Device

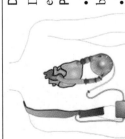

Description[17]

Device placed in the left ventricle and attached to an external pump drive.

Purpose[17]

• Helps a weakened heart ventricle pump throughout the body

• Used for client's following open-heart surgery or clients waiting for a heart transplant

• Used for long-term support in terminally ill clients who cannot undergo a heart transplant

Precaution[17]

• Keep the machine plugged in or on a battery pack at all times.

Pacing

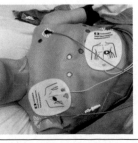

Description[17]

Electrodes attached to cardiac muscle or in the venous system that deliver electrical stimulation to the heart.

Purpose[17]

• External pacing delivers set rate of shocks per minute and is considered painful

• Internal pacing is connected to a controller and a heart, but does not cause pain

Precautions[17]

• Keep pacemakers attached to the controller.

• No exercise is allowed for external pacing.

(continued)

UNIT 3-95 INTERVENTION

UNIT 3-95 INTERVENTION

COMMON INTENSIVE CARE UNIT EQUIPMENT (CONTINUED)

CRANIAL EQUIPMENT

Intracranial Pressure Monitor

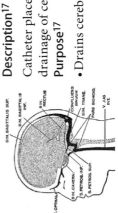	**Description**[17] Drain placed in ventricle, then attached to a transducer or a sensor placed in brain tissue, and then connected to a monitor. **Purpose**[17] • Measures ICP	**Precaution**[17] • Do not change the level of the bed.

Cerebral Venous Drainage

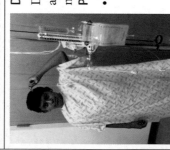	**Description**[17] Catheter placed in ventricle attached to a bag allowing for drainage of cerebral spinal fluid. **Purpose**[17] • Drains cerebral spinal fluid	**Precautions**[17] • Report leaks to nursing staff. • Check the chart to verify angle restrictions.

(continued)

COMMON INTENSIVE CARE UNIT EQUIPMENT (CONTINUED)

Halo		
	Description[17] Device that encircles the head and is attached to the skull with screws. **Purpose**[17] • Provides head and neck immobility and stability	**Precautions**[17] • May limit client's mobility. • The client is at risk for falling.

DRAIN EQUIPMENT

Penrose		
	Description[17] Flat, wide latex drain placed in wounds to allow drainage. **Purpose**[17] • Used to drain deep wounds and incisions	**Precautions**[17] • Risk of blood-borne pathogens. • Report any large amount of leakage.

(continued)

UNIT 3-95 INTERVENTION

COMMON INTENSIVE CARE UNIT EQUIPMENT (CONTINUED)

Jackson-Pratt Drain

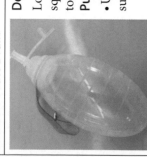

Description[17]

Long, thin tube attached to a bulb that is activated by squeezing and capping device. Provides gentle suction to area.

Purpose[17]

• Used commonly after surgery to drain fluids from surgical sites

Precautions[17]

• Do not pull on the drain; pin it to the gown if necessary.
• Pressure must remain constant in order to drain.
• Never open the plug, and report any open plugs.

Vacuum-Assisted Drainage

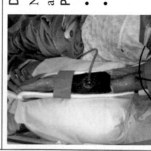

Description[17]

Negative pressure wound therapy with airtight seal attached to a collection device.

Purpose[17]

• Promotes wound healing
• Also known as a *wound vac*

Precautions[17]

• Leave the vacuum assisted drain plugged in.
• Keep occlusive dressing in place.

(continued)

COMMON INTENSIVE CARE UNIT EQUIPMENT (CONTINUED)

Pigtail

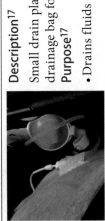

Description[17]

Small drain placed in wounds then attached to a drainage bag for collection of fluids.

Purpose[17]

- Drains fluids

Precautions[17]

- Do not pull on the drain.
- Report any drainage, leaks, or blood-soaked dressings.

RESTRAINT EQUIPMENT

Wrist

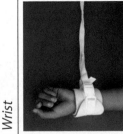

Description[17]

Soft wrist bands that attach to the bed frame or other non-moving structure.

Purpose[17]

- Used only when the client is a danger to self or others
- Most commonly used in Critical Care Units
- Requires a doctor's order with specific criteria for safety monitoring.

Precautions[17]

- Consult with nurse before loosening or removing the restraint.
- Monitor the client's hands closely whenever the restraints are removed.
- Tie the restraints to the frame of the bed, not the rail

(continued)

UNIT 3-95 INTERVENTION

COMMON INTENSIVE CARE UNIT EQUIPMENT (CONTINUED)

Mitt

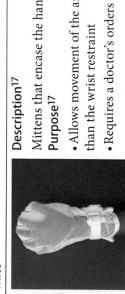

Description[17]

Mittens that encase the hand and are secure.

Purpose[17]

• Allows movement of the arms and is less restrictive than the wrist restraint

• Requires a doctor's orders

Precaution[17]

• Use caution whenever the mitts are removed.

Vest

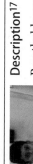

Description[17]

Breathable vests with straps that secure to bed frame or other non-moving structure.

Purpose[17]

• Used to prevent falls

• Restraint vests are rarely used today as the client has the right to fall

• Requires a doctor's order

Precautions[17]

• Place the client back into the restraint prior to leaving the room.

• Tie the restraint to the bed frame, not the rails

(continued)

COMMON INTENSIVE CARE UNIT EQUIPMENT (CONTINUED)

TRACTION EQUIPMENT

Weights

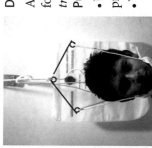

Description[17]

Attached to both the head and extremities to allow for reduction of bone and muscle. Also called *skeletal traction*.

Purpose[17]

- Used to straighten broken bones or relieve spinal pressure
- Weights are used to create gentle force

Precautions[17]

- Do not lift weights.
- Force must be applied consistently.

UNIT 3-95 INTERVENTION

Cardiovascular, Lymphatic, Respiratory, and Integumentary Systems Precautions and Contraindications

Therapy Guidelines With Cardiac Clients

Vital signs[1]	• Monitor before, during, and after therapy. • Heart rate during activity should not increase more than 20 to 30 beats/min above resting heart rate for the first few weeks after MI or surgery. • Notify physician if heart rate exceeds 125 beat/min with minimal effort. • If resting blood pressure is higher than 180/90 mm Hg, notify physician. • Vital signs may be altered due to medications; make note of signs of distress. Refer to Unit 1-82 in this section for information about vital signs.
Signs of exercise intolerance or cardiac arrest[1]	• Dizziness or light-headedness • Orthostasis • Excessive fatigue • Shortness of breath • Heart palpitations • Chest pain (burning, pressure, or heaviness) • Nausea or vomiting • Sweating • Confusion or anxiety
Avoid Valsalva maneuver[1]	• Holding breath slows heart rate and increases blood pressure.
Angina[1]	• Notify staff if angina is reported by a client with a percutaneous transluminal coronary angioplasty.

(continued)

CARDIOVASCULAR, LYMPHATIC, RESPIRATORY, AND INTEGUMENTARY SYSTEMS PRECAUTIONS AND CONTRAINDICATIONS (CONTINUED)

Sternal precautions (typically 6 to 8 weeks after surgery)[1]	• Do not lift arms over head; elbows should not go past the shoulders. • Do not reach or place hands behind the body. • Do not lift, push, or pull more than 5 pounds. • Do not use arms to push up from a seated position. • Do not lean on walker, and do not propel wheelchair. • Do not twist or turn torso when exercising. • Do not do resistive exercises for 6 weeks after surgery. • Do not push against bed rails with arms because of the force on the sternum. • Do not cross legs while sitting or lying in bed. • Avoid holding breath (eg, as seen with bowel movements). • Do not drive. • Consider using a cardiac pillow to hold and sit up without hands.
Pacemakers[1]	• After recent insertion of a pacemaker, do not lift the arm above 90 degrees.
Cardiac stents[1]	• Bed rest is required for 6 to 8 hours after the procedure. Obtain resume orders before mobilizing the client.
Left ventricle assist devices (LVADs)[1]	• Follow sternal precautions. • Do not do chest compressions. • Therapist should be LVAD-certified to evaluate and treat LVAD clients.
Edema management[1]	• Elevating upper and lower extremities above the level of the heart is contraindicated for patients with congestive heart failure.

(continued)

UNIT 3-96 INTERVENTION

CARDIOVASCULAR, LYMPHATIC, RESPIRATORY, AND INTEGUMENTARY SYSTEMS PRECAUTIONS AND CONTRAINDICATIONS (CONTINUED)	
Transplants[1]	• Follow strict neutropenic precautions. Use hand sanitizer for hand washing. • If you have had a respiratory illness recently, do not evaluate or treat a client who has had a transplant.
Chest tube management[1]	• Do not pull or tug on the chest tube. • Keep the chest tube chamber sitting upright. • Tipping the chest tube chamber may compromise the water seal. • Do not disconnect the chest tube from the wall suction without a doctor's authorization, as this may cause a pneumothorax. • Keep the chest tube chamber below insertion level to prevent backflow. • Safety-pin tubes to the client's gown, if needed, during bed mobility. • Use caution if placing a gait belt on the client. • If moving the client in bed, move to the side with the ventilator or shorter lines.

(continued)

UNIT 3-96 INTERVENTION

	CARDIOVASCULAR, LYMPHATIC, RESPIRATORY, AND INTEGUMENTARY SYSTEMS PRECAUTIONS AND CONTRAINDICATIONS (CONTINUED)

Lines[1]	• Arterial line:
	  ◦ Used in ICU clients to obtain a continuous blood pressure reading
	  ◦ Management example: If placed near wrist, do not aggressively test wrist flexion/extension
	• Central venous line:
	  ◦ May be placed in neck to deliver substances that are too toxic for peripheral infusion
	  ◦ Management example: Use caution when putting gown on client
	• Swan-Ganz catheter:
	  ◦ Placed in right side of heart for continuous monitoring
	  ◦ Do not raise arm more than 90 degrees; mobility will be limited
	• Femoral lines:
	  ◦ Do not get the client out of bed

Ventilator[1]	• If the ventilator becomes disconnected, keep calm. The nurse or other staff have enough time to walk into the room and reconnect it.

REFERENCES

1. Smith-Gabai H, Holm SE. *Occupational Therapy in Acute Care*. 2nd ed. Bethesda, MD: AOTA Press; 2017.
2. Jensen MSA, Thomsen JL, Jensen SE, Lauritzen T, Engberg M. Electrocardiogram interpretation in general practice. *Fam Pract*. 2005;22(1):109-113. doi:10.1093/fampra/cmh601
3. American Heart Association. Echocardiogram-Echo. American Heart Association. http://www.heart.org/HEARTORG/Conditions/HeartAttack/DiagnosingaHeartAttack/Echocardiogram---Echo_UCM_451485_Article.jsp#.WWGEw9MrLBJ. Published July 2015. Updated October 13, 2017. Accessed May 6, 2019.
4. Jette M, Sidney K, Blumchen G. Metabolic equivalents (METS) in exercise testing, exercise prescription, and evaluation of functional capacity. *Clin Cardiol*. 1990;13(8):555-565.
5. Ritche C. Rating of perceived exertion (RPE). *J Physiother*. 2012;58(1):62. doi:10.1016/S1836-9553(12)70078-4
6. National Pressure Ulcer Advisory Panel. NPUAP pressure ulcer stages/categories. National Pressure Ulcer Advisory Panel. http://www.npuap.org/wp-content/uploads/2012/01/NPUAP-Pressure-Ulcer-Stages-Categories.pdf. Published 2012. Accessed May 6, 2019.
7. Rohner-Spengler M, Mannion AF, Babst R. Reliability and minimal detectable change for the figure-of-eight-20 method of, measurement of ankle edema. *J Orthop Sports Phys Ther*. 2007;37(4):199-205. doi:10.2519/jospt.2007.2371
8. Gosselink R. Breathing techniques in patients with chronic obstructive pulmonary disease (COPD). *Chron Respir Dis*. 2004;1(3):163-172. doi:10.1191/1479972304cd020rs
9. National Pressure Ulcer Advisory Panel. Pressure injury prevention points. National Pressure Ulcer Advisory Panel. http://www.npuap.org/wp-content/uploads/2016/04/Pressure-Injury-Prevention-Points-2016.pdf. Published 2016. Accessed May 6, 2019.
10. Kligman L, Wong RK, Johnston M, Laetsch NS. The treatment of lymphedema related to breast cancer: a systematic review and evidence summary. *Support Care Cancer*. 2004;12(6):421-431. doi:10.1007/s00520-004-0627-0
11. Price KJ, Gordon BA, Bird SR, Benson AC. A review of guidelines for cardiac rehabilitation exercise programmes: is there an international consensus? *Eur J Prev Cardiol*. 2016;23(16):1715-1733. doi:10.1177/2047487316657669
12. Berry N. Appendix D: energy conservation and work simplification strategies. In: Smith-Gabai H, ed. *Occupational Therapy in Acute Care*. Bethesda, MD: AOTA Press; 2011:583-587.
13. Procter F. Rehabilitation of the burn patient. *Indian J Plas Surg*. 2010;43(suppl):S101-S113. doi:10.4103/0970-0358.70730
14. Reeves SU, Deshaies L. Burns and burn rehabilitation. In: Pendleton HM, Shultz-Krohn W, eds. *Pedretti's Occupational Therapy: Practice Skills for Physical Dysfunction*. 7th ed. St. Louis, MO: Elsevier; 2013:1110-1148.
15. Edgar D. Rehabilitation after burn injury. *BMJ*. 2004;329(7461):343-345. doi:10.1136/bmj.329.7461.343
16. Passy-Muir Inc. *Passy-Muir Tracheostomy & Ventilator Swallowing and Speaking Valve Instruction Booklet*. Irvine, CA; Passy-Muir Inc: 2014. http://www.passy-muir.com/sites/default/files/pdf/instructbklt.pdf. Published 2015. Accessed May 6, 2019.
17. Kovanis CA, Shivers E. Hospital equipment. In: Smith-Gabai H, ed. *Occupational Therapy in Acute Care*. 2nd ed. Bethesda, MD: AOTA Press; 2017:207.

Section Six

. . . .

Endocrine, Digestive, Urinary, and Reproductive Systems

Sit W, Neville M.
Handbook of Occupational Therapy for
Adults With Physical Disabilities (pp 429-466).
© 2020 SLACK Incorporated.

CASE

DIAGNOSIS: CANCER OF THE PROSTATE AND THE SKIN OF THE PENIS

A man in his 50s with a cancer diagnosis came to the hospital where I was working for an operation. Following the operation, he was assigned to my colleague's caseload. My colleague, quite alarmed, approached me about the referral. I was informed the client needed a cock-up splint—a typical wrist splint designed to counter wrist drop. I replied, "Okay, a cock-up splint," unsure why my colleague was acting so unusual. My colleague repeated, "No, a cock-up splint."

As it turned out, the referral was not for a typical wrist splint. The client's urology doctor transplanted the client's penis onto his forearm so that the blood supply to the penis would remain microscopically connected. The doctor referred the client to occupational therapy in order to create a splint that would hold the penis upright. The idea came from a splint we use for clients who have a spinal cord injury. The splint is propped between the client's legs and holds the penis in place for catheterization.

Chemistry Lab Values

Check your client's chart for his or her chemistry lab values. Understanding critical values and knowing when your client is unsuitable for therapy will keep the client safe. Always use your clinical judgment, and check with the nursing staff if you are unsure whether a client can participate in therapy.

(continued)

	CHEMISTRY LAB VALUES (CONTINUED)	
LAB	**NORMAL RANGE[1]**	**THERAPY IMPLICATIONS[1]**
Sodium (Na)	Normal range: 135 to 145 mEq/l • Hyponatremia (low sodium levels): ○ Symptoms include oliguria, nausea, abdominal cramps, weakness, confusion, apathy, tachycardia, and seizures. • Hypernatremia (high sodium levels): ○ Symptoms include mental status changes, confusion, agitation, tachycardia, oliguria, thirst, pulmonary edema, and dyspnea.	Critical values: • Below 120 mEq/l: Defer therapy. • Below 130 mEq/l: Client may become confused and disoriented. • Above 150 mEq/l: Client may become confused and disoriented. • Above 160 mEq/l: Defer therapy.
Potassium (K+)	Normal range: 3.5 to 5.0 mEq/l • Hypokalemia (low potassium levels less than 3.2 mEq/l): ○ This may lead to constipation, fatigue, leg cramps, paresthesias, sinus bradycardia, atrial tachycardia, atrioventricular block, ventricular tachycardia or fibrillation, and cardiac arrest: ¤ Do not see the client due to possible arrhythmia. • Hyperkalemia (high potassium levels greater than 5.0 mEq/l): ○ This may lead to abdominal cramps, nausea, diarrhea, flaccid paralysis, paresthesias, cardiac arrhythmias, tachycardia followed by bradycardia, and cardiac arrest.	Critical values: • Below 3.0 mEq/l: Defer therapy due to risk of cardiac damage. • Below 3.2 mEq/l: Defer therapy due to possible arrhythmia. • Above 5.0 mEq/l: Client may present with diarrhea or nausea. • Above 5.3 mEq/l: Defer therapy due to risk of cardiac damage.

(continued)

CHEMISTRY LAB VALUES (CONTINUED)

LAB	NORMAL RANGE[1]	THERAPY IMPLICATIONS[1]
Glucose	Normal range: 70 to 110 mg/dl fasting • Hypoglycemia (low glucose levels less than 60 mg/dl): ○ Avoid exercise before mealtime and after insulin. • Hyperglycemia (high glucose levels more than 250 mg/dl) • Pre-diabetes is indicated by glucose levels between 110 to 200 mg/dl. • Diabetes is indicated by glucose levels above 126 mg/dl.	Critical values: • Below 70 mg/dl: Defer therapy due to risk of dizziness and confusion. • Above 350 mg/dl: Defer therapy due to risk of blurry vision, nausea, and vomiting.
Troponin Proteins released with cardiac muscle injury or infarction	Normal range: Less than 0.35 ng/ml • Do not engage in therapy if troponin levels are elevated, due to possible cardiac issues. • Troponin I level peaks at 12 hours after injury and may remain elevated for 3 to 10 days.	Critical values: • Above 0.4 ng/ml: Defer therapy, as this level suggests a heart attack. • Above 1.5 ng/ml: Defer therapy due to possible cardiac complications.

(continued)

CHEMISTRY LAB VALUES (CONTINUED)

LAB	NORMAL RANGE[1]	THERAPY IMPLICATIONS[1]
Calcium (Ca+) blood level Involved in muscle contractions, cardiac conductivity, and bone formation	Normal range: 8.5 to 11 mg/dl • Levels not within normal ranges may cause abnormal heart rhythms.	Critical values: • Below 7 mg/dl: Defer therapy; indicates tetany (muscle contractions). • Above 12 mg/dl: Defer therapy; indicates coma.
Blood urea nitrogen (BUN) Measures amount of protein metabolized in the blood; measures kidney and liver function	Normal range: 7 to 20 mg/dl • Elevated BUN levels indicate renal impairment: ◦ May be present with congestive heart failure, diabetes mellitus, myocardial infarction, burns, and cancer. • Low BUN levels are uncommon and usually are associated with malnutrition, low-protein diet, overhydration, or liver disease.	Critical values: • Above 100 mg/dl: Defer therapy. • Elevated levels may present as confusion and disorientation.

(continued)

CHEMISTRY LAB VALUES (CONTINUED)

LAB	NORMAL RANGE[1]	THERAPY IMPLICATIONS[1]
Creatine phosphokinase or creatine kinase Measures kidney function	Normal range: 0.6 to 1.2 mg/dl (males); 0.5 to 1.1 mg/dl (females) • Levels rise with renal impairment.	Critical values: • No implications exist for participating in therapy.
CO_2 blood values Assesses status of electrolytes and pH level of blood	Normal range: 23 to 30 mEq/l • Elevated levels will cause patient to be confused, dizzy, and out of it.	Critical values: • Below 10 mEq/L: Defer therapy; indicates conditions associated with respiratory alkalosis or metabolic acidosis. • Above 40 mEq/L: Defer therapy; indicates conditions associated with respiratory acidosis or metabolic alkalosis.

SWALLOW ANATOMY AND DYSPHAGIA

Dysphagia is difficulty swallowing or the inability to swallow. Structures involved with swallowing, including cranial nerves, brainstem, cerebral cortex, and muscles, are outlined in the following table.[2] Dysfunction may occur in 5 stages of swallowing.[3]

SWALLOW ANATOMY AND STAGES OF SWALLOWING

Structures involved in swallowing[2,3]	• The following cranial nerves are involved in swallowing:
	     ◦ Trigeminal nerve (cranial nerve V)
	     ◦ Facial (cranial nerve VII)
	     ◦ Glossopharyngeal (cranial nerve IX)
	     ◦ Vagus (cranial nerve X)
	     ◦ Accessory (cranial nerve XI)
	     ◦ Hypoglossal (cranial nerve XII)
	 • The following brain regions are involved with swallowing:
	     ◦ Motor cortex
	     ◦ Sensory cortex
	     ◦ Cingulate gyrus
	     ◦ Prefrontal cortex
	 • 48 muscles are involved in swallowing.

Stages of swallowing[3]	• Pre-oral stage • Oral prep stage • Oral stage • Pharyngeal stage • Esophageal stage *(continued)*

SWALLOW ANATOMY AND DYSPHAGIA (CONTINUED)

DYSPHAGIA

Causes of dysphagia and related conditions[2,3]	• Dysphagia can be caused by upper motor neuron dysfunction, including cranial nerve dysfunction and pseudobulbar dysfunction.
	• Dysphagia may also be caused by lower motor neuron dysfunction, such as paralytic dysfunction.
	• Dysphagia is commonly associated with the following conditions:
	  ◦ Stroke
	  ◦ Guillain-Barré syndrome
	  ◦ Multiple sclerosis
	  ◦ Amyotrophic lateral sclerosis
	  ◦ Parkinson's disease
	  ◦ Myasthenia gravis
	  ◦ Brain injury
	  ◦ Tetraplegia (C5-level spinal cord injury and above)
	  ◦ Cancers of the head and neck
	  ◦ Pneumonia
	  ◦ Weakness
	  ◦ Tracheostomy
	  ◦ Sensory dysfunction
	  ◦ Cranial nerve dysfunction

(continued)

SWALLOW ANATOMY AND DYSPHAGIA (CONTINUED)	
DYSPHAGIA	

Signs and symptoms of dysphagia[2,3]	• A swallowing evaluation may be necessary if the following signs are observed in the client:
	  ○ Hoarseness of voice
	  ○ Coughing while eating
	  ○ Drooling or nasal regurgitation during eating
	  ○ Runny nose
	  ○ Tearing of eyes
	  ○ Requiring more time than normal to finish meals
	  ○ Choking
	  ○ History of pneumonia
	  ○ Changes in behavior at meal time, including pocketing of food, reported pain when swallowing, and loss of appetite
	  ○ Weight loss
	  ○ Avoidance of meals
	• Mild dysphagia may be undiagnosed in your client, so it is important to be familiar with the signs and symptoms of swallowing dysfunction in order to maintain client safety.

Problems related to dysphagia[2,3]	• Clients with dysphagia are at risk of poor nutrition and dehydration. • Safety concerns related to dysphagia include aspiration and penetration. • Aspiration occurs when food or liquid enters the client's airway. • Penetration occurs when food or liquid enters the client's airway above the vocal cords, but does not enter below the vocal cords. • Silent aspiration occurs when food or liquid enters the client's airway below the vocal folds, but the client does not exhibit coughing, choking, or other clinical signs. • Pneumonia may result from aspiration.

UNIT 2-100 EVALUATION

COMMON ASSESSMENTS ACROSS PRACTICE SETTINGS

ASSESSMENT	ACUTE	INPATIENT	HOME HEALTH	SNF	OUTPATIENT
Common Assessments Across Practice Settings					
Functional Independence Measure	✓	✓			
Pelvic Floor Distress Inventory (or Pelvic Floor Impact Questionnaire)		✓			✓
Pharmacology	✓	✓			
Swallow Assessment	✓	✓		✓	

SNF: skilled nursing facility.

(continued)

COMMON ASSESSMENTS
ACROSS PRACTICE SETTINGS (CONTINUED)

FUNCTIONAL INDEPENDENCE MEASURE

Refer to Section One, Unit 2-10, for information about the Functional Independence Measure.

PELVIC FLOOR DISTRESS INVENTORY (OR PELVIC FLOOR IMPACT QUESTIONNAIRE)[4]

- Purpose: Assesses life impact of pelvic floor disorders on women
- Context: Female clients with pelvic floor disorders
- Format: Pencil-and-paper questionnaire
- Time to administer: 5 minutes
- Materials: Paper form and pencil
- Cost: Free
- Website: http://www.3wpt.com/wp-content/uploads/2017/05/Pelvic-Floor-Distress-Inventory.pdf

UNIT 2-100 EVALUATION

UNIT 2-101 EVALUATION

PHARMACOLOGY

Pharmacology refers to the study of pharmaceutical drugs, while *polypharmacy* refers to 4 to 5 prescribed medications.[5,6] Clients of occupational therapy are likely to be on one or more medications; therefore, it is important to understand commonly prescribed medications, side effects, and drug interactions.[5]

Some medications increase a client's risk for falls, while others impact the client's motivation or ability to learn new information.[5] Familiarize yourself with common medications and be in the habit of reviewing your client's chart. Check with the physician or registered nurse if you have questions about a medication.

MEDICATION[5,7]	TREATMENT USE[5,7]	POTENTIAL THERAPY IMPLICATIONS[5,7]
Analgesics: • Aspirin • Tylenol (acetaminophen)	Treats moderate to severe pain	• Side effects may include dizziness, drowsiness, light-headedness, and nausea. • Client is at an increased risk for falls.
Angiotensin-converting-enzyme inhibitors/ hypotensives (end in "pril"): • Lotensin (benazepril) • Captopril • Enalapril • Prinivil, Zestril (lisinopril) • Norvasc (amlodipine) • Cardene (nicardipine)	Decreases blood pressure Administrated intravenously: Hypertensive emergency	• Side effects may include orthostatic hypotension, dizziness, light-headedness, headache, fatigue, nausea, tachycardia, peripheral edema, and paresthesias. • Client is at an increased risk for falls. • Clear activity with the nursing staff before therapy.

(continued)

PHARMACOLOGY (CONTINUED)

MEDICATION[5,7]	TREATMENT USE[5,7]	POTENTIAL THERAPY IMPLICATIONS[5,7]
Antibiotics: • Bactrim (sulfamethoxazale and trimethoprim) • Cipro (ciprofloxacin) • Keflex (cephalexin) • Macrodantin (nitrofuratoin) • Penicillin	Eradicates microorganisms to treat infections, commonly urinary tract infections (Bactrim) or respiratory infections (Cipro)	• Side effects may include dizziness, headache, fatigue, photosensitivity, paresthesias, nausea, nystagmus, hypotension, and brown/rust-colored urine.
Antidepressants (selective serotonin reuptake inhibitors, monoamine oxidase inhibitors, tricyclics): • Remeron (mirtazapine) • Prozac (fluoxetine) • Zoloft (sertraline)	Treats depression	• Side effects may include orthostatic hypotension, syncope, dizziness, drowsiness, headache, and abnormal gait.
Antidiabetics: • Insulin • Novolin	Treats diabetes	• Side effects may include seizures, anxiety, blurred vision, cold sweats, drowsiness, headache, nausea, slurred speech, weight gain, and fast heartbeat. • Client is at an increased fall risk. • Watch for signs of listlessness. Notify the nurse to check blood sugar if needed.

(continued)

UNIT 2-101 EVALUATION

UNIT 2-101 EVALUATION

PHARMACOLOGY (CONTINUED)

MEDICATION[5,7]	TREATMENT USE[5,7]	POTENTIAL THERAPY IMPLICATIONS[5,7]
Antiepileptics/ anticonvulsants: • Depakote (valproic acid) • Phenobarbital • Dilantin (phenytoin)	Treats seizures	• Side effects may include fatigue, nystagmus, ataxia, confusion, and numbness.
Anti-inflammatory drugs: • Decadron (dexamethasone)	Reduces inflammation	• Side effects may include dizziness and stomach irritation.
Antipsychotics: • Haldol (halperidol) • Risperdal (risperidone)	Treats psychosis	• Side effects may include orthostatic hypotension, agitation, tardive dyskinesia, nausea, ataxia, increased aspiration risk, and incontinence.
Antiseptics: • Hydrogen peroxide	Reduces bacterial growth to prevent infection	• Side effects may include redness of skin, irritation, or swelling.
Benzodiazepines/ antianxiety drugs: • Ativan (lorazepam) • Valium (diazepam)	Treats anxiety	• Side effects may include drowsiness, clumsiness, dizziness, and irritability.

(continued)

Pharmacology (continued)

Medication[5,7]	Treatment Use[5,7]	Potential Therapy Implications[5,7]
Beta blockers (usually end in "lol"): • Atenolol • Digoxin • Esmolol • Imdur (isosorbide mononitrate) • Metoprolol • Propranolol	Treats arrhythmias and heart failure, and decreases blood pressure	• A pulse below 60 indicates toxicity. • Side effects may include fatigue, agitation, weakness, headache, nausea, and vertigo. • Client is at an increased fall risk.
Blood thinners/ anticoagulants: • Coumadin (warfarin) • Plavix (clopidogrel)	Treats or prevents cerebrovascular accident and thrombophlebitis Plavix has a lower bleeding risk than Coumadin	• Side effects may include dizziness, syncope, weakness, headache, nausea, fever, and skin rash. • There is an increased risk for bleeding when on blood thinners.
Central acetylcholinesterase inhibitors: • Aricept (donepezil)	Manages Alzheimer's disease	• Side effects may include weakness, vertigo, aphasia, syncope, and paresthesia. • Signs of overdose include convulsions, increased sweating, low blood pressure, slow heartbeat, and increased muscle weakness. *(continued)*

UNIT 2-101 EVALUATION

UNIT 2-101 EVALUATION

Pharmacology (continued)

Medication[5,7]	Treatment Use[5,7]	Potential Therapy Implications[5,7]
Diuretics: • Dyazide (hydrochloroth and triamterene) • Lasix (furosemide) • Triamterene	Treats edema, congestive heart failure, and high blood pressure	• Side effects may include orthostatic hypotension and dizziness. • Client is at an increased fall risk. • Rare side effects include joint pain, painful urination, nausea, yellow eyes, and bruising. • Dry mouth, increased thirst, irregular heartbeat, mood changes, and/or weakness/tiredness indicate excess potassium depletion.
H2 blockers: • Ranitidine • Zantac (Ranitidine HCl)	Treats gastric or duodenal ulcers	• Side effects may include vertigo, headache, blurred vision, and angioedema.
Muscle relaxers/ antispastic agents: • Baclofen	Treats severe spasticity	• Side effects may include dizziness, drowsiness, headache, nausea, vomiting, and tiredness.
Opioids: • Darvocet (propoxyphene and acetaminophen) • Propoxyphene Hydrocodone • Vicodin (hydrocodone and acetaminophen)	Treats moderate to severe pain	• Side effects may include dizziness, drowsiness, light-headedness, and nausea. • Client is at an increased risk for falls.

(continued)

PHARMACOLOGY (CONTINUED)

Medication[5,7]	Treatment Use[5,7]	Potential Therapy Implications[5,7]
Potassium chloride	Counteracts potassium depletion when paired with diuretics	• Side effects may include confusion, numbness or tingling in hands/feet/lips, weakness, heaviness in legs, and irregular heartbeat.
Prokinetic agents: • Metoclopramide	Promotes gastric motility, and may be used for clients with diabetes	• Side effects may include diarrhea and drowsiness. • Symptoms of overdose include confusion, seizures/convulsions, and severe drowsiness.
Proton pump inhibitors: • Prevacid (lansoprazole) • Prilosec (omeprazole)	Treats gastric ulcers and gastroesophageal reflux disease (acid reflux)	• Side effects may include dizziness, headache, back pain, and increased risk of upper respiratory infection.
Steroids: • Prednisone	Treats multiple sclerosis, asthma, chronic obstructive pulmonary disease, and the geriatric population	• Side effects may include vertigo, paresthesias, headache, muscle weakness, aggravation, impaired wound healing, and spontaneous fractures.
Thyroid hormones: • Synthroid	Treats hypothyroidism	• Side effects may include nervousness, palpitations, insomnia, tremors, headache, and heat intolerance.

It is also important to provide occupational therapy intervention for medication management in preparation for discharge. Teaching the client to use a daily medication schedule, alarms, adaptive devices, or clear labels on pill bottles can be beneficial.

UNIT 2-101 EVALUATION

Swallow Assessment

A swallow assessment may be completed by an occupational therapist or a speech-language pathologist and may include data gathering, observation, bedside assessment, and imaging tests. Find out from your clinic how speech-language pathology and occupational therapy collaborate to address swallowing and dysphagia.

The American Occupational Therapy Association has a specialty certification available in feeding, eating, and swallowing.[8]

Data gathering[2,3]	• A physician must be consulted prior to evaluation. • Conduct a chart review of physical and medical history, onset, reason for hospitalization, review of system, and respiratory status. • Assess the client's behavior, responsiveness, current method of nutrition, and medication. • Conduct a client or family interview.
Supplies[3]	• Textures and consistencies for different diet levels. Refer to Unit 3-105 in this section for information about textures. • Cups • Several spoons • Tongue depressors • Cotton tip applicators • Thickener • Stethoscope • Flashlight or penlight • Laryngeal mirror • Gloves
Bedside assessment[3]	• Assess for cognition, trunk and head control, posture, and oxygen levels. • Observe the client eating or drinking different food and liquid consistencies.

(continued)

SWALLOW ASSESSMENT (CONTINUED)

Observation[3]	• Oral-prep stage:
	  ○ Check for lip closure when clearing the food from the utensil.
	  ○ Assess how the client masticates (chews) food. The client may chew in a rotary style or a munching style. Note the duration the client chews.
	• Oral stage:
	  ○ Assess client's sensation for touch, taste, and temperature.
	  ○ Check strength of facial muscles by observing facial expressions. These include smile, frown, grimace, pucker, and jaw movements.
	  ○ Oral reflexes to check include rooting, biting, sucking and swallowing, tongue thrust, and gag.
	  ○ Oral motor assessment includes tongue, swallow, hyoid elevation, laryngeal, and cough.
	• Pharyngeal stage:
	  ○ A pharyngeal assessment may be limited at the bedside.
	  ○ Observe the client initiate the swallow and for laryngeal elevation.
	  ○ Observe signs of aspiration, changes in vocal quality, cough, or complaints from the client.

Imaging and assessment instruments[3]	• Barium swallow test • Modified barium swallow test • Fiberoptic endoscopic evaluation of swallowing • Electromyography

UNIT 2-102 EVALUATION

UNIT 3-103 INTERVENTION

COMMON INTERVENTIONS ACROSS PRACTICE SETTINGS

Common Interventions Across Practice Settings

INTERVENTION	ACUTE	INPATIENT	HOME HEALTH	SNF	OUTPATIENT
Life legacy projects			✓		
Medication management		✓	✓	✓	✓
Nutrition and Feeding Tubes	✓	✓		✓	
Dysphagia Management	✓	✓		✓	
Managing Ostomies	✓	✓			✓
Managing Incontinence	✓	✓			✓
Addressing Sexuality	✓	✓	✓		✓
Endocrine, Digestive, Urinary, and Reproductive Systems Precautions and Contraindications	✓	✓	✓	✓	✓

(continued)

COMMON INTERVENTIONS ACROSS PRACTICE SETTINGS (CONTINUED)

LIFE LEGACY PROJECTS[9]

- Description: Life legacy projects are often used in hospice care and incorporate past learning, living in the present, and preparing for the future through journaling, creativity, and peer support.
- Approach: Summarize periods of the client's life through photos and descriptions of their meaning. Involvement from caregivers and loved ones is important. The client may create other projects for their loved ones to remember them following their passing.
- Precautions: Body donation must be initiated only by an organ procurement coordinator who is specially trained.
- Significance: Life legacy projects allow clients to summarize meaning in their life by developing their legacy.

MEDICATION MANAGEMENT

Refer to Section One, Unit 3-15, for information on medication management.

NUTRITION AND FEEDING TUBES

TUBE[10]	DESCRIPTION[10]	PRECAUTIONS[10]
Nasogastric tubes (NG tubes)	• NG tubes enter the nose and extend to the stomach. They allow for feeding or suctioning of stomach content. • Nutrition is delivered to the stomach. • NG tubes are temporary and do not require surgery.	• Report tubing that appears unsecured. • If the client has continuous tube feeding, then the head of the bed must stay at 30 degrees to prevent aspiration. • Pin the NG tube to the client's hospital gown if possible to reduce pulling.
Nasoduodenal tubes (ND tubes)	• ND tubes enter the nose and extend to the duodenum. • Nutrition is delivered to the duodenum. • ND tubes are temporary and do not require surgery.	• Feedings need to be given slowly over 18 to 24 hours.
Nasojejunal tubes (NJ tubes)	• NJ tubes enter the nose and extend to the jejunum. • NJ tubes are temporary and do not require surgery.	• Feedings need to be given slowly over 18 to 24 hours. *(continued)*

NUTRITION AND FEEDING TUBES (CONTINUED)

TUBE[10]	DESCRIPTION[10]	PRECAUTIONS[10]
Gastric tubes (G tubes)	• A G tube is a small feeding tube inserted directly into the stomach through an incision. • This is the most common type of feeding tube. • A G tube requires surgery to place. • There is no threat of aspiration with a G tube.	• Report leaking. • Prevent pulling or tugging.
Gastrojejunal tubes (GJ tubes)	• GJ tubes are used when a G tube is not tolerated by the client. • A GJ tube allows access to the stomach as well as the intestines.	• Tubes must be replaced at the hospital. • Feedings need to be given slowly over 18 to 24 hours.
Jejunal tubes	• Jejunal tubes deliver nutrition directly to the intestines.	• Feedings need to be given slowly over 18 to 24 hours.
Kangaroo pump	• A kangaroo pump is used for feeding through a tube. • A kangaroo pump allows for continuous or intermittent rate feeding.	• Report any pump alarms. • Never lay the client flat while the pump is in use.

UNIT 3-104 INTERVENTION

DYSPHAGIA MANAGEMENT

Practitioners can help manage a client's dysphagia by changing the consistency of food and liquids, which may increase client safety by reducing the risk of material entering the airway. Thickening agents may need to be added to liquids and foods in order to change the consistency. Other treatments include changing posture, strengthening, cueing, and introducing alternate methods of feeding.

Know what food and liquid consistencies are safe for your client to consume.

SOLIDS CONSISTENCY

Level 1: Pureed food[3]	• Pureed foods have a smooth, cohesive, and blended texture. Little to no chewing is required to consume pureed foods. • Pureed food includes the following examples: ◦ Pudding, applesauce, yogurt, and custard ◦ Pureed cooked meats, vegetables, and potatoes • The following foods are not safe to consume: ◦ Dry, crunchy, tough, and hard foods ◦ Raw vegetables and fruit skins *(continued)*

DYSPHAGIA MANAGEMENT (CONTINUED)

Level 2: Mechanically altered and semisolid food (also known as *mechanically altered ground*)[3]	• Mechanically altered and semisolid foods have a soft, moist texture. Some chewing is required to consume these foods.
	
	 • Mechanically altered and semisolid foods include the following examples:
	  ◦ Level 1 consistency foods
	  ◦ Hot cereal, scrambled eggs, and tofu
	  ◦ Soft macaroni and cheese, mashed potatoes, and soft cooked vegetables
	  ◦ Meatloaf, chicken/tuna/egg salad without large chunks, and chili with small pieces
	  ◦ Bread pudding, cobbler, soft bananas, and dunked or moistened cookies
	  ◦ Condiments including ketchup, butter, and gravy
	
	 • The following foods are not safe to consume:
	  ◦ Tough meats, hard cheeses, nuts, and seeds
	  ◦ Bread products and crispy or crunchy foods
	  ◦ Frozen, dried, and high-pulp fruits; and fibrous vegetables

Level 3: Advanced soft solid food (also known as *mechanically altered chopped*)[3]	• Advanced soft solid foods are moist and consumed in small pieces. More chewing is required to consume soft solid foods.
	
	 • Advanced soft solid foods include:
	  ◦ Level 1 and 2 consistency foods
	  ◦ Bread products if well moistened with jelly, syrup, or butter
	  ◦ Canned and cooked fruits, peeled fruits, and berries with small seeds
	  ◦ Thin-sliced and finely ground meats
	  ◦ Soft cookies and moist cakes
	
	 • The following foods are not safe to consume:
	  ◦ Tough meats, nuts, and seeds
	  ◦ Hard, crunchy, and crispy foods
	
	 (continued)

DYSPHAGIA MANAGEMENT (CONTINUED)

Level 4: Regular chewable food and mixed textures[3]	• All foods are safe for consumption. • Mixed textures include taking tablets with water.

LIQUIDS CONSISTENCY

Spoon-thickened[2]	• Spoon-thickened liquids have a viscosity of greater than 1750 cP. This is the thickest consistency.
Honey-like thickened[2]	• Honey-like thickened liquids have a viscosity of 351 to 1750 cP.
Nectar-like thickened[2]	• Nectar-like thickened liquids have a viscosity of 51 to 350 cP. • Examples of nectar-like thickened liquids include extra-thick milkshakes, strained creamed soups, V8 juice (Campbell Soup Company), and blended yogurt and milk.
Thin[2]	• Thin liquids have a viscosity of 1 to 50 cP. • Thin liquids include water, milk, ice cream, coffee, and Jell-O (Kraft).
	(continued)

Dysphagia Management (continued)

Intervention Guidelines

Pre-oral stage[2]	• Consider the client's context of eating. This includes:
	  ◦ Cultural considerations about food and utensils
	  ◦ Setting where eating takes place
	  ◦ Role of appetite
	• Consider the client's body functions. This includes:
	  ◦ Tactile sensations
	  ◦ Ability to see and locate food or utensils
	  ◦ Ability to use the upper extremity to bring food to the mouth
	• Emphasize the importance of oral hygiene to reduce the likelihood of bacterial aspiration.
	• Teach the client and the caregiver about proper thickener use.
	• Before eating, make sure the client is positioned upright at the edge of the bed or by raising the head of the bed.
	• Guide the client's awareness of food as needed by using the clock method or other cues.
	• If able, identify with the client the foods that are on the plate:
	  ◦ For example, ask the client to differentiate if a food item is mashed potatoes or bread.

Oral stage[2]	• Use oral motor exercises to increase the client's muscle strength for chewing and manipulating food in mouth with the tongue. • Use tactile or sensory cues to facilitate chewing: ◦ For example, massage the client's cheek to assist the weak side of the jaw. *(continued)*

Dysphagia Management (continued)

Compensatory swallow techniques for pharyngeal stage[2]	• Tucking the client's chin to the chest narrows the entrance to the larynx. • Rotating the client's head toward the weaker or hemiparetic side closes the weaker side of the pharynx. • Tilting the client's head toward the stronger side allows gravity to direct the bolus to the stronger side. • The client can swallow multiple times. • To do a supraglottic swallow, the client should take a deep breath, hold firmly while swallowing, and then cough prior to inhalation. • To do the Mendelsohn maneuver, the client should swallow while pushing the tongue into the hard palate (this is not used during solid or liquid intake). • The client can conduct a vocal quality check by monitoring his or her voice after swallowing. If wet, hoarse, or aphonic, the client should cough or clear his or her throat and swallow.
Alternate feeding[2]	• Alternate feeding methods include use of a NG tube or G tube, or parenteral feeding through a central line. • NPO (nil per os) indicates that the client should not ingest food or liquid by mouth.

MANAGING OSTOMIES

Emptying an ostomy pouch[11,12]	• The ostomy pouch should be emptied when it is one-third to one-half full of air or stool to prevent leakage or explosion. • Some pouches can be opened at the bottom for emptying. They can be emptied into a toilet, or, if measurement is needed, a plastic bag or container: ◦ If the client is emptying into a toilet, splashing can be prevented by placing toilet paper into the toilet first. The client can either stand facing the toilet to empty the pouch, or the client may sit and empty the pouch between the legs, depending on the client's preferences. • Some pouches are a closed system and are removed once filled. • Some clients may need to work on increasing their fine motor dexterity and strength to manipulate the pouch closure. • Daily cleaning of the pouch with water may help manage odors. • Some clients may choose to use a method other than a pouch for their ostomy, such as water irrigation.
Protecting the skin[11]	• The client should keep his or her skin clean of stool to prevent irritation. • The pouch should be changed regularly, about every 4 to 7 days, or if any leakage, itching under pouch, or burning sensation occurs. • Monitor skin for signs of allergic reaction to the pouch or any adhesive.
Dressing[11]	• Avoid tight waistbands directly on the stoma, but clothing can be chosen to conceal an ostomy. Pouch covers may also be worn. • Pouches are commonly tucked into underwear. • If belts are typically worn and lie directly on the stoma, suspenders may be an effective alternative. • Many clients report buying slightly larger clothing than normal to effectively conceal their pouch.

(continued)

UNIT 3-106 INTERVENTION

Managing Ostomies (continued)

Showering[11]	• The pouch can be covered with plastic wrap and taped to prevent leaking during showering.
	• The pouch can also likely be worn in the shower or during swimming, and dried using a hair dryer set on low and held at least 6 inches from the body.
Driving[12]	• The client may need to use a seatbelt shield to protect the ostomy.
	• The client may need to follow special precautions such as not driving for 3 weeks after surgery.
Exercising, engaging in sports[12]	• The client may need to follow special precautions such as no heavy lifting (more than 10 pounds) for 6 weeks after surgery.
	• Contact sports, such as football, may need to be avoided, or the client should discuss adaptations with a doctor.
	• Activities that involve bending over or using a golf swing may be more difficult depending on the client's stoma location.
	• Clients can participate in swimming. It is suggested that they empty their pouch before engaging in swimming.
Eating/diet[11]	• Diet may be modified after surgery from liquids to low-fiber foods for the first 6 to 8 weeks after surgery.
	• Avoid skipping meals, which can increase gas and watery output; in addition, drinking water can help prevent constipation.
	• Clients may find that eating frequent, smaller meals throughout the day helps control output. Clients may develop their own modified diets based on foods that they find cause different levels of gas or odor, or the effect of timing throughout the day.
Addressing psychosocial concerns[11]	• Address the client's psychosocial concerns to managing the ostomy, which may include handling fears about odors, managing their ostomy in public, dealing with sexuality, and using coping strategies such as relaxation.
	• Packing extra ostomy supplies and clothing may help manage anxiety during public outings or long-distance travels.

MANAGING INCONTINENCE

Incontinence is the loss of control of bladder or bowel that presents as involuntary urine or stool leakage.[1]

Prevalence of urinary incontinence after a stroke ranges from 37% to 79%, and thus is an important area to address in this population.[13] It should also be addressed in any other clients who struggle with incontinence.

Risk factors[13]	• Being female • Obesity • Smoking • Family history • Constipation or straining • Heavy lifting
Occupational therapy intervention[1]	• Address psychosocial concerns such as fear of embarrassment or odor, limitations in social or work activities, and depression. • Teach toilet transfer skills. • Provide clothing management training or adapted clothing fasteners. • Ensure hygiene and skin protection. • Reduce fall risks. • Schedule or prompt toileting (timed voiding). • Provide adaptive equipment use and training (eg, raised toilet seat, bedside commode, intermittent self-catheterization, or use of adapted handles for suppository insertion). • Educate on types of medications and their effects on continence. • Educate on the importance of preventing dehydration.
Advanced occupational therapy intervention[1]	• Urge suppression • Bowel and bladder retraining • Biofeedback • Modifications in diet and fluids • Pelvis floor muscle (Kegel) home exercise program

ADDRESSING SEXUALITY

Sexuality includes one's body image, self-concept, self-esteem, dress, social roles, sexual preferences, and more.[14]

Sexual expression can be affected by changes commonly present in clients, a few of which include sensory loss, spasticity, pain, bowel or bladder incontinence, medications, amputations, postoperative precautions, and cognitive changes.

The role of occupational therapy may include educating the client on the nature of the disability, providing educational resources, improving bowel and bladder management, teaching energy conservation, ensuring range of motion, or modifying the environment.[14]

The PLISSIT (permission, limited information, specific suggestions, intensive therapy) model describes levels of intervention.[15]

Permission[15]	All practitioners can allow clients an opportunity to discuss their sexual concerns and be reassured that their feelings are acceptable. Not all clients will feel comfortable discussing their sexual concerns. The practitioner can ask questions such as: "Many people who have this injury/condition wonder how it will affect their sexual activities. Is this a concern of yours? Would you like to talk about it?" Be sensitive to timing and location when bringing up sexuality with clients.
Limited information[15]	Knowledgeable practitioners can provide educational information regarding the client's condition and dispel myths. Therapists can provide factual information through handouts or other resources. For example, an occupational therapist can educate clients that spinal cord injuries affect male fertility but not female fertility.
Specific suggestions[15]	This level of intervention is aimed at solving a specific problem. Clinicians are required to have advanced knowledge and skill. For example, specific suggestions may involve recommendations about specific sexual positioning.
Intensive therapy[15]	This level of intervention requires specific training beyond occupational therapy. Clients are referred to sex therapy or psychotherapy.

UNIT 3-108 INTERVENTION

ENDOCRINE, DIGESTIVE, URINARY, AND REPRODUCTIVE SYSTEMS PRECAUTIONS AND CONTRAINDICATIONS

Gait belts	• Place the gait belt around the chest instead of the abdomen when there are abdominal incisions, percutaneous endoscopic gastrostomy (PEG) tubes, ostomy bags, or drains.
Urinary catheters	• Keep the leg bag and tubing below the pelvis at all times to prevent backflow of urine.
Ostomy bags	• Empty the ostomy bag before the pouch is full of stool or gas to prevent leakage or possible explosion.
Gastroesphageal reflux disease[16]	• Avoid positions that increase intra-abdominal pressure, such as coughing, bending, wearing tight clothing, and high-intensity exercise. • The client should sit up during and after meals to help minimize reflux.
Feeding tubes	• Keep the head of bed elevated while feeding tubes are on. If necessary or if the client is supine, ask the nurse if the feeding tube may be turned off to avoid risk of aspiration. • NG tube can be pulled out. Check the marking of the tube for positioning and contact the nurse if the tube needs to be repositioned. • A PEG tube allows liquid nutrition to be delivered directly to the stomach through an abdominal tube. An abdominal binder may be used to keep it in place, but do not place the gait belt directly over a PEG tube.
Dysphagia	• Follow the client's dysphagia dietary guidelines. • Be aware of the client's thickener requirements during occupational therapy treatment if the client needs water. • Maintain client's oral hygiene. • Turn off any tube feedings prior to lowering the head of the bed or lying the client back down.

(continued)

UNIT 3-109 INTERVENTION

ENDOCRINE, DIGESTIVE, URINARY, AND REPRODUCTIVE SYSTEMS PRECAUTIONS AND CONTRAINDICATIONS (CONTINUED)	
Clostridium difficile[17]	• Wash hands with soap and water to kill bacteria or use a non–alcohol-based hand rub. • Use contact precautions. Wear a gown and gloves.
Continuous venovenous hemodialysis	• A continuous venovenous hemodialysis allows for continuous bedside dialysis for patients with acute renal failure or multiple organ failure • Obtain approval from a nurse prior to therapy and perform only bed-level activity.
Oncology[16]	• Always monitor vital signs, be aware of lines and drains, and verify blood counts (see sections on hematology and chemistry). • Defer therapy when client has implanted radioactive seeds.
Breast surgery: DIEP (deep inferior epigastric perforators) and TRAM (transverse rectus abdominis) flap	• Use a log roll to avoid straining abdominal muscles during bed mobility. • In a seated position, the back should be reclined with hip flexion at 90 degrees or more and knee flexion. • In a walking position, the waist should be flexed forward 45 degrees to protect the incision and muscles. The client may need to use a rolling walker for support. • Do not lift more than 5 to 10 pounds on the ipsilateral side to prevent injury and lymphedema. • Avoid scapular retraction. • Do not perform repetitive bilateral upper extremity movement unless cleared by physician. See the physician's guidelines for range of motion limitations. *(continued)*

ENDOCRINE, DIGESTIVE, URINARY, AND REPRODUCTIVE SYSTEMS PRECAUTIONS AND CONTRAINDICATIONS (CONTINUED)

Bone metastases[16]	• Do not use massage techniques (biothermal) on any extremity with an active tumor. • Consult the physician before mobilizing a client with bone cancer, and be aware of weightbearing status. • Manual muscle testing may be contraindicated with multiple myeloma or bone metastases due to risk of fracture.
Head/neck surgery	• Keep the head of bed elevated at least 30 degrees. • For clients without reconstruction, the clinician can perform gentle neck exercises, as tolerated, to the point of pain. • For clients without reconstruction, avoid extensive neck exercises for 3 weeks. Keep the head in a neutral position as much as possible. Refer to weightbearing status with flap of origin (eg, trapezius, pectoralis, forearm, fibula).

REFERENCES

1. Smith-Gabai H, Holm SE, eds. *Occupational Therapy in Acute Care.* 2nd ed. Bethesda, MD: AOTA Press; 2017.
2. Avery W. Dysphagia. In: Smith-Gabai H, Holm SE, eds. *Occupational Therapy in Acute Care.* 2nd ed. Bethesda, MD: AOTA Press; 2017:583-598.
3. Smith J, Jenks KN. Eating and swallowing. In: Pendleton HM, Schutlz-Krohn W, eds. *Pedretti's Occupational Therapy: Practice Skills for Physical Dysfunction.* 7th ed. St. Louis, MO: Elsevier Mosby; 2013:679-717.
4. Barber MD, Chen Z, Lukacz E. Further validation of the short form versions of the Pelvic Floor Distress Inventory (PFDI) and Pelvic Floor Impact Questionnaire (PFIQ). *Neurourol Urodyn.* 2011;30(4):541-546. doi:10.1002/nau.20934
5. Stoops K. Fundamentals of pharmacology for occupational therapy. In: Smith-Gabai H, Holm SE, eds. *Occupational Therapy in Acute Care.* Bethesda, MD: AOTA Press; 2011:175-182.
6. Masnoon N, Shakib S, Kalisch-Ellett L, Caughey GE. What is polypharmacy? a systematic review of definitions. *BMC Geriatrics.* 2017;17:230. doi:10.1186/s12877-017-0621-2
7. Riedinger V, Glad K. Top ten medications prescribed in skilled nursing facilities—revisited. https://www.asha.org/Events/convention/handouts/2007/0637_Riedinger_Vicki/. Published 2007. Accessed May 7, 2019.
8. American Occupational Therapy Association. Specialized knowledge and skills in feeding, eating, and swallowing for occupational therapy practice. *Am J Occup Ther.* 2007;61(6):686-700. doi:10.5014/ajot.61.6.686
9. American Occupational Therapy Association. The role of occupational therapy in end-of-life care. *Am J Occup Ther.* 2016;70:S66-S75. doi:10.5014/ajot.2016.706S17
10. National Collaborating Centre for Acute Care (UK). Nutrition support for adults: oral nutrition support, enteral tube feeding and parenteral nutrition. In: *NICE Clinical Guidelines, No. 32.* London, United Kingdom: National Collaborating Centre for Acute Care (UK); 2006.
11. United Ostomy Associations of America, Inc. Colostomy guide. United Colostomy Associations of America, Inc. http://www.ostomy.org/uploaded/files/ostomy_info/ColostomyGuide.pdf?direct=1. Published 2011. Updated 2015. Accessed May 7, 2019.
12. Davis F, Campbell C. The role of occupational therapy in ostomy management for clients with cancer-related impairments. *Am Occup Ther Assoc Phys Disabil Spec Interest Sect Q.* 2015;38(4):1-4.
13. Dumoulin C, Korner-Bitensky N, Tannenbaum C. Urinary incontinence after stroke: identification, assessment, and intervention by rehabilitation professionals in Canada. *Stroke.* 2007;38(10):2745-2751. doi:10.1161/STROKEAHA.107.486035
14. American Occupational Therapy Association. Fact sheet: sexuality and the role of occupational therapy. American Occupational Therapy Association. https://www.aota.org/~/media/Corporate/Files/AboutOT/Professionals/WhatIsOT/RDP/Facts/Sexuality.pdf. Published 2013. Accessed May 7, 2019.
15. Annon J. The PLISSIT model: a proposed conceptual scheme for the behavioral treatment of sexual problems. *J Sex Educ Ther.* 1976;(2):1-15. doi:10.1080/01614576.1976.1 1074483
16. Smith-Gabai H. *Occupational Therapy in Acute Care.* Bethesda, MD: AOTA Press; 2011.
17. Kerrigan DA. Infectious diseases and autoimmune disorders. In: Smith-Gabai H, ed. *Occupational Therapy in Acute Care.* Bethesda, MD: AOTA Press; 2011:443-470.

APPENDIX A

Conversions

Sit W, Neville M.
*Handbook of Occupational Therapy for
Adults With Physical Disabilities* (pp 467-468).
© 2020 SLACK Incorporated.

VOLUME

1 ml = 16 minims
1 ml = 1 cc
1 ml = 15 gutta (gtt)
5 ml = 1 teaspoon
15 ml = 1 tablespoon
30 ml = 1 oz
240 ml = 8 oz (1 cup)
1000 ml = 1 L (1 qt)

WEIGHT

1 mg = gr 1/60
30 mg = gr ½
60 mg = 1 grain (gr)
1000 mg = 1 g
1000 g = 1 kg

Pounds (lbs) = g x 0.0022
lbs = kg x 2.2
kg = lbs x 0.45

LENGTH

1 inch (in) = 2.54 cm
1 cm = 10 mm
1 m = 100 cm
1 m = 39.4 in

in = cm / 2.54
cm = in x 2.54

TEMPERATURE

°F = (°C x 1.8) + 31
°C = (°F – 32) / 1.8

APPENDIX B

. . . .

Rehabilitation Abbreviations

Sit W, Neville M.
*Handbook of Occupational Therapy for
Adults With Physical Disabilities* (pp 469-477).
© 2020 SLACK Incorporated.

A

a	before
Ⓐ	assistance
AAA	abdominal aortic aneurysm
AAROM	active assistive range of motion
AC	acromioclavicular
Ach	acetylcholine
ACLS	Allen Cognitive Level Screening
ACTH	Adrenocorticotropic
abd	abduction
ABI	acquired brain injury
add	adduction
ad lib	as desired
ADL	activities of daily living
AFO	ankle-foot orthosis
AKA	above knee amputation
A-ONE	Arnadottir OT-ADL Neurobehavioral Evaluation
ALSAR	Assessment of Living Skills and Resources
AM-PAC	Activity Measure for Post Acute Care
AMPS	Assessment of Motor and Process Skills
AROM	active range of motion
AusTOMS	Australian Therapy Outcome Measure
AV	atrioventricular
AVM	arteriovenous malformation
AWP	Assessment of Work Performance

B

Ⓑ/bil	bilateral
BADL	basic activities of daily living
BAFF	both arm forearm fracture
bid	twice a day
BiVABA	Brain Injury Visual Assessment Battery for Adults
BMT	bone marrow transplant
BP	blood pressure
BSC	bedside commode

C

c	with
CA	cancer
CABG	coronary artery bypass graft
CAD	carotid artery disease/coronary artery disease
CA-ICU	Confusion Assessment Method for the Intensive Care Unit
CBC	complete blood count
CGA	contact guard assist
CHF	congestive heart failure
CHI	closed head injury
CHIEF	Craig Hospital Inventory of Environmental Factors
CIQ	Community Integration Questionnaire
CJD	Creutzfeldt-Jakob disease
CK	creatine kinase
CN	cranial nerves
c/o	complains of
COPD	chronic obstructive pulmonary disease
COTA	certified occupational therapy assistant
CP	chest pain
CPAx	Chelsea Critical Care Physical Assessment Tool
CPK	creatine phosphokinase
CPT	Cognitive Performance Test
crani	craniotomy
CVA	cerebrovascular accident
CVL	central venous lines
CVVHD	continuous venovenous hemodialysis

D

D/dep	dependent
DA	dopamine
DASH	Disabilities of the Arm, Shoulder and Hand
D/C	discharge
DJD	degenerative joint disease

DLOTCA	Dynamic Loewenstein Occupational Therapy Cognitive Assessment
DVT	deep vein thrombosis
dx	diagnosis

E

EADL	electronic aid for daily living
ED	extensor digitorum
EMS	electrical muscle stimulation
EOB	edge of bed
eval	evaluation
ex	exercise
ext	extension/extremities

F

FABER	flexion, abduction, and external rotation test
FADIR	flexion, adduction, and internal rotation test
FDP	flexor digitorum profundus
FDS	flexor digitorum superficialis
FEES	fiberoptic endoscopic evaluation of swallowing
FES	functional electrical stimulation
FFWB	foot flat weightbearing
FIM	Functional Independence Measure
flex	flexion
FSH	follicle-stimulating hormone
FSS-ICU	Functional Status Score for the Intensive Care Unit
FWB	full weightbearing
fx	fracture
fx'l	functional

G

GABA	gamma-aminobutyric acid
GERD	gastroesophageal reflux disease
Glu	glutamate

H

HA	headache
HCT	hematocrit
HEAP	Home Environment Assessment Protocol
hemi	hemiplegic
HEP	home exercise program
HGB	hemoglobin
HHA	handheld assist
HOB	head of bed
HR	heart rate
5-HT	serotonin (5-hydroxytryptamine)
HVPGS	high-voltage pulse galvanic stimulation
hx	history

I

Ⓘ	independent
IGF-1	insulin-like growth factor 1
IMS	ICU Mobility Scale
IP	interphalangeal
IVIG	intravenous immunoglobin therapy

J

J tube	jejunal tube
JP drain	Jackson-Pratt drain

K

KAFO	knee-ankle-foot orthosis
KELS	Kohlman Evaluation of Living Skills

L

Ⓛ	left
LAD	left axis deviation
lat	lateral
LE	lower extremity
LH	luteinizing hormone

M

MAEW	moves all extremities well
MAOI	monoamine oxidase inhibitor
max	maximum
MCA	middle cerebral artery
MCP	metacarpophalangeal
mCTSIB	Modified Clinical Test of Sensory Interaction on Balance
MI	myocardial infarction
MIDCAB	minimally invasive direct coronary artery bypass surgery
min	minimum
MMSE	Mini-Mental State Examination
mod	moderate
MQE	Measure of the Quality of the Environment
MS	multiple sclerosis
MVA	motor vehicle accident
MVC	motor vehicle collision
MVPT	Motor-Free Visual Perception Test

N

NE	norepinephrine
NG tube	nasogastric tube
NIHSS	National Institutes of Health Stroke Scale
NKDA	no known drug allergies
NPO	nothing by mouth
NRB	non-rebreather mask
NWB	nonweightbearing

O

O_2	oxygen
O_2 sat	oxygen saturation rate
OOB	out of bed
ORIF	open reduction internal fixation
ortho	orthopedics
OSA	obstructive sleep apnea

OSH	outside hospital
OT	occupational therapy
OT-DORA	Occupational Therapy Driver Off-Road Assessment
OTR	occupational therapist registered

P

p	after
PCA	patient-controlled analgesia pump/ posterior cerebral artery/posterior communicating artery
PCT	patient care technician
PFIT	Physical Function in Intensive Care Test
PICC	peripherally inserted intravenous central catheter lines
PLOF	prior level of function
Plts	platelet
PNS	peripheral nervous system
po	by mouth
prn	as needed
PROM	passive range of motion
PT	physical therapy
PVC	premature ventricular contraction
PVD	peripheral vascular disease
PWB	partial weightbearing

Q

q	every
qd	every day
qh	every hour
qod	every other day

R

®	right
RA	rheumatoid arthritis
RAD	right axis deviation
RCVA	right cerebrovascular accident
rehab	rehabilitation

ROM	range of motion
RPE	rating of perceived exertion
RSD	reflex sympathetic dystrophy
RT	recreation therapy/respiratory therapy
Rx	prescription
RW	rolling walker

S

s	without
S/sup	supervision
SAAFA	Structured Anchored Approach to Functional Assessment
SAH	subarachnoid hemorrhage
SBA	stand by assistance
SCD	sequential compression device
SCIM	Spinal Cord Independence Measure
SHA	superficial heat agent
SLUMS	St. Louis University Mental Status Examination
SNF	skilled nursing facility
SOB	shortness of breath/side of bed
SOMS	Surgical Intensive Care Unit Optimal Mobilisation Score
s/p	status post
SPADI	Shoulder Pain and Disability Index
SSRI	selective serotonin reuptake inhibitor
ST	speech therapy
stat	at once
STEMI	ST elevated myocardial infarction
SW	standard walker/social worker
sx	surgery

T

TBI	traumatic brain injury
TEA	Test of Everyday Attention
TENS	transcutaneous electrical nerve stimulation
t/fer	transfer

THR	total hip replacement
TIA	transient ischemic attack
tid	3 times a day
TKR	total knee replacement
TLSO	thoracic lumbosacral orthosis
tol	tolerated
TSH	thyroid-stimulating hormone
TTB	transfer tub bench
TTWB	toe-touch weightbearing
tx	treatment

U

UE	upper extremity
UFOV	Useful Field of View Test
UTI	urinary tract infection

V

V.O.	verbal order

W

WBAT	weightbearing as tolerated
WBC	white blood cells
W/C	wheelchair
WEIS	Work Environment Impact Scale
WeHSA	Westmead Home Safety Assessment
WFL	within functional limits
WNL	within normal limits

APPENDIX C

Resources

Sit W, Neville M.
*Handbook of Occupational Therapy for
Adults With Physical Disabilities* (pp 479-482).
© 2020 SLACK Incorporated.

Use the following pages to add resources that you come across in your practice.

CATEGORY	RESOURCE
Adaptive equipment	AOTA's OT Practice Buyer's Guide: http://www.aota.org/Publications-News/Advertise/BuyerGuide.aspx
Driver rehabilitation	Locate a Certified Driver Rehabilitation Specialist (CRDS) in your area: http://aded.site-ym.com/search/custom.asp?id=2046 Locate CarFit Events for Older Adults: https://www.car-fit.org
Ergonomics	OSHA Workstations Checklist: https://www.osha.gov/SLTC/etools/computerworkstations/checklist.html
Job accommodations	Job Accommodation Network: AskJan.org
Referral services	Dial 211 to inquire about available services in your city

CATEGORY   **RESOURCE**

CATEGORY   **RESOURCE**

Index